Acupuncture Research

Strategies for Establishing an Evidence Base

For Elsevier

Commissioning Editor: Karen Morley, Claire Wilson
Development Editor: Kerry McGechie
Project Manager: Kerrie-Anne Jarvis
Designer: Charles Gray
Illustrator: Ian Ramsden
Illustration Manager: Gillian Richards

Acupuncture Research

Strategies for Establishing an Evidence Base

Edited by

Hugh MacPherson PhD

Research Director
Foundation for Traditional Chinese Medicine, York, UK
Senior Research Fellow, Department of Health Sciences
University of York, York, UK

Richard Hammerschlag PhD

Dean of Research
Oregon College of Oriental Medicine, Portland, OR, USA
Adjunct Professor of Neurology
Oregon Health & Science University, Portland, OR, USA

George Lewith MA, MD, FRCP, MRCGP

Reader in Complementary Medicine
University of Southampton Medical School, Southampton, UK

Rosa Schnyer LicAc

Research Associate
Osher Institute, Harvard Medical School, MA, USA
New England School of Acupuncture, MA, USA

CHURCHILL
LIVINGSTONE

ELSEVIER

EDINBURGH   LONDON   NEW YORK   OXFORD   PHILADELPHIA   ST LOUIS   SYDNEY   TORONTO   2007

CHURCHILL LIVINGSTONE
ELSEVIER

An imprint of Elsevier Limited

First published 2007

ISBN: 978-0-443-10029-1

British Library Cataloguing in Publication Data
A catalogue record for this book is available from the British Library

Library of Congress Cataloging in Publication Data
A catalog record for this book is available from the Library of Congress

Notice
Knowledge and best practice in this field are constantly changing. As new research and experience broaden our knowledge, changes in practice, treatment and drug therapy may become necessary or appropriate. Readers are advised to check the most current information provided (i) on procedures featured or (ii) by the manufacturer of each product to be administered, to verify the recommended dose or formula, the method and duration of administration, and contraindications. It is the responsibility of the practitioners, relying on their own experience and knowledge of the patient, to make diagnoses, to determine dosages and the best treatment for each individual patient, and to take all appropriate safety precautions. To the fullest extent of the law, neither the Publisher nor the Editors assume any liability for any injury and/or damage to persons or property arising out or related to any use of the material contained in this book.

The Publisher

ELSEVIER your source for books, journals and multimedia in the health sciences

www.elsevierhealth.com

Working together to grow libraries in developing countries
www.elsevier.com | www.bookaid.org | www.sabre.org

ELSEVIER **BOOK AID** International Sabre Foundation

The Publisher's policy is to use **paper manufactured from sustainable forests**

Printed in China

Contents

Contributors

Alan Bensoussan

Alan Bensoussan is Director of the Centre for Complementary Medicine Research at the University of Western Sydney. Professor Bensoussan has been in clinical practice for over 20 years. He works in an advisory capacity for both government and industry, including as an expert panel member to the Complementary Medicines Evaluation Committee of the Australian Therapeutic Goods Administration, and frequently serves as a short-term consultant to the World Health Organisation. He sits on a number of relevant journal editorial committees, has published two books including *A Review of Acupuncture Research* (1990) and a major government report on the practice of traditional Chinese medicine in Australia (1996), which has led to the passage of the Victorian Chinese Medicine (Practitioner) Registration Act. Dr Bensoussan's research contributions, particularly his clinical trials and public health research in Chinese medicine, have been widely reported and recognised.

Stephen Birch

Stephen Birch has been practising acupuncture for 25 years. He is co-author of seven books and multiple papers on acupuncture. After studying with Yoshio Manaka he started pursuing further research studies. He completed his PhD at Exeter University focusing on the methodology of 'placebo-controlled' acupuncture trials. He helped establish the Society for Acupuncture Research in the early 1990s in the US, chaired the basic science panel at the 1994 US FDA workshop on acupuncture and was one of the presenters at the US NIH Consensus Development Conference on Acupuncture in 1997. He worked on clinical trials at Harvard and Yale Medical Schools and has consulted for a number of other studies including the recent large GERAC migraine study. As well as participating in workshops such as that which preceded the publication of this book, he is working towards the development of an integral research approach for acupuncture as a holistic therapy.

Mark Bovey

Prior to his acupuncture career Mark Bovey gained a MSc in animal breeding and worked as a geneticist for an international agri-business company. In 1983 he received his licentiate from the College of Traditional Acupuncture in the UK; since then he has been in private practice in Oxford, where he lives. Half of his working week is spent as co-ordinator of the British Acupuncture Council's Acupuncture Research Resource Centre, based first at Exeter University and then Thames Valley University. He is the author of a number of acupuncture research articles and currently a co-investigator on studies of acupuncture for Parkinson's disease and on the effects of cupping on inflammatory markers. He teaches at the College of Integrated Chinese Medicine, Reading, where he also has helped to develop the research module.

Claire M. Cassidy

Claire M. Cassidy earned her interdisciplinary doctorate in human biology at the University of Wisconsin, and completed post-doctoral programs at the Smithsonian Institution (anthropology) and the Johns Hopkins School of Medicine (history of medicine). She served on anthropology faculties of the Universities of Minnesota and Maryland, pioneering courses in cross-cultural and comparative human medicine; and carried out medical and nutritional anthropology research in Mauritania, Sri Lanka, Belize and the US, focusing on mother and child nutrition. In 1991 she became Research Director at the Traditional Acupuncture Institute (now TAI-Sophia), near Baltimore, Maryland. There she performed the first US national survey of acupuncture users, and was active in the early work of what became the NIH National Center for Complementary and Alternative Medicine. In 1997 she entered Chinese medicine school in Bethesda, Maryland, graduated in 2001, and has since worked as a clinician. Dr Cassidy is an Associate Editor of the Journal of Alternative and Complementary Medicine. Her research interests include qualitative and narrative research of medical practitioners and patients, and questionnaire design.

Richard Hammerschlag

Richard Hammerschlag, PhD, currently serves as Dean of Research at the Oregon College of Oriental Medicine (OCOM), Portland, Oregon, and Adjunct Professor in Neurology, Oregon Health & Science University. He received a doctorate in biochemistry from Brandeis University and was a biomedical researcher in neurobiology for 25 years, mainly at the Beckman Research Institute of the City of Hope in Duarte, California, where he served as Associate Chair of the Division of Neurosciences. A long-term interest in acupuncture and its unique challenges for research led to a career change and a move to Portland to create a research department at OCOM, where he has been coordinating NIH/NCCAM-funded acupuncture and Oriental medicine clinical trials in collaboration with Oregon Health & Science University, Kaiser Permanente Center for Health Research, and the University of Arizona. He was recently awarded one of the first NIH/NCCAM grants to complementary and alternative medicine (CAM) colleges to enhance research education. He served from 1997 to 2003 as co-President of the Society for Acupuncture Research and is a Senior Editor for the Journal of Alternative and Complementary Medicine.

Hélène M. Langevin

Hélène M. Langevin received an MD degree from McGill University, followed by a post-doctoral research fellowship in neurochemistry at the Medical Research Council's Neurochemical Pharmacology Unit in Cambridge, England; a residency in internal medicine and fellowship in endocrinology and metabolism at John Hopkins Hospital in Baltimore, Maryland. She studied acupuncture at the Tristate Institute of Acupuncture, Stamford, Connecticut and at the Worsley College of Classical Chinese Acupuncture in Leamington Spa, England and Miami, Florida. She currently is a Research Associate Professor in the Departments of Neurology, Orthopedics and Rehabilitation at the University of Vermont and is the Principal Investigator of two NIH-funded studies investigating the mechanism of action of acupuncture and the effect of acupuncture on connective tissue in low back pain. She is the past co-President of the Society of Acupuncture Research.

Lixing Lao

Lixing Lao, is a Professor of Family Medicine and the Director of Traditional Chinese Medicine (TCM) Research Program in the Center for Integrative Medicine, University of Maryland Baltimore (UMB), School of Medicine. He is currently a guest professor in the Shanghai University of Traditional Chinese Medicine, Shanghai, China. Dr Lao graduated from the Shanghai University of TCM in 1983 after 5 years' training in acupuncture, Chinese herbal medicine and Western medicine. He completed his PhD in physiology at UMB in 1992. As a licensed acupuncturist, Dr Lao has practised acupuncture and Chinese medicine for more than 20 years. Dr Lao has conducted and participated in several clinical trials including a recently published large clinical trial on the effect of acupuncture on knee osteoarthritis. He established the laboratory of TCM research in UMB in 1999 to conduct basic

science studies on acupuncture and Chinese herbal medicine and leads a laboratory research team. He is currently the elected co-President of the Society for Acupuncture Research. He became a board member of the National Acupuncture Foundation in 2006.

George Lewith

George Lewith is a qualified physician who has practised and researched within complementary and alternative medicine (CAM) for the last 30 years. His first degree at Trinity College, Cambridge was in biochemistry; he then qualified in medicine in 1974 and obtained his MRCP in 1977, MRCGP in 1980, PhD in 1994 and FRCP in 1999. He trained in acupuncture in China in 1978. He now works as a Physician practising integrated medicine (acupuncture, homeopathy, nutritional medicine and conventional medicine) for 2 days a week and for the remaining 3 days is at the University of Southampton where he leads an internationally respected CAM research group within the Department of Primary Medical Care. He has raised over £4 million in research funds in the last 10 years and has published over 200 peer-reviewed articles as well as making contributions to over 30 books. Dr Lewith is currently President of the International Society for Complementary Medicine Research (ISCMR) and has acted as a consultant and/or committee member to many government agencies, funding bodies and charities in the UK and overseas.

Klaus Linde

Klaus Linde was born in Munich, Germany in 1960. From 1981 to 1982 he studied German literature at the University of Freiburg, Germany. From 1983 to 1990 he trained at medical schools in Bologna, Italy and Munich. His MD thesis was on dose-dependent reversal effects at the Institute for Pharmacology and Toxicology of the Ludwig-Maximilians-University, Munich in 1990. His PhD in epidemiology was achieved at the Humboldt-University Berlin in 2002. From 1991 to 1997 he was a Researcher at the Project for Integration of Natural Healing Procedures into Research and Teaching at the Ludwig-Maximilians-University, Munich. Since 1998 he has been Deputy Director of the Centre for Complementary Medicine Research, Department of Internal Medicine II, Technical University, Munich. He has conducted large-scale randomised trials, observational studies, and systematic reviews of acupuncture for chronic pain.

Hugh MacPherson

Hugh MacPherson attained a PhD in fluid mechanics and then trained in acupuncture and Chinese herbal medicine. He continues to practise at the York Clinic for Complementary Medicine in York, UK. He founded the Northern College of

Acupuncture, based in York, and steered the college towards the first acupuncture degree course in the UK. His interest in research led to him setting up the Foundation for Traditional Chinese Medicine and the Acupuncture Research Resources Centre in the 1990s. More recently his research interests have led him to join the Department of Health Sciences, University of York as a Senior Research Fellow, funded by the UK Department of Health. His research focus is varied, and includes evaluating the safety and effectiveness of acupuncture as well as neuroimaging to explore underlying processes of acupuncture in action. He also is coordinator of the STRICTA initiative involving an international group of experts with the aim of improving standards of reporting of clinical trials of acupuncture.

Charlotte Paterson

Charlotte Paterson is an experienced General Practitioner, and a Senior Research Fellow at the Peninsula Medical School, Universities of Exeter & Plymouth, UK. Her 10-year research programme into complementary medicine has combined qualitative and quantitative methods and has focused on the patients' perspective and how to define and measure patient-centred outcomes. She has been funded by the Medical Research Council as a Special Training Fellow in Health Services Research for a research programme entitled 'Developing patient-centred research methods for complex interventions: acupuncture for people with chronic disease'. She has developed and validated an individualised outcome questionnaire: 'Measure Yourself Medical Outcome Profile (MYMOP)'. She is a Trustee of the Research Council for Complementary Medicine and is on the research subcommittee of the British Acupuncture Council. Her work informs the debate about the 'integration' of complementary and conventional care and the value of holistic therapies and packages of care for people with long-term health problems.

Rosa N. Schnyer

Rosa N. Schnyer is an acupuncturist and Chinese herbalist in private practice. She is also a Research Associate at the Osher Institute at Harvard Medical School and at the New England School of Acupuncture (NESA). In addition, she serves as a Consultant to the Department of Psychiatry at Stanford University and the Department of Pediatrics at the University of Arizona. She is Co-Investigator of several National Institute of Health-funded research projects investigating acupuncture and co-President of the Society for Acupuncture Research. Rosa is the author of 'Acupuncture in the treatment of depression: a manual for research and clinical practice', 'Curing depression with Chinese medicine', several book chapters and articles on acupuncture research methodology. She began her East Asian medicine education in shiatsu and graduated from the now Tri-State College of Acupuncture in 1987. She is a doctoral student in the Doctor of Acupuncture and Oriental Medicine (DAOM) programme as well as a Research Fellow at Oregon College of Oriental Medicine.

Karen J. Sherman

Karen Sherman, PhD, MPH is a Scientific Investigator at the Group Health Center for Health Studies where she specializes in evaluating various types of complementary and alternative medicine (CAM), including acupuncture, for common health conditions. She received her Ph.D. in Behavioral Biology from Cornell University in 1983 and her MPH in Epidemiology in 1986 from the University of Washington. She worked as a cancer epidemiologist before becoming the Research Director at the Northwest Institute of Acupuncture and Oriental medicine, Seattle, Washington USA in 1996. In this position, she developed the clinical research programme, coordinated the development of acupuncture clinical protocols for two randomized trials and recruited and trained over 25 acupuncturists for various studies. She also taught Research Design to acupuncture students for five years. She has been the PI on four US National Institutes of Health funded clinical trials of CAM therapies and has been involved in the design of more than 10 randomized trials of CAM therapies, including both pragmatic and explanatory trials. She currently serves as Treasurer for the Society of Acupuncture Research.

Kate Thomas

Kate Thomas is Professor of Complementary and Alternative Medicine Research at the School of Healthcare, University of Leeds. Kate has undertaken research into complementary and alternative therapies, including acupuncture, for a number of years. During this time she has worked closely with colleagues at the Foundation for Traditional Chinese Medicine in York, and with them she has recently completed a large pragmatic trial of acupuncture for patients with low back pain being treated in primary care. This study found acupuncture to be cost-effective treatment for this group of patients and recommended its consideration for inclusion in National Health Service (state-funded) provision. Her current research interests are in the clinical and economic evaluation of complementary therapies for use in the UK National Health Service, the evaluation of different models of service delivery, and population/patient group patterns of use and access to complementary therapies. Her methodological research interests include the design of clinical trials for complex interventions and whole systems of healthcare, the application of mixed quantitative and qualitative research methods, and the development of appropriately patient-centred outcome measurement.

Peter Wayne

Peter Wayne, PhD, is an Instructor in Medicine and the Director of Tai Chi Research Programs at Osher Institute, Harvard Medical School. Dr Wayne's research focus is on the design and conduct of randomised trials of acupuncture and Tai Chi. Dr Wayne received his PhD in evolutionary biology from Harvard University in 1992, and remained there through to 2000 conducting research on the evolution of plant physiological traits. In 2000, pursuing his personal interest in Tai Chi and Chinese medicine, he founded the faculty research program at New England School of Acupuncture (NESA), served as its Director through to 2006, and continues to serve as the Principal Investigator for the NIH-funded NESA Acupuncture Research Collaborative Developmental Center grant jointly awarded to NESA and Harvard Medical School. Dr Wayne is also an active board member of the Society for Acupuncture Research. In addition to research, Dr Wayne is a long-term practitioner of Tai Chi and Qigong, and Director of the Tree of Life Tai Chi Center in the Boston area.

Adrian White

Adrian White is a conventionally trained doctor who developed an interest in acupuncture after seeing successful results in his patients in general practice. After training as an acupuncturist, he practised for 12 years before making the change to train as a researcher. He has conducted several clinical trials on the safety and effectiveness of acupuncture, and has completed several systematic reviews on different subjects including acupuncture for smoking cessation, for back pain and for osteoarthritis of the knee. His published papers were the basis of his thesis for his doctorate which was awarded in 2004. He is currently working on musculoskeletal pain, particularly myofascial pain and the pain of osteoarthritis. He runs a small acupuncture practice, holds a UK Department of Health Research Capacity Award in Complementary Medicine, and is also Editor of the journal *Acupuncture in Medicine*.

Peter White

Peter White trained as a physiotherapist in the UK and ultimately specialised in musculoskeletal outpatients in a National Health Service setting. He became interested in acupuncture in 1995 and used this alongside other conventional treatment modalities in his clinical practice. He started his research career in late 1998 when he began his PhD at the University of Southampton, a project designed to test the efficacy of acupuncture for neck pain. Since then Peter has written many papers on various aspects of acupuncture. He has been an advisor to the World Health Organisation on compiling guidelines for acupuncture research. He continues to conduct clinical trials and mechanistic studies on acupuncture at the University of Southampton and is particularly interested in utilising functional imaging to push this line of enquiry forward.

Foreword

The authors and editors of *Acupuncture Research: Strategies for Establishing an Evidence Base* are all pioneers who have a long track record of making significant contributions to our fundamental understanding of acupuncture and acupuncture research. They have now brought together their collective experience, knowledge, and wisdom into a single landmark book that represents the best and most insightful reflection on the state of acupuncture research in the Western world.

Some of the authors began their careers as practitioners of acupuncture. Instead of only accepting the familiar thought and behavioural patterns of East Asian medicine such as resonance (*gang ying*) or the reliability of sensory awareness, they decided to actively engage such biomedical notions as linear causality and the need for objective measurement. As a result, they have changed and expanded the conversation of the East Asian tradition. Some of the authors were originally trained in scientific research or Western medicine. But instead of pursuing only the straight and narrow trajectory, they decided to explore what was once called the 'margins' of healthcare. And, like their acupuncturist colleagues, they changed the boundaries of the permitted. From their different points of departure, each of these authors has become a unique and exemplary cross-cultural scientist-researcher-philosopher. They are solid in their traditions but competent and even fully qualified in an adopted framework. These researchers are bursting with creativity and new ideas. Bringing such individuals together into a single volume is a rare opportunity for a thoughtful reader to ponder important questions with the leading Western acupuncture researchers.

The authors and editors of this volume ask both the often-avoided broad questions and confront the details of more focused questions. The broad questions they ask include: why do Western-style research? What is it that we seek to learn by bringing the tools of science to Asian medicine? Does East Asian medicine need the validation of evidence-based biomedical approaches? Who gives the final answer on validity? How can one incorporate the patient's perspective and Asian medicine outcomes in Western research? How can the unique and often difficult-to-categorise experiences of patients be captured in research? How can qualitative and quantitative research support one another?

They also ask the necessary focused questions: what can be learned without control groups? How should experiments be designed to compare acupuncture with other types of healthcare? What are the different components of acupuncture treatment that need to be controlled in randomised trials? What should the placebo control be in explanatory randomised controlled trials of acupuncture? How should we judge the evidence presented in systematic reviews and meta-analyses? What do we know about the safety of acupuncture? What is the relationship of acupuncture basic science experiments to clinical research? How does one standardise an acupuncture intervention when there are so many different forms of acupuncture and when most clinical approaches involve constant adjustments and fine tunings?

Acupuncture Research does not give final answers to any of these questions. Rather the authors know that it is more important to build a framework for a collective discussion and look for answers to unfold in a long process of engagement and reflection.

Biomedical research often involves unanticipated outcomes and difficult-to-accept answers. Previous deeply held convictions are challenged. Research is about uncovering the unexpected. Each of the authors of this volume has been involved in research that has produced unexpected results. The authors have learned to sit with such experiences, meditate on them and gradually develop innovative responses. They know that the process is likely never to be complete and likely to remain tentative. They know that they have to rely on colleagues for new insights, conceptions, feedback and criticism. They have learned that science is a collective enterprise that, besides some competition, more importantly provides intellectual, academic, career and even emotional support. Their sense of collegiality infuses this volume and one gets the sense that ultimately the authors are actively in dialogue and learning from each other as they inform and engage the reader. They reach out to us to become colleagues.

The volume explores the interface where acupuncture and biomedicine meet in evidence-based acupuncture research and it ultimately raises the question of what is the purpose of this encounter. Why take the risks the authors of this volume have undertaken? It may not be obvious. Is the purpose to incorporate acupuncture (or those acupuncture protocols that pass for specific indications) into biomedicine? Is the purpose to have acupuncturists accept or reject aspects of acupuncture that are supported or not supported by evidence-based research? Are we creating a new domain called evidence-based acupuncture? Is the purpose to 'prove' acupuncture works and win the respect of the Western medicine establishment? Is the purpose to debunk acupuncture's claims? Will this research provide an additional set of evaluative eyes to ponder what is acupuncture? Is this an adventure to the unexplored? Will acupuncture and/or Western medicine develop new insights and healing capacities from this encounter? Will acupuncturists read classical texts or treat patients differently after they read reports of randomised clinical trials? Will biomedicine develop new ideas on how to incorporate patient perspectives and qualitative approaches into experimentation or healthcare? Who stands to gain? Will patients gain? Will society gain? Clearly, there are potential benefits and risks. Exactly what will happen is unclear. Discussions on contested frontiers are always loaded with the unknown and fear. Multiple strategies and outcomes — cooptation, assimilation, cooperation, pluralism or self-destruction — are all on the table. Despite these risks, the cross-cultural adventure has already begun and will undoubtedly continue to move forward. This volume has created an important framework for honest discussion and invites all people interested in East Asian medicine to join in this unique and unpredictable exploration.

Honest discussion ultimately concerns ethics. It is important to remember that honesty and ethics are complex value judgements often influenced by culture.

In this cultural encounter between Asian medicine and biomedicine, whose ethics should prevail? How does one accommodate potentially conflicting ethics or value judgements? A few examples might be helpful to illustrate the dilemma. Since the 1960s, biomedicine has developed an ethics that asserts that, ideally, legitimate healing and its social acceptability should be based on an improvement that is 'more than what happens in the placebo arm of a randomised controlled trial'. Legitimacy originates in a comparison with a bogus ritual. Asian medicine historically believes that the legitimacy of an intervention is derived from whether it helps improve a person's health. Legitimacy is comparison of outcome with a patient's earlier status or baseline. Results are important, not the method. Which ethical judgement should prevail?

Another example: modern medicine privileges objective measurement over subjective reporting or sensory awareness. Asian medicine privileges the subjective report and sensory impressions over any objective marker. Whose value judgements should prevail?

A final example: Asian medicine claims that the non-replicable experience of a patient is the ultimate ontological entity of healthcare. All treatments must be modified to capture this unique configuration. The alterations and adjustments are the critical details. Modern medicine believes that the standardised, replicable and statistically represented 'average person' is a more genuine reality. Whose values should prevail? *Acupuncture Research*, with its honest discussion of the big and small questions provides an important basis for contemplating such fundamental examination of ethics and paradigm.

The dialogue that *Acupuncture Research* initiates will clearly benefit all practitioners — East and West — and has the potential to enrich both. Discoveries, new awareness and sensibility await the results of research and the give and take of opinions and perspectives. This volume only increases the debt of appreciation all readers already have for the bravery of these pioneering authors.

Ted J. Kaptchuk
Harvard Medical School
Boston, USA

Preface

This book represents the first comprehensive overview of the key issues in acupuncture research and explores relevant strategies to develop a stronger evidence base for this traditional system of healthcare. The idea for the book had been brewing for many years; its time has now come. The reason for 'why now?' is because the field has reached an appropriate level of maturity to reflect on what has been achieved, as well as sufficient clarity about what remains to be done. We offer this book in the hope that it will be a useful guide for those who for whatever reason are puzzled, curious, and intrigued about acupuncture. It is also for those who are asking questions about how and why it works, for what conditions it is most effective, and wish to explore the reasons for its increasing popularity. It is also written for those who are sufficiently motivated to pursue answers to these questions, whether their primary focus is acupuncture practice or research. We also hope the book will be of interest to a wider audience, beyond the boundaries of professional practice and academic disciplines. For those with an interest in researching other complementary therapies, we hope the book will provide useful crossover perspectives. From a broader perspective, however, we are aware that this book does not have all the answers. Developing the evidence base for acupuncture is inevitably an ongoing process, and our aim has been to provide supportive signposts for the way ahead. In putting forward a strategic approach that has breadth and depth, we hope to make sense of the evidence to date, so that we can build on and broaden the existing evidence base in a way that is appropriate for the medicine.

The process of writing this book has been unusual. Almost all the authors attended a 3-day workshop in York in July 2006 where we brainstormed the ideas and methods that form the core chapters. Those invited to attend had a track record of conducting research in the field and were sufficiently open-minded regarding styles of acupuncture and breadth of appropriate research methods to be likely to be able to work collaboratively. Our intention was to bring together people with different backgrounds, in order for the book to benefit from the collective breadth of experiences. Our backgrounds in research included epidemiology, sociology, anthropology, neurobiology, immunology and health services research. Our backgrounds in acupuncture included a range of styles, including traditional Chinese medicine, Five Element acupuncture and Japanese acupuncture as well as Western styles such as trigger point acupuncture. Rather than a collection of stand-alone chapters, it was intended that the chapters of this book addressed a spectrum of issues within an overall structure. The chapters were designed to fit together like a jigsaw puzzle, each interlocking with the others to make an integrated whole. We also hoped for a consistent and accessible style, with frequent use of actual research examples to provide practical illustrations. As a group, we had prepared for the workshop by having the lead author of each chapter prepare a draft that was pre-circulated beforehand. At the workshop the themes underlying each chapter were discussed and debated. We were inspired by the new ideas that emerged, the fresh insights that were contributed, and the potential to synthesise these in our emerging chapters. Back home we pulled together what we had learned, and rewrote and revised our chapters into their present form. Inevitably we have not exhaustively covered every aspect of acupuncture research. We hope however that we have set out the broad strategies that will be helpful for the field and that the issues raised will inspire you to think about and engage in research in creative ways, whether as patients, as practitioners or as researchers. As you will see from what we have written, we hope that you will join us in integrating what is best about the practice of acupuncture with the core principles of good research and appropriate evidence-based medicine, evidence based in the context of what is relevant for the field.

Acknowledgements are due to those who have supported creation of this book and helped with the associated workshop in York. The initial ideas for the book were discussed with many people, and in particular with co-editors Richard Hammerschlag in Norway and Portland and with George Lewith in London. At Elsevier, we have had useful ideas and practical support from Inta Ozols, Karen Morley, Kerry McGechie and Claire Wilson. Inspiration for the overall style came from Kate Thomas and Mike Fitter's chapter in the book 'Clinical research in complementary therapies', edited by Lewith et al (2002), especially the way they used examples of research from the field. Professor Trevor Sheldon provided helpful ideas on the structure of the chapters, as of course did many of the contributors to this book. Anne Burton was instrumental in organising the workshop, co-coordinating arrangements for accommodation and travel. She also helped with the preparation of the manuscripts for several chapters. Mike Fitter helped construct the programme for the event, and provide a calm and thoughtful presence facilitating the first 2 days of the event. Val Hopwood and Richard Blackwell also attended the workshop, and they provided us with support and help in creating the content and style of the chapters. In the editorial group that included Rosa Schnyer, Richard Hammerschlag and George Lewith we brainstormed how to turn the workshop output into an accessible and inspiring book. Thanks are due to the staff at the Knavesmire Manor Hotel who looked after us so well and to the crew of the *River Countess* for our evening boat trip down the river. A number of people helped with reviewing and proof reading chapters at various stages, including Volker Scheid, Stephanie Prady and Sara Robin.

Financial support for the workshop came from many sources, and their confidence that we would use their support wisely is appreciated. We gratefully acknowledge funding from the Medical Research Council's Health Services Research Collaboration (with Charlotte Paterson taking the lead for this grant), Elsevier Ltd (in part as a result of George Lewith's generosity in waiving a contribution to an annual conference that had been held in Southampton), Stichting for Traditional East Asian Medicine, the Acupuncture Research Resources Centre (who provided funds left over from an international workshop organised by Stephen Birch in Exeter in 2001), and Richard Hammerschlag (who generously donated his air miles). A personal award in complementary and alternative medicine that I received from the UK's Department of Health is also gratefully acknowledged. Finally, the Foundation for Traditional Chinese Medicine has also provided considerable support for the workshop and the book, both financially and administratively.

Hugh MacPherson
Foundation for Traditional Chinese Medicine &
Department of Health Sciences, University of York,
York, 2007

Glossary of research terminology

Allocation concealment: in randomised controlled clinical trials, the concealment of the allocation to groups is required in order to be confident that researchers or those providing treatment do not (unconsciously or otherwise) influence who gets allocated to which group at randomisation. By helping prevent selection bias, the procedures ensure the benefits of randomisation.

Audit: a process used in clinical practice to identify whether certain standards are met, such as sending out letters to referring physicians, or reporting of side effects. An audit is often conducted at specific intervals to enable consideration of whether changes should be made to practice on the basis of findings. A less common use of the term 'audit' is in the context of collecting data, usually retrospectively, on patients attending a particular clinic. This might be more accurately described as patient or service monitoring.

Blinding/blinded: randomised controlled trials are fully blinded if all the people involved are unaware of the treatment group to which trial participants are allocated, until after the analysis of the results. It is not feasible for acupuncturists to be blinded in controlled trials, as they will usually be aware of the treatment that they are delivering. In explanatory randomised controlled trials with a control group, efforts are made to keep the patients blind to whether they are receiving the real or the control intervention. It is good practice to assess the success of blinding by checking if patients were aware of which group they had been allocated to. In randomised trials that compare two or more different interventions, where patients are aware of the treatment they are receiving, it is essential to blind the assessor of treatment outcome. In addition, it is possible for the statistician to be blind to allocation when conducting the analysis. The terms 'single blind' and 'double blind' are not used consistently in the literature.

Case series: repeated observations of more than one patient, often with data collected to identify whether there is an association between treatment and improvement. This also may help establish whether particular patients or treatments are associated with a relatively better (or poorer) outcome. Commonly all patients have the same condition. There is no control group.

Case study: a report based on clinical observation of one patient, usually with some assessment of outcome.

Cohort study: a study in which a group of people are identified who have something in common, for example, a new diagnosis of hepatitis C, and followed over time to observe the outcome, without any treatment or other intervention. The term is not usually used for a study of outcome from treatment, for which a 'case series' is usually the correct term.

Complex intervention: a description of a treatment that comprises multiple components or modalities and where it is not clear how to separate out individual components of treatment in order to measure specific effects. In any complex intervention it may be that some of the components are 'active' and others are not. It is possible that the sum of all the components are synergistic, interacting in such a way that the whole can be expected to be more effective than the sum of the parts.

Confidence interval (CI): a statistical calculation presenting the 'best guess' of the effect of an intervention (e.g. a mean) with a range of likely effects known as the confidence interval. Typically the 95% confidence interval is presented and we interpret this to mean that there is a 95% chance that the true (but not exactly known) size of the effect falls within the confidence interval. A 95% confidence interval provides the range within which the P value is less than 0.05 (see P value below).

Controlled trial: a comparison between two or more different treatment groups, for example one group receiving acupuncture and another group acting as a control, who might receive usual care, some other treatment, or sham acupuncture. The term 'controlled trial' is often used for trials without random allocation to groups, in which case there is potential selection bias due to groups not being equivalent. Non-randomised controlled trials will have weaker findings due to possible bias. When the method of allocation to groups is by random selection, the study is referred to as a randomised controlled trial (RCT) (see RCT below).

Correlation: a correlation is a quantification of the strength of an association between two variables. A correlation will not indicate whether there is causation (see mechanism below).

Cost-effectiveness: an analysis undertaken alongside a clinical trial to determine the costs of producing a change in a particular health outcome. Measures may include cost of treatment, days lost from work and surgeries avoided. When health outcomes are expressed in terms of costs for increased quality of life (typically 'quality adjusted life years' or QALYs, see below), the analyses are known as 'cost-utility analyses'.

Cross-sectional study: a study design that involves surveying a population at a single point in time. It can be used for assessing the prevalence of utilisation of treatment or of a specific condition in the population.

Delphi study: a consensus process designed to elicit expert opinion by asking participants to provide quantitative ratings, for example of the criteria for judging whether an acupuncture intervention is adequate. There may be several rounds of ratings, with confidential feedback to participants between rounds of both their rating and the group average rating. By giving equal weight to the views and ratings of each participant there is less risk that individuals or sub-groups will dominate. This type of consensus approach is frequently used to develop criteria or guidelines where the literature-based evidence is inadequate. Another consensus process with similarities to the Delphi approach is the nominal group technique.

Ecological validity: the extent to which the patients, practitioners and style of acupuncture within a study reflect the context of normal practice. This is similar to external validity (see below).

Effectiveness trial: a trial to measure the therapeutic effect of an intervention when it is delivered as it would be in practice in the real world. Effectiveness trials are usually simpler in design than efficacy trials as they may include flexible treatment protocols and broader inclusion criteria. Effectiveness trials in general have better external validity than efficacy trials.

Effect size: a measure of the size of the difference in effect between two variables. It is commonly quantified as the standardised mean difference (see below). Effect sizes can be used as a measure of mean change between groups, or within one group between baseline and outcome. Effect sizes can also be measured using rate ratios, responder ratios (see below) and odds ratios.

Efficacy trial: a trial to measure the therapeutic effect of an intervention in a rigorously controlled setting with 'optimal' administration of treatment. Efficacy trials are designed to include participants willing to adhere to the treatment regimen so they can determine whether the treatment works among those who receive it. It is worth noting that the use of 'sham' or 'placebo' controls does not itself constitute an efficacy study.

Equipoise: a genuine uncertainty on the part of the practitioners and researchers about the comparative therapeutic merits of each arm of a clinical trial. As an ethical principle, clinical equipoise provides a clear requirement that the healthcare of subjects should not be disadvantaged by research participation.

Explanatory trial: a trial undertaken to establish the specific component(s) by which a therapy such as acupuncture may work. It controls for non-specific elements in order to evaluate the specific effects associated with the 'active ingredients' of a treatment. Explanatory trials of acupuncture typically evaluate the effects of needling 'in the correct location' compared to some form of 'sham' acupuncture. Typically, these trials have stringent inclusion criteria and 'objective outcomes' if possible. These design characteristics lead to high internal validity.

External validity (generalisability): a measure of the validity of the results of a trial beyond that trial. For example, a study is externally valid and generalisable to regular clinical practice if its results are applicable to people encountered in regular clinical practice. This depends on the population from which the trial population was drawn, not just the entry requirements for the trial. External validity is enhanced when the acupuncture provided within a trial is representative of the acupuncture that is normally provided in routine practice.

Forest plot: a graphical method used in meta-analyses to show the variation in outcome between the individual studies under review. The plot also provides an estimate of the overall effect based on combining the results of all relevant studies.

Generalisability: see external validity above.

Heterogeneity: a term used in the context of meta-analyses as a measure of the dissimilarity between studies. Statistical heterogeneity occurs when the results of studies differ by more than chance alone. This dissimilarity can be due to the use of different statistical methods. Or it can result from differences in the patient populations, treatment characteristics or outcome measures, known as clinical heterogeneity. Pooling of data in meta-analyses may be unreliable or inappropriate when the trials are too heterogeneous.

Intention to treat (ITT) analysis: the method used to analyse the data for all participants based on the group to which they were (randomly) allocated, whether or not they ceased or changed treatment during the trial. The analysis is not based on whether they completed the per-protocol course of treatment.

Internal validity: a study is internally valid if it is designed and carried out in a way that provides results that are unbiased and gives an accurate estimate of the effects associated with the intervention.

Kappa: known as Cohen's Kappa, this statistic is used when two (or more) people provide a rating on a scale. On the basis that some agreement will occur by chance, the Kappa is a measure of the agreement between raters beyond chance: a Kappa of 1 is 100% agreement while a Kappa of 0 means no agreement beyond chance.

Manualisation: the development of guidelines for the implementation of an intervention for a clinical trial, with sufficiently accurate descriptions for it to be delivered appropriately and replicated if required. There is scope for flexibility in providing individually tailored treatments, while maintaining standardisation within a predefined treatment style.

Mechanism of action: the series of (physiological) events by which a cause induces an effect. In the case of acupuncture, the process by which needling induces changes in outcome. To be distinguished from correlation which identifies association rather than causation.

Meta-analysis: a quantitative method used to summarise the results of several clinical trials in a single estimate, weighted on the basis of the size or quality of each trial. This is different from, and is often performed subsequent to, a systematic review which is an explicitly systematic search and appraisal of the literature.

Model validity: a measure of the extent that the assumptions underlying the research design are congruent with the practice or intervention being tested. Good model validity or 'fit' is reflected in research methods that adequately address the unique healing theories and therapeutic contexts.

Natural history of a condition: the tendency of the severity of a condition to wax or wane over time. For many chronic conditions, patients often consult at a time when their symptoms are more severe, and the natural history of the condition may result in recovery over time, regardless of the intervention. Sometimes such changes over time are called 'non-specific' or 'placebo effects'.

Non-specific effects: in clinical trials, the non-specific effects are the contributions to outcome from anything other than the specific component that is being tested. What constitute non-specific effects will vary depending on the hypothesis. In acupuncture trials, needling at designated locations is often considered the specific or 'active' component, in which case the non-specific effects include those effects that result from anything but this needling, e.g. physiological effects associated with sham needling. When acupuncture is considered as a more complex intervention, there might be potentially active components beyond needling that are specific to acupuncture and therefore would contribute to the specific effects (see below).

P value: when comparing the effects of two interventions, the P value is the probability that an observed difference occurred by chance, assuming there is no real difference between the effects. The result is conventionally regarded as being 'statistically significant' if this probability is less than one chance in 20, i.e. a P value less than 0.05. A difference with a P value of less than 0.05 falls within the range of a 95% confidence interval (see above). As a guide, P values can indicate the strength of evidence of a difference as follows: greater than 0.1 = little or no evidence; between 0.05 and 0.1 = weak evidence; between 0.01 and 0.05 = evidence of a difference; less than 0.01 = strong evidence; less than 0.001 = very strong evidence.

Pilot study: any study that is specifically designed as a small-scale forerunner of a larger, more definitive study, for example a randomised controlled trial (RCT), to help develop and design it. Pilot studies usually address numerous feasibility aspects of the research design, e.g. will patients agree to be randomised to real acupuncture vs. sham acupuncture, and so sometimes are given the generic name feasibility studies.

Placebo: in explanatory clinical trials, 'placebo' is the term used in drug trials to describe the substance that is given to the control group. Ideally the placebo is identical in appearance, taste and feel to the intervention and physiologically inert. Moreover it must not have any of the specific (active) effects that are associated with the experimental treatment. In acupuncture trials, placebo treatments are often referred to as sham treatments. Placebos are not the same as giving no treatment, as they are expected to mirror all aspects of the experimental intervention except those that are associated with the specific (and presumed active) component(s) being tested. Therefore placebos cannot be assumed to be inert and, as in sham acupuncture trials, can be expected to have some level of physiological impact.

Pragmatic trial: a clinical research design, also known as a practical trial or management trial, which assesses the overall benefits of a routine treatment, providing results that are directly applicable to normal practice. Unlike the explanatory randomised controlled trial (to evaluate efficacy under rigorously controlled conditions), pragmatic randomised controlled trials do not aim to separate the treatment into specific and non-specific components, and usually compare a treatment to another accepted treatment (i.e. an active control), for example to standardised care, or to no treatment. Pragmatic randomised controlled trials aim to recruit a population that is representative of those who are normally treated, so these trials tend to employ broader inclusion criteria. Results are analysed on an 'intention-to-treat' basis (see above). Pragmatic trial designs are useful when conducting cost-effectiveness analyses (see above).

Prospective studies: any research design that is based on a pre-defined set of outcome measures to be assessed over a specific period of time. Prospective studies can be contrasted with retrospective studies (see below).

Psychometrics: the methods used to develop and test an outcome questionnaire to ensure that it performs well, is sensitive to change and measures what it is designed to measure.

Qualitative study: an investigation that provides non-numerical data on qualities, for example an investigation into the experience of an acupuncture consultation, from the perspectives of patients or acupuncturists. Qualitative data can be collected to provide information on perceptions of patients, acceptability of treatment, factors associated with satisfaction, etc., all of which can complement results based on quantitative data.

Quality adjusted life years (QALYs): a defined measure that combines the quantity and quality of life on the basis that 1 year of perfect health and life expectancy is worth 1, and anything less than perfect health and life expectancy is worth less than 1, i.e. between 1 and zero (equivalent to death). QALYs can be used to quantify benefits gained from a treatment in terms of quality of life for the patient. Although QALYs gained are a fairly crude measurement, they can be compared across different conditions and across different interventions. Pre-defined thresholds can be set based on a consensus regarding acceptable levels for cost-effectiveness. They are therefore useful for guiding decisions on the allocation of resources.

Quantitative study: an investigation that provides data on measured numerical quantities rather than qualities. Quantitative data lends itself to statistical analyses.

Quasi-randomised controlled trials: trials where the method of allocating participants to different treatments is not truly random, for example, allocation by day of the week, by date of birth, or by alternating the order in which participants are included in the study. The limitation of this method is that the allocation is not adequately concealed (see above) compared with randomised controlled trials.

Randomised controlled trial (RCT): a test for differences in outcome between two (or more) groups. In a parallel arm trial, one group receives the intervention to be tested and another receives a control or comparison procedure. The allocation to groups is randomised so that patient groups are expected to be equivalent at baseline. This design provides for an assessment of the relative benefits of interventions based on whether there are statistical differences in outcomes. The purpose of the randomisation and control are to minimise bias in order to better ascribe any differences in outcome to the intervention. The allocation to groups should be concealed (see allocation concealment above) from those providing treatment, so as to minimise potential interference with the random nature of the allocation process. Randomisation is likely to have been successful if the different treatment groups have the same characteristics at baseline, e.g. there should be the same number of men and women, or older and younger people, or degrees of disease severity and duration. (For descriptions of explanatory and pragmatic randomised controlled trials, see above.)

Regression to the mean: a statistical artefact whereby pre-selected extreme values when measured again later tend to regress towards the mean. In theory the effects of regression are balanced out in randomised controlled trials.

Reliability: a measure of the consistency of measurement when repeated over time, or consistency between different people measuring that same thing, or consistency between different measures.

Responder ratio (RR): a ratio of the response rate among those receiving an intervention to the response rate of those in the control group. The response needs to be defined in a valid way, such as 50% reduction in pain. In acupuncture trials for example, if more patients respond to acupuncture than to the control, then the responder ratio is greater than 1, however if more patients respond to the control then the responder ratio is smaller than 1.

Retrospective studies: a general type of research design based on previously collected data. Retrospective studies can be contrasted with prospective studies (see above).

Sham acupuncture treatment: a control procedure that, ideally, is identical in appearance and experience to acupuncture but lacks any of the presumed treatment-specific effects. Various types of sham acupuncture have been used as controls: superficial needling at the same acupuncture points, superficial or deep needling at non-acupuncture points, skin tapping with cocktail sticks, stage dagger needles (that retract inside the handle of the needle), etc. Sham acupuncture is sometimes categorised as either penetrating (invasive) or non-penetrating (non-invasive) in the belief that there might be more physiological effects with penetration. A general weakness of sham interventions is the lack of a generally accepted delineation of the acupuncture-specific effects that one wants to exclude from the sham intervention.

Significant effects: a term that implies a statistical test has shown a significance level of less than 5% (i.e. a P value less than 0.05). This is the same as an observed difference between interventions that would only occur by chance one time in 20. This is considered identical to having a 95% confidence interval that does not include the value corresponding to no effect. The convention is that when the word 'significant' is being used, it is in this statistical sense. Differences that do not reach significance can be called trends. (For confidence intervals and P values and their interpretation, see above.)

Specific effect: in clinical trials, the 'specific' effect under examination will depend on the hypothesis being tested, and so the specific effect can vary from study to study. In acupuncture trials, the specific effects are often assumed to be the therapeutically active effects resulting from the insertion of acupuncture needles at precise points with correct stimulation. When acupuncture is considered as a more complex intervention, there might be potentially active components beyond needling that are specific to acupuncture and therefore would contribute to the specific effects.

Standardised mean difference: a measure of a difference in means with the standard deviation as a denominator to provide a dimensionless measure of an effect. For example when comparing two interventions, the standardised mean difference is the mean difference in outcomes divided by the standard deviation. This is also known as an effect size (see above for other measures of effect sizes). The standardised mean difference can be helpful for making decisions about the size of an effect: 0.2 is a small effect, 0.5 is a moderate effect and 1.0 is a large effect.

Stratification: a procedure used to generate equal numbers of participants with a characteristic that is likely to be a predictor of outcome in each arm of a trial. Stratification is usually performed by using a separate randomisation for those with and those without the characteristic.

Systematic review: a type of review in which pre-specified search and assessment criteria are employed to address a defined research question. In this approach, a set of research studies, usually randomised controlled trials, are systematically identified, appraised, and summarised.

Introduction: acupuncture and the emerging evidence mosaic

Hugh MacPherson and Kate Thomas

THE PURPOSE OF THIS BOOK

Over the past two decades, we have seen an unprecedented growth in the practice of acupuncture in the West (Eisenberg et al 1998). This major shift in people's healthcare-seeking behaviour has had some important consequences, not the least of which has been the parallel growth in expectation that acupuncturists should produce evidence that what they practise actually works and is safe, as well as identify a plausible mechanism of action. This has been fuelled by the recent upsurge of, and widespread support for, the theory and practice of evidence-based medicine (Sackett et al 1996) as well as the rising standards of quality required for published research (Plint et al 2006).

However, acupuncturists often work in isolation, rarely possessing the resources, skills and expertise necessary for such a challenging research endeavour. Much research activity to date has been conducted by well-meaning experts from other fields, who have often underestimated or even overlooked the knowledge base within the traditions of acupuncture, the complexity of the field, and the subtle nuances required for good practice. As a consequence, the developing evidence base of acupuncture research has been patchy, with many clinical trials evaluating acupuncture that is not representative of everyday practice, or research that is insufficiently funded to provide unequivocal results. Reviews of existing data from acupuncture research repeatedly bemoan both the small scale and poor quality of published studies, and frequently conclude that evidence of effect requires more and better studies to be conducted.

In contrast, acupuncturists who treat patients on a daily basis regularly see obvious benefits resulting from the treatments they provide. Their conviction that acupuncture 'works' is based on careful observation and experience. They know that anyone joining them for a day at their clinic and hearing their patients' stories would be convinced that their patients experience real benefits. Acupuncturists welcome the sceptics who come for treatment, knowing that it is sometimes among this group of patients that the most dramatic results occur. Former sceptics can become enthusiastic about acupuncture and its benefits! Acupuncturists and patients alike would be forgiven for thinking that the current state of research evidence for acupuncture relates to a different therapy. How can it be that such good results are seen in the clinic and yet the evidence base is so weak?

Acupuncturists react in various ways to this weak evidence base for acupuncture. Some maintain that research is simply not needed, while others would maintain that most research to date is inappropriate or fatally flawed in some way. Others assert that the funding for research in this discipline has been so small that one could not expect much of an evidence base anyway at this stage of what is a relatively new profession in the West. Nevertheless there remain cogent arguments that we do need to know more about acupuncture, how it is practised, whether it is safe, and for what conditions is it effective. Only by building up an evidence base can we begin to map acupuncture's strengths and weaknesses, and whether it is possible to develop those areas of clinical practice that are most promising. Instead of writing off acupuncture research, there are valid arguments that it could be conducted better, and from this perspective, there are opportunities and imperatives to get involved (Fitter & Thomas 2005). Only by involvement can we really understand the types of research that can be conducted, the assumptions underlying the methods used, and the ways in which research could better reflect the medicine being practised. The current challenges in acupuncture research, and potential strategies for addressing them, form the core content of this book.

Our aim, then, is to identify the state of acupuncture research, the background to today's situation, and the current challenges in the field. These challenges relate to the nature of acupuncture, the potential of research, and the strategies most likely to bridge the gap between current research evidence and the actual experiences of acupuncturists in the field. We trust these strategies will be based on a better understanding of acupuncture and the complexity inherent in its practice, whether this is based on traditional principles or the more modern variants. By incorporating a more sophisticated understanding of the field, this book details a range of strategies aiming to develop the evidence base with the utmost rigour. It is the first book on acupuncture research to take this unique view, integrating the very best of evidence-based medicine with a genuine sensitivity to the discipline of acupuncture, from its traditional and holistic roots to its more modern practices.

WHY DO RESEARCH?

If conducting research into acupuncture is a challenge, then motivation is a major factor in undertaking it. For some, the spur is curiosity — about acupuncture, how it works, the conditions for which it is effective, and the aspects of the discipline that are more associated with benefits. Beyond curiosity, there are two further prime motivators: to 'prove' acupuncture works, and to 'improve' practice (Thomas & Fitter 2001). 'Proving' whether acupuncture, as a relatively new health technology in the West, is safe and effective for specific conditions is seen as essential for ethical patient care. The desire to explore the potential role of acupuncture in patient care often has to do with increasing its social acceptability and widening its access to those for whom it would not otherwise be affordable. It is also likely that a substantive evidence base is a prerequisite for an expanded role for acupuncture in funded health-care systems and insurance reimbursement schemes.

Establishing acupuncture's effectiveness, and therefore 'proving' whether it works or not, for specific conditions and in defined contexts is no small challenge. There are huge learning opportunities on the way for those who, for personal or professional reasons, are enthusiastic enough to become involved in research. The learning curve is one that is of value for those who see limited career pathways for the professional acupuncturist. Such research can involve exploring and validating the patient perspective, an important dimension to the field, given that, by and large, it is patients who have driven the expansion of acupuncture across the West. Also of importance is the practitioner perspective. For acupuncturists, an important interest has been how to optimise the benefits of treatment, and how to ensure that the qualities and approaches integral to the way that they practise are not lost in a research process designed to evaluate outcome. Practitioners' motivations can extend to a desire to be at the centre of research collaborations, not just to be invited to deliver a proscribed treatment within a clinical trial. Wanting to be at the centre of research collaborations is a response to the desire to shape the field, to set out more clearly what acupuncture involves, to emphasise the subtlety required to practise it well and to incorporate the flexibility needed to match treatment to the inherent variability of patients and their often complex conditions.

For many, 'improving practice' is the key reason for getting involved in research. How can we refine our techniques, better understand the dynamics of acupuncture in practice, improve results by changing treatment, or identify aspects of the therapeutic relationship that can better facilitate patients' active involvement? It should be stressed that these motivations need not necessarily always be wholly altruistic. Desires for intellectual challenge and career development may be very beneficial to the individual and field.

Acupuncture has also held a remarkable fascination for researchers with backgrounds from a range of disciplines. It poses a specific and as yet unanswered challenge to the dominance of biomedicine (Lupton 2003). It is clear that acupuncture has a fundamentally different understanding of the body than conventional medicine, one that can lead to a remarkable resonance with the experiences of the patient. Such a contrasting perspective is a compelling challenge to explore and investigate, potentially leading to a deeper and richer understanding of how healing processes can be triggered as well as a broader evidence base. Sociologists, anthropologists and historians of medicine have all been intrigued by acupuncture and taken up the challenges of research in the field. Many have a fascination with patients' stories, their experiences, and their insights based on these experiences. Investigating these perspectives, with rigorous and systemic research, has provided a useful qualitative background to counterbalance the evidence from those researchers who focus primarily on numbers. A range of scientists from a more quantitative background, including statisticians, health service researchers, health economists and methodologists have also become engaged with acupuncture research, providing support for the more technical aspects of surveys, trial designs and their analysis. Their motivation is often 'to do good science', and they are attracted by the fresh opportunities arising in a relatively new field of research.

One of the key characteristics of a profession is the ownership of a unique body of knowledge that informs professional practice and is constantly reviewed, renewed and augmented by the profession itself. It is clear that acupuncturists already have this body of knowledge, and that they need to engage in the ongoing creation of more knowledge, in order to keep the profession contemporary and vibrant. The key challenge for acupuncturists is to keep an open mind when collaborating and conducting research with others. Much can be learned from scientists who pride themselves on their 'professional' scepticism, a position that is least likely to bias the outcome of research. Needless to say, for those of us who primarily identify as researchers there is also a challenge to let go of the often tacit assumption that 'I know best' or 'I know which methods are best'. Where researchers and acupuncturists meet, there will inevitably be a creative tension. On the one hand, both bring different perspectives and important dimensions to potential collaborations; on the other hand, it would be a mistake to allow one or the other to have complete control of the creation of new knowledge. For those of us who work as both practitioners and as researchers, these tensions are likely to reside within, tensions that can impel us to seek resolution through insight and creativity. It is at the boundaries that we often see the development of a leading edge, the reframing of positions, and the extension of knowledge and understanding. It is the aim of this book to focus on this creative edge.

WHY ACUPUNCTURE IS A CHALLENGE TO RESEARCH

Acupuncture is a complex intervention that has its roots in China. In part, it has been an oral tradition, and in part text based, which has led to a proliferation of styles and schools of practice (Unschuld 1985). This diversity might be problematic for Westerners who would like a more definitive explanation of acupuncture and how it should be practised. However, within China such diversity has been seen as normal. The culture allows for mutually contradictory ideas to hold sway simultaneously. An example of competing traditions was during the Warring States period (480 BCE to 221 BCE) when there were four dominant 'schools', each of which had a coherent theoretical framework for guiding treatment (Unschuld 1985). More recently in China, we have seen a systematisation that has resulted in what some call a 'Westernised' style of acupuncture, which has been taught in the colleges of traditional Chinese medicine since the 1950s (Hsu 1999, Taylor 2004a). The limiting aspects of this systematisation have been widely discussed, with little sign that the debates are resolving (Scheid 2002). The point to be made here is that in China over the last two millennia there never has been a consistent and agreed framework for the practice of acupuncture.

Acupuncture as a practice has been transmitted to the West in a number of ways. Early on, Europeans studied acupuncture extensively in China, returning to Europe with a substantial body of knowledge which they passed on in books (Soulie de Mourant 1972). Other individuals have made a substantial contribution to the literature in English through translation. Furthermore, we have seen acupuncture being adapted in this process of transmission, with charismatic individuals blending their own unique view of acupuncture's potential, and new forms of acupuncture seamlessly created, which are usually passed off as 'traditional' without acknowledging what precisely is based on Chinese medicine and what is really a fresh interpretation (Taylor 2004b). In the independent sector, acupuncture is usually practised by individuals with no institutional affiliations. These acupuncturists are free to build their own repertoire, with personal adaptations to fit life experiences and temperament. Added to this diversity are the developments within specific professional groupings, with healthcare professionals using acupuncture as an adjunct to their existing practices. In these developments, we see components of acupuncture that are perceived to be of most value being extracted, and in some cases adapted, so that the new variant better fits the theoretical framework of the existing profession. For example the acupuncture practised by anaesthetists in pain clinics is likely to be very different from that practised by 'traditional' acupuncturists in private clinics. In effect, the acupuncture practised in the West today bears only a partial resemblance to that practised in China in previous years, and is now very diverse in terms of style, type of practitioner and setting for delivery. This becomes an issue for acupuncture research because it is extraordinarily difficult to know what is authentic, with the very real possibility that seeking the essential or core components will never bring a resolution that is acceptable to all.

This brings us to one of the key aspects of research into acupuncture, namely that acupuncture incorporates a potentially complex range of components, which together contribute to its practice. These components divide roughly into two main areas, the first of which is needling, a feature common to all styles of acupuncture. Acupuncturists make many judgements about the diagnosis that directs the overall treatment plan. Related judgements are made about the number of needles, insertion points, depth of insertion, obtaining the needle sensation of *De Qi* (Bovey 2006), the stimulation method used, the directing of *Qi* in a specific way, and so on. The second area of acupuncture practice is the non-needling aspect of care, an area particularly important in the more traditional styles of acupuncture. This area might include: diagnostic procedures such as palpation which enhance clinical judgements about managing the case; explanations based on acupuncture theory that help patients make sense of their conditions; and facilitating patients' active involvement so that they can make changes to their lifestyles (MacPherson et al 2006). These can be expected to be driven by a theoretical framework consistent with the knowledge base of acupuncture. These different components of practice are not independent of each other; both will influence each other in the iterative process of treatment and diagnosis that constitutes acupuncture care (Paterson & Dieppe 2005).

This complexity of practice is not unique to acupuncture. It is a well-recognised issue for research in many areas of conventional care (Medical Research Council 2000) as well as other traditional practices, such as homeopathy (Weatherley-Jones et al 2004). In all these areas of healthcare, complex interventions raise multiple questions at every turn. Is it possible to test each potentially active component of practice as if they operate in isolation? Or should we accept the interrelatedness of the various components, the whole being greater than the sum of the parts, and start with a multi-component approach to evaluation? This alternative approach takes the view that acupuncture is a complex intervention where it is neither feasible nor sensible to isolate every potential active ingredient.

Here we arrive at one of the major challenges that inspires this book, namely how best to conduct research into acupuncture in a way that is fair to the medicine. Acupuncture as it is currently practised raises all manner of questions about which style, which practitioner, and which theoretical frameworks are legitimate, as well as which setting is most appropriate for its delivery. If we aim for the simplification of acupuncture in order to reduce variability, then this will help us know more precisely what one can attribute any changes (if any) in outcome to. However, the greater the simplification of treatment, the greater the likelihood that results of such research will be dismissed on the basis that the acupuncture is unrepresentative of real practice. This is just one of many challenges to be addressed in this book, in which we hope to outline creative solutions and positive strategies for developing the field.

USING RESEARCH TO MOVE FROM EXPERIENCE TO EVIDENCE

The dream of science is to find explanations and answers for everything, and the simpler these explanations are, the better. The preference has often been for idealised solutions, abstract theories, objective facts, and hierarchical organisational structures and models. This has led much medical science headlong down a reductionist path, where workable rules and justifiable explanations become easier as we explore the parts that make up the whole. This tendency has produced a circularity, whereby finding rules or explanations using particular scientific methods renders these rules and explanations scientific! However, if researchers have too narrow an agenda then they may be in danger of losing sight of the whole. The human body, and the multifarious ways it deals with disease, is extraordinarily complex. Explanations from a reductionist perspective tend to be partial, especially where chronic disease is concerned. In contrast, in this book we take the broader position that medical science can also have a more holistic path, as it does in many other scientific disciplines, one that will support researchers in addressing the complexity of the human condition. We also draw on some of the traditions within science which recognize the merit in valuing and evaluating the potential whole with its interconnected parts, where the whole may be more than the sum of the parts.

Our desire in writing this book is to expand the way science is used to set standards in medicine, so that it is more geared towards complexity and diversity (Walach et al 2006). Instead of an evidence hierarchy, where there is only one way that is the most 'scientific', we would argue for an evidence mosaic (Reilly & Fitter 1997), which would incorporate evidence to answer different research questions, using appropriate methodologies and taking into account the needs of stakeholders with an interest in the answers. The origins of 'evidence-based medicine' were more patient centred, requiring 'a bottom up approach that integrates the best external evidence with individual clinical expertise and patients' choice' (Sackett et al 1996). It is hoped that this book will illustrate how, in developing an evidence mosaic for acupuncture, only some research questions can be answered using the methods of randomised controlled trials and meta-analyses.

One of the questions repeatedly asked about acupuncture, is 'does it work?'. This, of course, depends on what is meant by 'work'. The question is, in itself, ambiguous and poorly formulated, and can be deconstructed into issues of: whether acupuncture has a measurable active ingredient; whether it is better than some standard care; whether patients are sufficiently satisfied to continue treatment; whether it saves money or is cost-effective; and so on (Cassidy 1998a, 1998b). While the appropriate research method depends largely on the question, for each research question there can be a number of methods. This pluralistic approach, which has been called 'horses for courses' (Fitter & Thomas 1997, Thomas & Fitter 1997), is useful in providing us with a broader choice. Instead of a possible 'hierarchy', with a 'best' method sitting at the top, we need to adopt the methods that most properly fit our research question (Walach et al 2006). Research is often driven by the priorities embedded in social and institutional settings. Given limited resources, such prioritisation will help to focus research activity. An example of such an approach is the recent model developed by Fønnebø for the field of complementary and alternative medicine, an approach that is worthy of consideration for acupuncture (Fønnebø et al 2007). The model operates on the assumption that there should be a different prioritisation of research questions for pharmaceutical medicines still undergoing extensive testing and monitoring prior to general release to the public, as opposed to those therapies (or interventions) already in extensive use and outside national healthcare or regulatory systems. In the case of new pharmaceutical medicines, the conventional order of priority is sequenced as follows:

- mechanism and toxicity studies (often with animals)
- small-scale feasibility trials with humans
- large-scale efficacy trials
- trials comparing the intervention with a form of standard care
- general release to the public
- safety monitoring based on pharmacovigilance.

In contrast, for therapies that are already in widespread use (like acupuncture), the order of priority proposed by Fønnebø (2007) is sequenced as follows:

- map the field, and explore levels of utilisation
- investigate the public health issue of safety
- establish clinical (and cost) effectiveness of routine care
- evaluate the components of the therapy, assuming it has been found to be effective
- explore the mechanism for those components most strongly associated with efficacy.

For many, this alternative framework, which is illustrated in Chapter 13 (Fig. 13.2) seems eminently more suitable for ordering priorities than the drug model. The model has, to some extent, informed the ordering of chapters in this book.

ABOUT THE STRATEGIC APPROACH OF THE BOOK

This book consists of a series of integrated chapters each written by a small team of authors. Many of us have a professional background in acupuncture along with an abiding interest in research. Others amongst us have specialist research skills in another discipline and an ongoing commitment to harnessing these skills in close collaboration with acupuncturists to better evaluate the medicine. As a group we met for a 3-day workshop to plan and develop our ideas for this book. As a result of the considerable cross-fertilisation of information, ideas and inspiration, the content of this book has evolved to be very much a collective endeavour.

Underpinning the chapters of this book are several themes that have, to a lesser or greater extent, informed the strategic direction we have taken, including:

1. an understanding that the field of acupuncture research is a developing one; we have come so far already, but we have further to go
2. an excitement about the opportunities to learn from what has gone on before, rather than always having to reinvent the wheel
3. a respect for rigorous methods of clinical evaluation
4. a commitment to inclusivity — in the styles of acupuncture to be investigated, in the breadth of appropriate methods that might be suitable, and in the range of investigators that we encourage to engage in research in this field
5. a sensitivity to the medicine, the tradition, and the orientation to acupuncture being a unique and person-centred approach
6. a creativity that identifies current challenges and opportunities as well as possible future strategic directions
7. a recognition of the potential of research to improve clinical practice
8. an acknowledgement of the imperative for research to be informed by clinical practice.

In Chapter 2, we outline the background to acupuncture research, particularly as it pertains to the West. We offer a brief history of acupuncture as a way of introducing the diversity of current practice. We then explore some key cultural and philosophical differences between oriental and Western approaches to developing a knowledge base. We flag up the potential for mismatches, for example where a reductionist methodology might not be appropriate in the evaluation of a holistic medicine. Following this brief introduction to acupuncture research, the chapter concludes by identifying some useful perspectives for understanding the complexity of acupuncture and the diversity of the field. These include the need for research studies to be designed in a way to accurately reflect the patients, the practitioners and the style of acupuncture being tested.

In Chapter 3, we set out the research strategies used to map patterns of utilisation and the experiences of acupuncture patients. We are interested in research that focuses on not just *who* is using acupuncture, but *why* they are doing so. This calls for more in-depth investigation, where qualitative methods, such as interviews, can reveal patients' perceptions and experiences and what they particularly value about the treatment process. The case is put forward for multiple perspectives, with no one research method providing answers to all research questions. Strategies for research in this area may involve collecting either qualitative data or quantitative data, and sometimes a mixture of both. In this chapter we particularly stress the importance of the patient's perspective and the potential value this has if it can permeate all types of research into acupuncture.

In Chapter 4, we explore approaches to researching acupuncture safety, assuming that acupuncture can only be shown to be safe when we have robust evidence from real-world clinical practice. In this context we set out the key methods that have been used to identify and quantify the levels of risk associated with acupuncture. Given the current level of evidence, it is increasingly accepted that acupuncture can be considered safe in competent hands, but there remain a number of challenges. These include exploring the inherent variability and sensitivity of patients in their reactions to acupuncture, and the relationship between short-term reactions, which may include aggravations to treatment, and health outcomes. The goal of much of this research endeavour is to improve the safety of routine practice, and further research is likely to enhance this process.

In Chapter 5, we move on to the question of how best to measure the outcomes and processes of acupuncture from the patient's perspective. Our premise is that the patient should be central to the measuring process, and there is a need to identify what patients actually value about treatment, which often includes broader changes than those related to the primary presenting symptom. These broader changes can include whole person effects, and even a shift in social and personal identity. This chapter explores how these changes can be captured by specific outcomes measures, and opens up the opportunity of mapping change in this way in larger-scale studies and clinical trials.

Chapter 6 is the first of three chapters in which we investigate the 'effectiveness' of acupuncture. In this chapter we focus on studies where treatment effects and outcomes from routine acupuncture care are explored, but without the benefit of a control group for comparative purposes. We set out a range of appropriate research methods, ranging from single and multiple case series to surveys and qualitative studies. We also include an overview of the potential of pilot studies to assess the feasibility of larger-scale studies and clinical trials of acupuncture. While these uncontrolled studies are not 'definitive' in the way that randomised controlled trials can be said to be, they present some challenging aspects. We stress that the quality of the research methods is always important, and that feasibility studies are an excellent way of informing the key design features of more definitive studies of treatment effects and outcomes.

Chapter 7 concerns the comparison of treatment effects of acupuncture with other types of healthcare. Methods are explored by which we can ascertain whether acupuncture is more or less effective when weighed against a reasonable comparison. We set out a field guide for such research, clarifying the differences between effectiveness and efficacy, and between pragmatic and explanatory trials. The chapter focuses more on pragmatic and effectiveness studies, providing examples of how these studies have contributed to the evidence base for acupuncture. This approach lends itself well to studies of cost-effectiveness, an important concern in times of limited healthcare resources and when decisions have to be made about their allocation. We also explore some of the challenges posed, for example the potential limitations imposed when the acupuncture is constrained in a trial treatment protocol.

In Chapter 8, we explore research designs to investigate the efficacy of components of acupuncture. In contrast to the previous chapter, methods here are concerned with establishing efficacy *per se*, using explanatory trials. As with effectiveness studies, efficacy studies require a design that will produce as little bias as possible. Potential sources of bias are explored, and in particular for efficacy studies, the role of a sham or placebo arm for comparative purposes is described. A range of sham techniques that have been used in placebo-controlled studies are presented, as well as an assessment of their limitations. One concern is that placebo or sham acupuncture seems not to be physiologically inert, as would be ideal in a control. We ask whether it is actually possible to fully control for 'placebo' effects, especially when acupuncture is practised as a dynamic and interactive intervention. Nevertheless, we argue that there continues to be a need for rigorous methods that minimise bias, for establishing how well acupuncture works and for identifying the components of acupuncture to which any putative benefit can be ascribed.

In Chapter 9, acupuncture is described as a complex treatment intervention which has developed from a rich and diverse history. We set out the breadth of current approaches and styles of acupuncture, based on the traditions from Asia. Such diversity raises unique challenges when conducting studies to evaluate the clinical impact of acupuncture. This chapter addresses a range of questions, such as: How specific are the actions of the acupuncture points? How reliable are acupuncturists' diagnoses? How far can acupuncture be standardised without compromising the integrity of the intervention? We suggest some useful pointers for developing research strategies that combine the intellectual rigour of good science with a focus on evaluating the impact of acupuncture as a dynamic and interactive intervention.

Chapter 10 examines how research into the biological correlates and physiological mechanisms of acupuncture has developed, explaining the differences between correlations and mechanisms. Correlations are simply associations between some aspect of acupuncture and a biological measure, which could occur at any stage along the causal pathway. Mechanisms, in contrast, are the fundamental processes of acupuncture that initiate and drive physiological change. Knowledge of these can be helpful for many reasons. We illustrate how clinical practice can inform the direction of research into physiological mechanisms, and also how mechanism research can inform clinical practice. We provide an overview of research methods to establish correlations and mechanisms, assessing the strength and limitations of these approaches, and provide suggestions for advancing the evidence in the field. The importance of this type of research is stressed, not least as it may well provide a challenge to the dominant biomedical model of health and disease, with the potential for furthering the credibility for acupuncture.

Chapter 11 sets out the processes by which we can bring evidence together and systematically synthesise it in reviews and meta-analyses. Systematic reviews are explained, along with their clear research questions, explicit methods for identification and selection of relevant studies from literature, and criteria for critical appraisal of these studies. A short history of systematic reviews of acupuncture is provided, highlighting how differing interpretations can lead to different conclusions. This research endeavour presents us with several challenges, such as the variability of study designs used in acupuncture trials, as well as the variability in the styles of acupuncture that have been under scrutiny. Given the diversity of current acupuncture practice, assessing the adequacy of the treatment provided in clinical trials is a major issue. Nevertheless, there continues to be an important role for synthesising clinically relevant evidence in systematic reviews as an important approach to building the evidence base.

In Chapter 12 we explore the process by which acupuncturists can become involved in research. We are aware that the language and activities of research can be daunting, and so in this chapter we set out how research can be tackled by working with others. Research projects can, for example, be initiated at acupuncture schools and colleges, and we provide a number of examples where small-scale projects have led to useful understanding and fresh perspectives. Guidelines for conducting such studies, including having a clear research question, building a team of collaborators, and obtaining the necessary ethics permissions, are outlined. In this chapter we also argue that acupuncturists have an essential role in supporting projects initiated by established research groups. The expertise of practising acupuncturists can inform research designs and help set up appropriate treatment protocols so that the acupuncture evaluated is clinically relevant. In conclusion, we argue that acupuncturists have an essential role in promoting acupuncture research and helping ensure a respect for the integrity of the medicine.

In Chapter 13, we offer a 'blue skies' perspective, covering a range of ideas and thoughts about the future of acupuncture research. In particular, we focus attention on the need for a clearer strategic direction if we are to see advances in the field. Key dimensions emerge, including the therapeutic importance of acupuncture points, the value of incorporating the patient's perspective, the need to consider both qualitative and quantitative methods, the role of the consultation process, the importance of seeing acupuncture as a dynamic and interactive treatment modality and the cost-effectiveness perspective. A number of challenges lie ahead, including whether it is possible to establish a placebo control that is sufficiently inert to unequivocally identify which components of acupuncture work.

References

Bovey M 2006 De Qi. Journal of Chinese Medicine 81:18–29

Cassidy C M 1998a Chinese medicine users in the United States. Part I: Utilization, satisfaction, medical plurality. Journal of Alternative and Complementary Medicine 4(1):17–27

Cassidy C M 1998b Chinese medicine users in the United States. Part II: Preferred aspects of care. Journal of Alternative and Complementary Medicine 4(2):189–202

Eisenberg D M, Davis R B, Ettner S L et al 1998 Trends in alternative medicine use in the United States, 1990-1997: results of a follow-up national survey. Journal of the American Medical Association 280(18):1569–1575

Fitter M, Thomas K 1997 Evaluating complementary therapies for use in the NHS: 'Horses for Courses'. Part 1: the design challenge. Complementary Therapies in Medicine 5:90–93

Fitter M, Thomas K 2005 Duty, curiosity, and enlightened self-interest: what makes acupuncture practitioners participate in national research studies? Journal of Alternative and Complementary Medicine 11(2):227–228

Fønnebø V, Grimsgaard S, Walach H et al 2007 Researching complementary and alternative treatments – the gatekeepers are not at home. BMC Medical Research Methodology 7:7

Hsu E 1999 The transmission of Chinese Medicine. University of Cambridge, Cambridge

Lupton D 2003 Medicine as culture: illness, disease and the body in Western societies. Sage, Thousand Oaks, CA

MacPherson H, Thorpe L, Thomas K J 2006 Beyond needling - therapeutic processes in acupuncture care: a qualitative study nested within a low back pain trial. Journal of Alternative and Complementary Medicine 12(9):873–880

Medical Research Council 2000 A framework for development and evaluation of RCTs for complex interventions to improve health. Medical Research Council, London

Paterson C, Dieppe P 2005 Characteristic and incidental (placebo) effects in complex interventions such as acupuncture. British Medical Journal 330(7501):1202–1205

Plint A C, Moher D, Morrison A et al 2006 Does the CONSORT checklist improve the quality of reports of randomised controlled trials? A systematic review. Medical Journal of Australia 185(5):263–267

Sackett D L, Rosenberg W M, Gray J A et al 1996 Evidence based medicine: what it is and what it isn't. British Medical Journal 312(7023):71–72

Scheid V 2002 Chinese medicine in contemporary China: plurality and synthesis. Duke University Press, North Carolina

Soulie de Mourant G 1972 Chinese acupuncture (L'Acupuncture Chinois). Maloine, Paris

Taylor K 2004a Chinese medicine in early communist China (1945–1963): medicine in revolution. Routledge, London

Taylor K 2004b Divergent interests and cultivated misunderstandings; the influence of the West on modern Chinese medicine. Social History of Medicine 17(1):93–111

Thomas K, Fitter M 1997 Evaluating complementary therapies for use in the NHS: 'horses for courses'. Part 2: Alternative research strategies. Complementary Therapies in Medicine 5:94–98

Thomas K J, Fitter M 2001 Evaluating complementary medicine: lessons to be learned from evaluation research. In: Lewith G, Jonas B J, Walach H (eds) Clinical research in complementary therapies: principles, problems and solutions. Churchill Livingstone, London, UK

Thomas K J, Fitter M 2002 Possible research strategies for evaluating CAM interventions. Jonas and Lewith (eds) Clinical research methods in complementary therapies; principles, problems and solutions. Churchill Livingstone, Edinburgh

Unschuld P 1985 Medicine in China. A history of ideas. University of California Press, Berkeley

Walach H, Falkenberg T, Fonnebo V et al 2006 Circular instead of hierarchical: methodological principles for the evaluation of complex interventions. BMC Medical Research Methodology 6:29

Weatherley-Jones E, Thompson E A, Thomas K J 2004 The placebo-controlled trial as a test of complementary and alternative medicine: observations from research experience of individualised homeopathic treatment. Homeopathy 93(4):186–189

Acupuncture research: the story so far

Stephen Birch and George Lewith

INTRODUCTION TO THE HISTORY OF ACUPUNCTURE

While acupuncture may have its roots elsewhere, the first texts of acupuncture appeared in China a little over 2000 years ago, circa 200 BCE (Unschuld 1985). The theories and methods of acupuncture that were first described at this time already reflected considerable variety. This was to be expected since the early texts were themselves collections of many different people's ideas from different places and times (Birch & Felt 1999, Lu & Needham 1980, Unschuld 1985). Subsequent ideas and methods used in the practice of acupuncture continued changing as a consequence of China's evolution and also as acupuncture migrated to, and was adopted as, an effective treatment in different Asian and European countries and cultures. Consequently there are often many contradictory ideas about acupuncture that can be found in historical and modern literature (Birch & Felt 1999, Lu & Needham 1980).

Acupuncture is thus a broad and diverse field of medical practice. Much of what has been described about the clinical practice and use of acupuncture over the last 2000 years can appear confusing and even contradictory. This is reflected in the past and present diversity in the expression, models of theory and practice, and understanding of acupuncture. It has also added to the difficulty in interpreting acupuncture's clinical literature (Birch & Felt 1999). These historical facts are relevant to the discussions of acupuncture research in this and later chapters.

Acupuncture is a multi-faceted and multi-modal therapy. It may combine many different ideas and theories with the clinical application of those theories in diagnosis and treatment selected from amongst a range of very different 'acupuncture' techniques (Birch & Felt 1999, MacPherson & Kaptchuk 1997). Additionally, the therapist may use Chinese traditional medical theory to advise the patient, for example by explaining and justifying lifestyle, and dietary changes, as well as employing an evolving therapeutic

15

intervention involving needling, moxibustion, cupping, herbs and massage. It is wise not to approach acupuncture as though it were a single simple therapy around which there is expert consensus, but rather as a complex intervention (Medical Research Council 2000). One of the challenges that acupuncture research faces is the development of appropriate methods that are able to capture and investigate this complexity (Paterson & Dieppe 2005, Verhoef et al 2005). Another important challenge is the development of a more complete understanding of the nature of acupuncture, including the inherent diversity derived from its philosophical and cultural roots.

OVERVIEW OF IMPORTANT PHILOSOPHICAL AND CULTURAL CONTEXTS OF ACUPUNCTURE

Acupuncture arose in quite different cultural contexts from Western medicine and the scientific method encapsulated in the 'Enlightenment'. Therefore there are important cultural and philosophical differences between acupuncture and modern bio-medicine. Highlighting some of these differences illustrates some of the problems that researchers face when trying to investigate acupuncture using scientific methods.

One of these differences is the historical East Asian trend of seeing body, mind, emotions as one, rather than distinct (Birch & Felt 1999, Ikemi & Ikemi 1986, Roth 1999, Shen 1986). Since the time of Rene Descartes, Western science has been struggling with its tendency to see the body, mind and emotions as separate, especially in the fields of biology and medicine (Foss & Rothenberg 1987).

Another important difference lies in the virtual absence of the 'either-or' logical assumptive approach in ancient China and other Asian cultures. While this dominates modern Western scientific thinking, its virtual absence in ancient Asian philosophies is often overlooked. Unschuld argues that this is probably a by-product of science having developed in a monotheistic culture (Unschuld 1987). In the either-or assumptive model, one cannot accept the validity of competing ideas; if one idea is right a contradictory one must be wrong. The scientific method for establishing 'truth' is a clear example of the either-or approach. Scientific truth is developed using methods that assume this to be axiomatic. However, the traditional literature on acupuncture is full of contradictory ideas, even within the same texts. This was not a problem for early authors since they did not assume that if one approach was right the other had to be wrong. Rather ideas and assumptions of all kinds coexist at many different 'levels' of interpretation with no attempt or indeed any reason to derive an absolute truth (Unschuld 1985, 1987, 1992). This is reflected in acupuncture being more than a single uniform therapy; it is, and always has been, defined by diversity of ideas and methods (Birch & Felt 1999, Scheid 2002, 2006). This creates problems for scientists when they assume a 'Western' truth model as well as uniformity in acupuncture theories and try to formulate testable hypotheses on the basis of their (rather than acupunctures') assumptions.

Systemic differences

Much of the early evolution and development of acupuncture was based on practitioners collecting their own experiences during their clinical lifetime and learning from it, and passing that information on to their pupils as their wisdom. The perspective of objectivity that underlies the scientific approach did not develop in Asia until it was gradually imported from the West after the seventeenth century (Birch & Felt 1999). This is not to say that acupuncture did not follow a systematic approach in making observations and then further developing theories based on those observations, but it did so with empiricism and respect for the wisdom of the experienced individual physician, in much the same way as medicine evolved in Europe before the Enlightenment. Today we speak of 'evidence-based medicine' as helping provide a standardised medical care based on research. In a parallel way we can speak of acupuncture as 'experience-based medicine', relying on systematic use of empirical and pragmatic observations. The latter can be said to rely strongly on three basic steps, while the former uses the same three steps but then adds two more steps in order to make the process more objective (see Table 2.1).

Of course practitioners of experience-based medicine also published and discussed their cases and observations, which, over time constituted a peer-review process. But in the evidence-based approach these last

Table 2.1 Iterative stages in the process of development of evidence-based medicine and experience-based medicine

Stages	Evidence-based medicine	Experience-based medicine
(i)	models of theory and practice	models of theory and practice
(ii)	process of inquiry	process of inquiry
(iii)	experience of the patients and practitioners as well as the case history literature	experience of the patients and practitioners as well as the case history literature AND then iterative feedback from Stage (iii) to Stages (i) and (ii) to develop and improve the models of theory and practice
(iv)	verifiable observations and planned experiments	
(v)	peer review of observational and experimental literature AND iterative feedback from Stages (iii), (iv) and (v) to Stages (i) and (ii) to develop and improve the models of theory and practice	

two stages are highly formalised, following strict guidelines. For example publication is preceded by peer review rather than vice versa. Verification of observations and experiments includes the use of validation processes and objective measurements, each of which is tested and verified before being acceptable. Thus Stages (iv) and (v) in an evidence-based approach are more rigorous and formalised than in the experience-based approach.

Cultural-philosophical differences

Acupuncture developed in China mostly under Confucian and Daoist philosophical influences (Lo 2001, Unschuld 1985). Asian historical cultural processes and their primary philosophical and cultural contexts were based on a very different world view than that which predominates today in Western scientific thinking (Birch & Felt 1999). Important features of these East Asian thought processes were to see the body and mind as necessarily interconnected and inseparable, and to see the connections and interactions of everything as equally if not more important than the individual elements of an illness or pathological process. In modern scientific thinking we frequently but not invariably consider the minutiae of specific organ-based pathologies as primary because of the dominance of Cartesian mind–body dualism and reductionist thinking (Birch 1995, Birch & Felt 1999, Foss & Rothenberg 1987, Unschuld 1987, 1992). These are useful generalisations as they highlight some of the challenges researchers face (Birch 1998, Birch & Felt 1999). Table 2.2 summarises the differences in philosophical and cultural tendencies between traditional and historical forms of acupuncture medicine and modern scientific medicine.

Table 2.2 Differences in philosophical and cultural tendencies between traditional East Asian medicine and Western scientific medicine

Western scientific medicine	Traditional East Asian medicine
General adoption of an 'either-or' assumptive approach	General adoption of a 'both-and' assumptive approach
Widespread effort at generating objective descriptions	Little to no effort at generating objective descriptions
Widespread adoption of mind–body dualistic thinking	Widespread adoption of mind–body integrative thinking
Widespread use of reductionist type thinking processes	General emphasis on holistic thinking processes

[For more discussion of these differences, see Birch (1995), Birch & Felt (1999), Unschuld (1987, 1992).

The importance of these philosophical and cultural differences becomes clear if we contrast the tendency in the West of making the 'tenuous distinctions between energy and matter and between mind and body' (Roth 1999, p 41). The lack of these divisions in China and subsequently traditional East Asian medicine is apparent within acupuncture (Birch & Felt 1999). Instead the ancient Chinese theoretical model posited the existence of '*Qi*' which is both the source of all material objects and all psychic and spiritual phenomena. In cosmological theory it was proposed as early as 140 BCE that *Qi* is the origin of heaven and earth and everything in between (Roth 1999, p 41), and circa 90 CE that just as water freezes to become ice, so too *Qi* condenses to become matter (Birch & Felt 1999, p 92). Likewise *Qi* was described in the early literature as lying at the heart of all emotional, mental and spiritual phenomena (Birch & Felt 1999, Roth 1999). There has thus been a distinct absence of Western mind–body duality and the reductionist tendencies of modern Western thinking in traditional East Asian medicine healthcare models (Birch & Felt 1999, Unschuld 1992). The concept of *Qi* lies at the heart of the more unified and holistic models of traditional East Asian medicine. These fundamentally different assumptions about the nature of the human being and the world remain unaddressed issues in the scientific investigation of acupuncture.

Given these important philosophical and cultural differences between Western ways of approaching and understanding the body and the more historically based approaches from Asia we can expect to find important challenges confronting us when investigating acupuncture. Three examples highlight some of the important challenges researchers face investigating acupuncture.

How helpful or relevant is it to use the placebo-controlled randomised clinical trial (placebo RCT) for assessing acupuncture's clinical effects? This kind of clinical trial may assume that the components of the treatment that contribute to the overall treatment effects are separable and do not interact so they can be reduced to discrete components. However the validity of these assumptions has been questioned in the context of acupuncture research (Foss & Rothenberg 1987, Kaptchuk 1996, Paterson & Dieppe 2005). If the traditional model of practice that is being assessed is more holistic, meaning that it does not assume a mind–body duality and does not permit isolation of part of the whole process and is not based on an either-or logical assumptive approach, then the RCT must be designed around this assumption. It will then only be able to assess the 'whole system', rather than evaluate the effects of various components within that system. This may mean that we require more pragmatic studies (see Chapter 7), even though such studies will tell us nothing about the contribution from contextual factors, sometimes labelled the 'placebo' effects (see Chapter 8).

Likewise, how can the mechanisms of acupuncture's treatment effects be identified using laboratory research methods? If we ask, for example, how acupuncture is able to treat pain, this tends to lead into an examination of known analgesic mechanisms in the body and how acupuncture may affect them (Birch & Felt 1999). How do we separate mechanisms from a whole system of interacting effects and meaningfully discuss those with reference to acupuncture? What theoretical model of acupuncture was used for the research question — one based on known Western analgesic mechanisms or one based on traditional acupuncture theories and methods? Sometimes it appears that the varied traditional theories of acupuncture are ignored in these studies in favour of current Western physiological understanding (Kim 2006). It is certainly possible to address these issues but it requires sensitivity and sophistication as well as an understanding of the historical evolution of acupuncture.

A third example of these difficulties lies in the influence of the 'either-or' assumptive model. Today the most popular theoretical model underpinning acupuncture in the West has become that of 'TCM' (traditional Chinese medical) acupuncture, sometimes loosely called 'traditional' or 'classical' acupuncture. Since this has now become misnamed but synonymous with all traditional forms of acupuncture (Birch 1995, Birch & Felt 1999) it is then assumed that it not only covers all forms of traditional acupuncture but that other forms (if they exist) may be 'incorrect' (Birch 1995) as they are not real TCM. However TCM is not the monolithic system it has been portrayed to be in the West and is itself a mix of diverse traditions (Scheid 2002). Further, it is not representative of all the other traditional forms of acupuncture (Birch & Felt 1999, MacPherson & Kaptchuk 1997). But researchers have assumed that if they are testing what they consider to be 'TCM', 'traditional' or 'classical' acupuncture they have investigated all forms of 'traditionally based systems of acupuncture' (Birch 1997). There is a major problem with attempting to generalise about traditional forms of acupuncture under the misnamed and misunderstood rubric of 'TCM', 'traditional' or 'classical' acupuncture.

While we can expect that science and scientific methods will be used to investigate traditional medical practices, it is vital to understand and attempt to deal with these philosophical and cultural issues when we wish to conduct such research and interpret the results. Calls for further research into the more traditional methods and ideas of acupuncture (Acupuncture 1998) require that efforts be made to address these fundamental issues.

THE ACCULTURATION OF ACUPUNCTURE: A HISTORY OF CLINICAL RESEARCH ON ACUPUNCTURE

The situation for understanding acupuncture and modern iterations of traditionally based systems of acupuncture is further complicated by the fact that modern Western ideas have been penetrating and influencing Chinese, Japanese and Asian cultures over the last 300 years (Birch & Felt 1999, Lu & Needham 1980, Unschuld 1985). Equally, traditional Asian ideas have been penetrating into Western cultures for the same period of time. Thus, for many forms of acupuncture we can no longer look only to the traditional ideas and methods of thinking, we find many new culturally based 'blends' that merge East and West, explicitly or implicitly combining the different approaches.

Sometimes traditional ideas are translated in modern texts in terms that seem familiar to us in the West, often as a result of modification of those terms in light of modern scientific concepts. This problem is encountered both when modern Asian authors have attempted to translate historical ideas into modern language and concepts (Sivin 1987) and even more so when Westerners attempt to translate the historical and modern Asian texts into Western European languages (Wiseman & Feng 1997). This complicates the process of developing accurate models of acupuncture that are to be tested (Stage (i) in Table 2.1). It is also difficult to establish congruence of terms between different traditions of practice (Stage (iii) in Table 2.1). A debate has been occurring about how to translate Asian medical texts into Western languages for the last 20 years and is still unresolved (Bensky et al 2006, Birch & Felt 1999, Reid 2006, Wiseman & Feng 1997). This raises difficult questions about how to interpret the acupuncture theories and ideas that are available to us in the West when we initiate research into the methods of practice on which they are based. The difficulties are considerable and are not simply limited to trying to find a one-to-one translation of seemingly similar terms such as '*gan*' to 'Liver' or '*xin*' to 'Heart'. Traditional acupuncture is full of terms and concepts that are completely foreign to Western scientific cultures, with no obviously equivalent terms or concepts available for translation. The most obvious being the term '*Qi*' variously translated as 'energy', 'vital energy', 'breath', 'vapours' and 'influences'. These problems challenge clinicians and research scientists (Birch & Felt 1999). Many invalid cultural assumptions are honestly but unwittingly made by practitioners and researchers when they translate acupuncture into terms and concepts familiar to them (Lu & Needham 1980, p 11–12, Unschuld 1987, 1992, p 55).

Sometimes the traditional ideas are reframed in the context of a modern scientific model of the body. This also complicates the processes of inquiry, observation, the interpretation of findings and designs intended to improve the model and process of inquiry (Stages (i)–(iii) in Table 2.1). Three examples are outlined below.

Currently the most popular form of acupuncture in the West is some form of the TCM approach following developments in China after the communists took over. Starting in the early 1950s under Mao's rule, traditional medicine was encouraged to continue in China provided it was adapted to fit within the socio-political systems of the day. Traditional forms of medicine were called '*zhong yi*', literally 'centre medicine' or 'Chinese medicine' to distinguish them from '*xi yi*' or 'Western medicine'. The process of adaptation involved blending acceptable forms of traditional theory and methods from the diverse traditions of acupuncture, herbal medicine and massage with a modern Western medical model (Birch & Felt 1999, Unschuld 1985, p 250–251, 1992, Scheid 2002,

Sivin 1987, p 17, Taylor 2004, Wang & Zhao 2007). With an eye to Western interests in China, the first publications to label it as 'traditional Chinese medicine' or TCM appeared in 1955 (Taylor 2004). This occurred alongside a desire to project China as contributing to the modern scientific world and with the beginnings of a research agenda that projected TCM to 'be a showpiece of the progress of science' (Taylor 2004). What is widely known as TCM acupuncture in China and the West reflects this combination of traditional Chinese and modern Western thinking, raising questions about its claims of historical validity (Ogawa 1996, Unschuld 1998) and concerns about the survival of traditional theories and methods (Freuhauf 1999, Kaptchuk 1985).

Acupuncture developed quite differently in Japan from the late 1800s. During the push to modernisation of the Meiji Restoration, modern biomedicine was adopted as the 'standard' of healthcare. Acupuncture was relegated to a technique that modern physicians (using Western medicine) or blind practitioners could practise. The practice by blind practitioners was eventually restricted by eliminating all traditional concepts from their training (Manaka et al 1995, p 14). This led to a backlash and the development of a growing traditional style of acupuncture known as 'keiraku chiryo' — 'meridian therapy' (Fukumoto 2006, Shudo 1990). This new traditionally based model developed with the explicit goal of re-establishing traditional acupuncture methods, with unnecessary and impractical ideas stripped out to allow it to survive in the modern Western Japanese environment (Birch & Felt 1999). After 1948 acupuncture had become standardised in the licensing curriculum but with increasing diversity of approaches in post-graduate education and clinical practice. Here purely 'traditional' schools, purely 'scientific' schools and all kinds of other combinations were allowed to develop (Birch & Felt 1999). Some schools of acupuncture combined biomedical with traditional ideas and methods, while some attempted only traditional or only scientific approaches. Just as we find a broad diversity of approaches to the practice of acupuncture today in China (Scheid 2002) we also find a broad diversity of approaches in Japan (Birch & Felt 1999, Lock 1980). This suggests that acupuncture is not a single entity.

A third example of the attempted integration of modern Western ideas into traditional approaches can be found in those models that have incorporated modern Western psychological theories and concepts into their systems of acupuncture practice (Hammer 1990). Just as psychoanalytic theory was new for Western medicine in the twentieth century, it was very new for East Asian cultures and their medicines. Western practitioners familiar with both systems have found unique ways of combining them (Hammer 1990, Seem 1987). These combinations muddy the waters further for the researcher attempting to investigate acupuncture as they tend to create more confusion about its nature and practice (Birch 1998).

Sometimes, the Western student is searching for an alternative to the dominant Western medical model and picks out only those 'holistic' sounding ideas and methods as representing 'traditional acupuncture'.

One consequence of this is the construction of very selective approaches to acupuncture in the West that possibly fit better to the assumptions and desires of the Western student and practitioner than the traditional model or practice (Unschuld 1987, 1992). This complicates the processes of development, inquiry, observation and patient experience (Stages (i)–(iii) in Table 2.1).

So far we have examined how acupuncture has been acculturated in the modern period. But, science and modern medicine have also been adopted in and acculturated into East Asian cultures. As we will see, this has consequences for how East Asian and Western scientific investigations of acupuncture have proceeded.

SCIENTIFIC INVESTIGATIONS OF ACUPUNCTURE

Early research

Early investigations of acupuncture were more speculative than scientific, focusing on trying to understand this traditional medicine. These occurred both in Asia as well as the West. Following Sugita Gempaku's publication of a Japanese translation of a Dutch anatomical text in 1774, Western-based anatomical and physiological concepts began influencing the understanding and practice of acupuncture in Japan (Lu & Needham 1980, Kuriyama 1992). Less than 25 years later in France in 1798, Rougement speculated that acupuncture was a kind of 'counter-irritation' therapy, thus invoking current physiological understanding. This model was reiterated by Japanese physician Tesai Okubo in 1894 (Lu & Needham 1980). Today there are well-developed models of 'counter-irritation therapy' such as that of 'diffuse noxious inhibitory control' with scientific evidence of the analgesic mechanisms involved and proposals that they may help us understand some of the effects of acupuncture (Le Bars et al 1988). These and other writings of the eighteenth and nineteenth centuries focused on the use of acupuncture for pain relief, often in rheumatic diseases (Lu & Needham 1980).

There were also some important innovations during this time that set the stage for later scientific investigations. For example in 1825 Sarlandiere in France started applying electrical stimulation to the inserted needles to see how this altered treatment effects (Lu & Needham 1980). But in general, acupuncture did not make sufficient inroads in Western countries to warrant much attention from scientists. However, following the Meiji Restoration in the latter part of the nineteenth century, Japan was modernizing rapidly. After Western-style medical practice was adopted as the standard of healthcare in Japan, a number of physicians and scientists turned to studying acupuncture and its related moxibustion therapy. This in turn led to the establishment of a research movement in 1905 led by Kinnosuke Miura (Manaka et al 1995, p 349). Then, beginning in 1912, studies exploring the biological and physiological basis of moxibustion therapy were published. Historically moxibustion was rolled into small pieces and burnt on the skin, leaving small blisters on the acupoints. While this style of moxibustion has become less popular in modern China, it is still common in Japan where the method is called 'okyu'. At the beginning of the twentieth century this style of moxibustion had developed the reputation for curing serious infectious diseases such as tuberculosis. Thus one of the early foci for the physiological investigations of okyu was into its immunological effects (Hara 1929, Tamura 1934). Between 1912 and 1941 more than 45 studies were completed showing the probable physiological and immunological basis of okyu moxibustion therapy (Manaka et al 1995, p 353–354). For example studies found that this kind of moxibustion stimulated red blood cell production (Hara 1927) while acupuncture needling generally did not — leading to a clinical differentiation still taught in many Japanese acupuncture schools (Manaka et al 1995, p 353). Other researchers suggested a physiological model of moxibustion as a kind of stimulation therapy similar to the counter-irritation therapy, focusing on the zones of Head (Goto 1914).

Reductionist science and electrodermal measurement

In the 1950s in France, Niboyet and colleagues began the first studies of the acupuncture points and channel systems using electro-dermal measurement methods (Lu & Needham 1980, Zhu 1981). This work provided the first circumstantial evidence that the acupuncture points and channels may exist and were scientifically measurable. This innovative work was capitalised by others who developed commercial applications. In the 1950s Yoshio Nakatani started measuring the acupuncture channels and points using an electro-dermal measurement technology that he acknowledged measured the galvanic skin response. He assumed that this measured the state of the autonomic nervous system (Nakatani & Yamashita 1977). This was accompanied by the development of the Ryodoraku diagnosis and treatment system which claimed to focus on the autonomic nervous system (ANS), a system that many Japanese believe to be central to acupuncture (Oda 1989). Parallel developments occurred in Germany with the work of Voll who also investigated the electro-dermal properties of acupuncture points and channels developing the system known as 'Electro-acupuncture according to Voll' or EAV (Voll 1975). This, like Nakatani's system, involved commercial developments in the form of a diagnostic instrument with treatment protocols. However, differences in how the electro-dermal measurements were made and simultaneous interest in more Western medical therapies such as homeopathy led to completely different approaches to those used in Ryodoraku. There were different models and social pressures in Germany leading to more of an integrated approach, where acupuncture (the new therapy) was integrated with homeopathy (an already established and accepted Western therapy). The basic approach in Japan was one of trying to validate traditional ideas and treatments in a modern social and scientific context.

The issue of how to measure electro-dermal properties of the skin, acupoints and channels re-emerged in the 1970s with questions about pressure, electrochemical artefacts, appropriate voltage and current parameters (McCarroll & Rowley 1979, Noordergraaf & Silage 1973, Omura 1975). American researchers Reichmanis and Becker made important contributions to this debate with their landmark studies in the mid 1970s (Becker & Selden 1985, Reichmanis et al 1975, 1976). While theoretically important it has been difficult to demonstrate the immediate clinical relevance of this work to the scientific community, which, naturally, is more interested in understanding acupuncture in biomedical terms, through the accepted physiological systems in the body. Tiller provides the most comprehensive discussion of electro-dermal research in acupuncture for those wishing to enter this debate more completely (Tiller 1989).

The physiology and biochemistry of pain

The physiological basis of acupuncture was investigated by research teams in China and Japan from the 1950s onwards. In the West, following James Reston's now famous 1971 article about receiving acupuncture for post-appendectomy abdominal pain, physiological studies of acupuncture developed momentum. Ji Sheng Han was conducting important research in Beijing (Han & Terenius 1982), but it was the developments in the West that seem to have dominated this research. In particular, the Western fascination with pain control played a major role in much of the physiological research. How does acupuncture act on the body to block pain during surgery? Researchers acknowledge that in order to do this research more rigorously it was necessary to standardise the research protocols by using electrical stimulation of the needles with fixed settings (frequency, amplitude) rather than manual handling and manipulation of the needles. In part acupuncture was a useful tool for researching pain mechanisms (Anon 1988). This focus led in the 1970s to the important discovery that acupuncture influences the body's natural opiate systems, for example endorphins. Bruce Pomeranz was one of the investigators involved in this important work (Pomeranz & Chiu 1976) and has summarised the findings of these lines of investigation (Pomeranz & Berman 2003). Since the early work in the 1970s, significant progress has been made in mapping out the analgesic mechanisms of acupuncture and other physiological effects (Bowsher 1998) (see Chapter 10 for more details of physiological studies on acupuncture).

Controlled clinical trials

The first clinical trials of acupuncture began in Japan in the 1960s with the arrival of 'biostatistics' and the methodologies such as randomisation that are fundamental to controlled clinical trials (Shichido 1996, Tsutani et al 1990). Prior to this the more common approach for examining clinical treatment effects was one of observation and case history reporting. Historically, within acupuncture and traditional East Asian medicine in general, case history reporting has been the most important tool for communicating information about the effectiveness of treatments (Chace 1992, Chen & Wang 1988). This can be done systematically and rigorously and is still used in modern medical research as a tool for communicating initial or exceptional clinical findings. Bio-medicine sees careful observation as an important early phase of clinical research, one that sets the stage for more detailed scientific clinical studies such as the RCT. All clinical investigations have their origin in a desire to define clinical effects and communicate these observations to the world of practice. This begins with a case description and in modern medicine results in a multi-disciplinary research team that delivers a large-scale RCT (Berman et al 2004, Scharf et al 2006). The concepts and methodologies involved in the various types of modern clinical trials, such as pragmatic and explanatory studies, are discussed elsewhere (Chapters 7 and 8).

In terms of using modern biomedical methods for investigating the clinical effects of acupuncture, not only were the first RCTs of acupuncture conducted in Japan in the 1960s by Kinoshita and Okabe (Shichido 1996), but the earliest attempts at 'inter-rater' reliability studies were also Japanese (Debata 1968, Matsumoto 1968, Ogawa 1978).

Tensions reflected in different research agendas

Acupuncture has been socially accepted in Japan for some time. Starting in 1948 practitioners have been licensed and obtain life-long licenses after completing their 3–4-year training. Acupuncture receives almost no social insurance reimbursement. Practitioners are thus under no pressure from the government, insurance or healthcare systems to prove themselves, so why develop a research agenda? Acupuncture and moxibustion therapies in Japan are quite diverse (Birch & Felt 1999). Over the last two centuries, since Gempaku's revelations, there has been an increasing trend towards accepting modern anatomical and scientific models of the body. This created pressure on traditional Japanese medical systems like acupuncture and herbal medicine (Kampo), both during the Meiji Restoration in the early 1900s and again post 1945, to align themselves with modern science (Birch & Felt 1999, p 40). The scientific establishment in Japan tried to ban or limit acupuncture, but failed. There has been a long-standing tension in the acupuncture community between the more scientifically oriented and the more traditionally oriented practitioner groups. Yoshio Manaka and Kodo Fukushima both spoke about this development in the 1960s (Y Manaka, personal communication, 1986, K Fukushima, personal communication, 1990). The scientific acupuncture community saw the possibility of challenging the more traditional acupuncture community using new biostatistical methodologies. Some senior figures such as Manaka were concerned about whether those methodologies were appropriate for investigating the complex systems of practice that are used in acupuncture, especially traditional acupuncture. They therefore considered how they might develop different investigative approaches (Manaka & Itaya 1986, Manaka et al 1995). Others in the practitioner community were put off by the arguments from the scientific community about the supposed failures of traditionally oriented acupuncture in clinical research (K Fukushima, personal communication, 1990). This tension still exists in Japan today and mirrors the worldwide debate in acupuncture between researchers and practitioners.

Over the last five decades research has also been conducted in China but has been influenced by different pressures than in Japan and the West. Like Japan, acupuncture was already socially and politically accepted, but unlike Japan it was also government supported and sanctioned as part of the solution to a massive public health crisis. As a result of this public health role most research on acupuncture was not focused on trying to prove that it works, rather on how to understand it within the existing healthcare system and how to promote it as part of the whole field of TCM. Thus while research in China was conducted partly for internal political consumption, it was also intended to help show the West something of the development of China, both modern and traditional. Research was informed by perceived needs to achieve that goal, allowing for significant influences from the West both on the formulation of the medical systems of TCM (Taylor 2004) and how models of understanding and practice were constructed (Scheid 2006), thus some aspects of the research agenda influenced this newly developed approach to acupuncture. One of the major trends in the last five decades in mainland China has been the development of an integrated medical system, bringing together traditional and modern biomedical ideas into a single system (Scheid 2002, 2006, Sivin 1987, Taylor 2004, Unschuld 1985). One such example has been the effort to find correlations between traditional ideas and modern biomedical concepts, for example studies seeking correlations between traditional diagnostic signs and biomedical markers in the blood (Chen 1988, Fu 1988, Xie 1988), as well as investigating the correlations between traditional pathological conditions such as Kidney *Yang* Vacuity and the biomedical condition of adrenal insufficiency (Scheid 2006). Clinical trials often focused more on demonstrating to an accepting audience that the treatments could be used within the public health system rather than in a real search for new information. There was little interest in demonstrating that acupuncture works, as this was and is accepted wisdom. Fulfilling this social and political need has often allowed methods of investigation to be used that would not be acceptable to scientists outside of China because they were asking different questions. Therefore much of this research is not cited in high-quality scientific publications;

for example few mainland Chinese clinical trials are of the required quality to be included in systematic reviews of acupuncture.

Since the end of the cultural revolution in China (1976) scientific research in China has increased. In 1978 the first WHO Western group of conventional doctors to learn about acupuncture in China was taught the newly developed integrated approach to TCM (Lewith & Lewith 1981). Western diagnoses were used as the 'entry criteria' to understand the traditional approach and then an appropriate differentiation of syndromes occurred based on a *zangfu* diagnosis with specific tradition functions ascribed to many of the important acupoints. This allowed the conventional physician learning acupuncture to 'know where to start' and to develop a simple approach in order to access the wisdom and centuries of experience of the traditional acupuncturist. The major research institutions in Shanghai and Beijing were fundamentally physiology and biochemistry laboratories using Western methods to investigate traditional approaches such as acupuncture and herbal medicine. In recent years collaborations have sprung up between many modern Chinese research institutions and Western research environments that have led to further developments. A recent example is the collaborative project that is working to develop a sham moxibustion research model (Zhao et al 2006).

The social and political needs for investigating acupuncture in the West have, on the whole, been quite different than in Japan and China. Acupuncture is relatively new in the West and uses terminology and models that sound exotic. It is often practised in countries where insurance reimbursement is available so research has a different focus to that in Asia. On the one hand it must prove itself to be effective following accepted models of research, such as the placebo-controlled randomised clinical trial; and on the other hand it must also demonstrate itself to be cost-effective to warrant insurance reimbursement or health service provision (Bovey 2005, Cherkin 2001, Sherman & Cherkin 2003, Wonderling 2006). It must demonstrate that its mechanisms are consistent with a Western scientific understanding of biology; if it is to be acceptable, it must be plausible. Thus the understanding of acupuncture in the scientific community has tended not to focus on traditional concepts or methods, rather it has often been forced to ignore them. These different social concerns have recently surfaced as acupuncture has been shown to be a more complex intervention (Paterson & Dieppe 2005) with different research needs (Medical Research Council 2000, Verhoef et al 2005), including the particular need to include its own traditional explanations, concepts, theories and clinical methods within the research paradigm (Acupuncture 1998).

Western clinical trials of acupuncture

Clinical trials of acupuncture in the West began soon after US President Richard Nixon's visit to China in 1972. The first trials started appearing in 1973 (Scarognina et al 1973). They naturally focused on trying to test the effectiveness of the methods that had been observed in hospitals in China. During Nixon's visit the Chinese showcased their developments of acupuncture during surgery, which triggered much interest and excitement in the Western scientific community. The first trials were thus related to this use of acupuncture as an analgesic. This focus on the analgesic effects of acupuncture in clinical trials follows the pattern of the understanding of acupuncture from the eighteenth and nineteenth centuries in the West (Lu & Needham 1980). It also parallels the focus on understanding the analgesic mechanisms of acupuncture that have dominated physiological studies of acupuncture in the West (Pomeranz & Berman 2003). Hundreds of clinical trials have been conducted in Western countries since the early 1970s. Since the late 1980s meta-analyses and systematic reviews of these RCTs have been conducted with an evolving consensus about which medical conditions acupuncture appears to help (Birch et al 2004). (See also Chapter 11 for more on systematic reviews and meta-analyses.)

Because the philosophical and cultural issues involved in applying Western-based methods to traditional East Asian systems were virtually ignored (Birch & Felt 1999), there remain a number of important methodological challenges for the researcher investigating acupuncture.

CHALLENGES FOR RESEARCHERS INVESTIGATING ACUPUNCTURE

Researching acupuncture in a way that is fair to the medicine has proven to be a difficult task. While hundreds of RCTs and thousands of basic science studies of acupuncture have been conducted, results are often equivocal and many challenges remain. Among these challenges, two relate to the important scientific concepts of external validity and model validity (sometimes called 'model fit validity'). The first of these, external validity, tells us how well results from studies are representative of actual practice. This challenge is also addressed in Chapter 11. The second challenge, model (fit) validity, is articulated by Cassidy in the context of a question: 'Are the assumptions underlying the design well understood and factored into the design so that the resultant data accurately represent the people or practice or intervention being tested?' (Cassidy 2002). Verhoef et al define model validity: it 'encompasses the need for research to adequately address the unique healing theory and therapeutic context of the intervention' (Verhoef et al 2005). Model validity must be considered in relation to many of the issues discussed in this chapter, and in particular, what is the model of theory and practice that is to be tested? Table 2.3 summarises some of the main challenges that researchers face in light of issues discussed in this chapter, and highlights the relevance of specific items in relation to external validity (EV) and model validity (MV).

Table 2.3 Challenges for acupuncture researchers and relevance to external validity and model validity

1. Mapping and investigating the diversity of acupuncture practice
    i. Historical developments, role of culture, politics, social & economic pressures on development and manifestations of models of practice (MV)
    ii. Cultural translational issues (MV)
    iii. Linguistic translational issues (MV)
    iv. Recognising differences in the nature of different systems of practice and being explicit about the specific approach that is being investigated (MV + EV)
    v. Developing better research methods for investigating traditionally based systems of practice (MV + EV)
    vi. Making valid generalisations from research (EV)

2. Addressing the bias of cultural assumptions about acupuncture and science
    i. Applicability of either-or logical assumptions when investigating acupuncture (MV)
    ii. Applicability of Cartesian mind–body duality model when investigating acupuncture (MV)
    iii. Applicability of reductionist approaches when investigating acupuncture (MV)
    iv. Recognising the validity of different investigational approaches: evidence-based medicine versus experience-based medicine (MV)

3. Modelling and assessing acupuncture
    i. Development of models of theory and practice and their assessment as complex interventions (MV + EV)
    ii. Development of models of theory and practice and their assessment as whole systems with holistic models and approaches (MV + EV)

EV = external validity; MV = model validity.

If we look to the scientific method itself, we can restate these challenges for both clinical and basic science research in another, perhaps more fundamental way:

The fundamental feature of the scientific method is that it does not prove a theory to be true. Rather, it disproves competing, alternate or opposite hypotheses. Thus any scientific experiment can only disprove competing hypotheses (hence the common use of the 'null hypothesis') and is consequently entirely dependent on the initial theoretical framework or model. Most experiments on acupuncture have had significant difficulties formulating, or have ignored, a valid model of 'acupuncture' based on a clearly articulated theoretical framework. This necessarily means that 'acupuncture', as we have discussed, has been neither proved nor disproved in most if not all scientific experiments. Until such time as better models of acupuncture theory and practice are formulated and included in clinical trial design, the theories and practices central to acupuncture will remain untested. We will simply be evaluating individual re-interpretations of acupuncture. This represents a significant challenge not only for the medical research community but also for acupuncture practitioners and researchers.

Research resources

Birch S, Felt R 1999 Understanding acupuncture. Churchill Livingstone, Edinburgh

Cassidy C 2002 Contemporary Chinese medicine and acupuncture. Churchill Livingstone, Edinburgh

Lu G D, Needham J 1980 Celestial lancets. Cambridge University Press, Cambridge

Stux G, Hammerschlag R (eds) 2001 Clinical acupuncture: scientific basis. Springer, Berlin

Unschuld P U 1985 Medicine in China: a history of ideas. University of California Press, Berkeley

References

Acupuncture 1998 Acupuncture: NIH consensus development panel on acupuncture. Journal of the American Medical Association 280(17):1518–1524

Anon 1988 Interview with Ji Sheng Han. Omni, February 1988, pages 81 and following

Becker R O, Selden G 1985 The body electric. William Morrow and Company Inc., New York

Bensky D, Blalack J, Chace C et al 2006 Toward a working methodology for translating Chinese Medicine. Lantern 3(3):10–14

Berman B M, Lao L, Langeburg P et al 2004 Effectiveness of acupuncture as adjunctive therapy in osteoarthritis of the knee: a randomized, controlled trial. Annals of Internal Medicine 141:901–910

Birch S 1995 Problems in the translation of Japanese medicine into contemporary America (in Japanese). Ido no Nippon Magazine 7(9):88–94

Birch S 1997 Testing the claims of traditionally based acupuncture. Complementary Therapies in Medicine 5(3):147–151

Birch S 1998 Diversity and acupuncture: acupuncture is not a coherent or historically stable tradition. In: Vickers A J (ed) Examining complementary medicine: the sceptical holist. Stanley Thomas, Cheltenham, p 45–63

Birch S, Felt R 1999 Understanding acupuncture. Churchill Livingstone, Edinburgh

Birch S, Keppel Hesselink J, Jonkman F A M et al 2004 Clinical research on acupuncture 1: what have reviews of the efficacy and safety of acupuncture told us so far? Journal of Alternative and Complementary Medicine 10(3):468–480

Bovey M 2005 Effectiveness and cost-effectiveness. British Acupuncture Council News November:16–17

Bowsher D 1998 Mechanisms of acupuncture. In: Filshie J, White A (eds) Medical acupuncture. Churchill Livingstone, Edinburgh, p 69–83

Cassidy C M 2002 Methodological issues in investigations of massage/bodywork therapy. American Massage Therapy Association Foundation, Evanston

Chace C 1992 Fleshing out the bones. Case histories in the practice of Chinese medicine. Blue Poppy Press, Boulder

Chen R J, Wang N 1988 Acupuncture case histories from China. Eastland Press, Seattle

Chen Z L 1988 Development of research on tongue diagnosis. Chinese Journal of Integrative Medicine 8(Special issue 2):104–108

Cherkin D C, Eisenberg D, Sherman K J et al 2001 A randomized trial comparing traditional Chinese medical acupuncture, therapeutic massage and self-care education for chronic low back pain. Archives of Internal Medicine 161:1081–1088

Debata A 1968 Experimental study on pulse diagnosis of rokubujoi. Japan Acupuncture and Moxibustion Journal 17(3):9–12

Foss L, Rothenberg K 1987 The second medical revolution. Shambhala Publications, Boston

Freuhauf H 1999 Chinese medicine in crisis. Journal of Chinese Medicine 61:1–9

Fu C Y 1988 Achievements of research on pulse-taking with integrated traditional Chinese and Western medicine. Chinese Journal of Integrative Medicine 8(Special issue 2):108–112

Fukumoto K 2006 From the perspective of meridian therapy. North American Journal of Oriental Medicine 13(38):7–9

Goto M 1914 Head's zones and acumoxa therapy. Kyoto Iggakai Zasshi 11:4

Hammer L 1990 Dragon rises, red bird flies. Station Hill Press, New York

Han J S, Terenius L 1982 Neurochemical basis of acupuncture analgesia. Annual Review of Pharmacology and Toxicology 22:193–220

Hara S 1927 Effect of moxa on hemoglobin and RBC count. Iji Shinbun 1219

Hara S 1929 Tuberculosis and moxibustion. Jiechi Ika to Rinsho 6:9

Ikemi Y, Ikemi A 1986 An oriental point of view in psychosomatic medicine. Advances 3(4):150–157

Kaptchuk T J 1985 Introduction to Wiseman N, Ellis A. Fundamentals of Chinese Medicine p xvii–xxxvii

Kaptchuk T J, Edwards R A, Eisenberg D M 1996 Complementary medicine: efficacy beyond the placebo effect. In: Ernst E (ed.) Complementary medicine: an objective appraisal. Butterworth Heinemann, Oxford, p 42–70

Kim J Y 2006 Beyond paradigm: making transcultural connections in a scientific translation of acupuncture. Social Science & Medicine 62(12):2960–2972

Kuriyama S 1992 Between mind and eye; Japanese anatomy in the eighteenth century. In: Leslie C, Young A (eds) Paths to Asian medical knowledge. University of California Press, Berkeley, p 21–43

Le Bars D, Willer J C, de Broucker T 1988 Neurophysiological mechanisms involved in the pain-relieving effects of counterirritation and related techniques including acupuncture. In: Pomeranz B, Stux G (eds) Scientific bases of acupuncture. Springer-Verlag, Berlin

Lewith G T, Lewith N R 1981 Modern Chinese acupuncture. Thorsons Publishers, Northampton

Lo V 2001 The influence of nurturing life culture on the development of Western Han acumoxa therapy. In: Hsu E (ed.) Innovation in Chinese medicine. Cambridge University Press, Cambridge, p 19–50

Lock M M 1980 The organization and practice of east Asian medicine in Japan; continuity and change. Social Science & Medicine 4B:245–253

Lu G D, Needham J 1980 Celestial lancets. Cambridge University Press, Cambridge

MacPherson H, Kaptchuk T J 1997 Acupuncture in practice. Churchill Livingstone, New York

Manaka Y, Itaya K 1994 Acupuncture as intervention in the biological information system. (Meridian treatment and the X-signal system). Address given at the annual assembly of the Japan Meridian Treatment Association, Tokyo, March 29–30, 1986. Published in English in the Journal of the Acupuncture Society of New York 1(3–4):9–18

Manaka Y, Itaya K, Birch S 1995 Chasing the dragon's tail. Paradigm Publications, Brookline

Matsumoto T 1968 Experimental study on fukushin (abdominal palpation). Japan Acupuncture and Moxibustion Journal 17(3):13–16

McCarroll G D, Rowley B A 1979 An investigation of the existence of electrically located acupuncture points. IEEE Transactions on Bio-medical Engineering 26(3):177–181

Medical Research Council 2000 A framework for development and evaluation of RCTs for complex interventions to improve health. Online. Available: http://www.mrc.ac.uk/pru/pdf-mrc_cpr.pdf 5 Oct 2005

Nakatani Y, Yamashita K 1977 Ryodoraku acupuncture. Ryodoraku Research Institute, Tokyo

Noordergraaf A, Silage D 1973 Electroacupuncture. IEEE Transactions on Bio-medical Engineering 20:364–366

Oda H 1989 Ryodoraku textbook. Naniwasha Publishing Company, Osaka

Ogawa T 1978 To establish new 'Chinese medicine': searching for the contemporary significance of the 'meridian controversy' (in Japanese). Chinese Medicine 1(2):151–158

Ogawa T 1996 Comparison of TCM and meridian therapy. North American Journal of Oriental Medicine 3(6):6–11

Omura Y 1975 Some historical aspects of acupuncture and important problems to be considered in acupuncture and electro-therapeutic research. Acupuncture and Electro-Therapeutic Research, the International Journal 1(1):3–44

Paterson C, Dieppe P 2005 Characteristic and incidental (placebo) effects in complex interventions such as acupuncture. British Medical Journal 330:1202–1205

Pomeranz B, Chiu D 1976 Naloxone blocks acupuncture analgesia and causes hyperalgesia. Life Sciences 19:1757–1762

Pomeranz B, Berman B 2003 Scientific basis of acupuncture. In: Stux G, Berman B, Pomeranz B (eds) Basics of acupuncture. Springer-Verlag, Berlin, p 1–86

Reichmanis M, Marino A A, Becker R O 1975 Electrical correlates of acupuncture points. IEEE Transactions on Bio-medical Engineering 22(6):533–535

Reichmanis M, Marino A A, Becker R O 1976 D.C. skin conductance variation at acupuncture point loci. American Journal of Chinese Medicine 4(1):69–72

Reid T 2006 Terminology in TCM. Lantern 3(1):16–19

Roth H D 1999 Original Tao – inward training (Nei Yeh). Columbia University Press, New York

Scarognina P, Gardiol E, Lanza U et al 1973 The value of chemical pre-anesthesia in acupuncture anesthesia. American Journal of Chinese Medicine 1(1):143–150

Scharf H P, Mansmann U, Streitberger K et al 2006 Acupuncture and knee osteoarthritis: a three-armed randomized trial. Annals of Internal Medicine 145:12–20

Scheid V 2002 Chinese medicine in contemporary China. Duke University Press, Durham

Scheid V 2006 Not very traditional, nor exactly Chinese, so what kind of medicine is it? TCM's discourse on menopause and its implications for practice, teaching and research. Journal of Chinese Medicine 82:5–20

Seem M 1987 Body mind energetics. Thorson's Publishers, Rochester

Shen G J 1986 Study of mind-body effects and qigong in China. Advances 3(4):134–142

Sherman K J, Cherkin D C 2003 Challenges of acupuncture research: study design considerations. Clinical Acupuncture and Oriental Medicine 3:200–206

Shichido T 1996 Clinical evaluation of acupuncture and moxibustion. Ido no Nippon Journal 8:95–102

Shudo D 1990 Japanese classical acupuncture: introduction to Meridian therapy. Eastland Press, Seattle

Sivin N 1987 Traditional medicine in contemporary China. Center for Chinese Studies, University of Michigan, Ann Arbor

Tamura S 1934 Effects of moxa on the functions of WBC in the human body. Kanazawa Ika-daigaku Juzenkai 39:11, 1936; 41:2

Taylor K 2004 Divergent interests and cultivated misunderstandings: the influence of the West on modern Chinese medicine. Social History of Medicine 17(1):93–111

Tiller W A 1989 On the evolution and future development of electrodermal diagnostic instruments; energy fields in medicine; a study of device technology based on acupuncture meridians and chi energy. The proceedings of a symposium sponsored by the John. E. Fetzer Foundation, Kalamazoo, May, p 257–328

Tsutani K, Shichido T, Sakuma K 1990 When acupuncture met biostatistics. Paper presented at the Second World Conference of Acupuncture and Moxibustion, Paris

Unschuld P U 1985 Medicine in China: a history of ideas. University of California Press, Berkeley

Unschuld P U 1987 Traditional Chinese medicine; some historical and epistemological reflections. Social Science & Medicine 24(12):1023–1029

Unschuld P U 1992 Epistemological issues and changing legitimation: traditional Chinese medicine in the twentieth century. In: Leslie C, Young A (eds) Paths to Asian medical knowledge. University of California Press, Berkeley, p 44–61

Unschuld P U 1998 Chinese medicine. Paradigm Publications, Brookline

Verhoef M J, Lewith G, Ritenbaugh C et al 2005 Complementary and alternative medicine whole systems research: beyond identification of inadequacies of the RCT. Complementary Therapies in Medicine 13:206–212

Voll R 1975 Twenty years of electroacupuncture diagnosis in Germany; a progress report. American Journal of Acupuncture 3:7–17

Wang Y L, Zhao Y L 2007 Contemporary education in Chinese medicine within a strategy of standardization. Thieme Almanac 2007: Acupuncture and Chinese medicine. Georg Thieme Verlag, Stuttgart, p 198–202

Wiseman N, Feng Y 1997 A practical dictionary of Chinese medicine. Paradigm Publications, Brookline

Wonderling D 2006 Acupuncture in mainstream health care. British Medical Journal 333:611–612

Xie Z F 1988 Researches on 'cold' and 'heat' in traditional Chinese medicine. Chinese Journal of Integrative Medicine 8(Special issue 2):93–96

Zhao B, Wang X, Lin Z 2006 A novel sham moxibustion device: a randomized, placebo-controlled trial. Complementary Therapies in Medicine 14(1):53–60

Zhu Z X 1981 Research advances in the electrical specificity of meridians and acupuncture points. American Journal of Acupuncture 9(3):203–216

Patient patterns of use and experience of acupuncture

Claire M. Cassidy and Kate Thomas

3

How and why people choose to use acupuncture medical care, and who uses it, are subjects of interest to many audiences, from patients, practitioners, and educators, to healthcare policy planners, and philosophers intent on designing a 'new' or integrated approach to medicine. Current research methods, when well applied, are largely sufficient to the task of gathering quality data. This chapter summarises the range of qualitative and quantitative methods that have been used to gather patterns of use and experiential data from patients, and identifies key areas that remain as challenges to doing 'best' research and best serving our audiences.

WHY ARE PATTERNS OF USE AND THE PATIENT EXPERIENCE IMPORTANT?

Knowing which segments of the whole population are drawn to use acupuncture care, and what experiences they have as a result, is important to acupuncturists themselves, to those who teach them, and to those who fund (or insure) medical care. The potential audience enlarges when we remember that a revolution in medical perception is in progress: acupuncture care is already supported by sufficient research and clinical data to be of marked interest to health policy planners and others concerned to develop more integrated, efficient and potentially lower-cost approaches to the mass delivery of quality medical care. But how integration is to take place remains largely unresolved (Luff & Thomas 1999, 2000). Having at hand a mass of quality experiential, demographic, and epidemiologic data will help support this move toward appropriate integration. Finally, public opinion indirectly guides policy development, and existing attitudinal data indicate that acupuncture popularity among users is strikingly high (Cassidy 1998a, 1998b, Gould & MacPherson 2001, Paterson & Britten 2004). Users typically praise acupuncture care for offering symptom relief, enhancing their ability to cope physiologically and emotionally, providing an alternative to pharmaceuticals and surgery, and offering a close patient–practitioner relationship during treatment. In Box 3.1, some quotes from patients illustrate this.

Box 3.1   Patients vote with their feet!*

'I still call acupuncture "voodoo," but it cured my chronic foot pain in just two treatments!'

Lawrence

'In the four short months that I've been getting acupuncture treatment, I've seen huge improvements in my overall health, immune system, and stress levels. My irritable bowel syndrome is gone! Each visit feels like an "internal" massage, and I leave feeling refreshed, renewed, and invigorated.'

Suzanne

'My practitioner: extremely knowledgeable, respectful, and accurate diagnostician. I first saw her when I was having illness undiagnosed by Western medicine – it turned out to be a thyroid problem which she both diagnosed and effectively treated...'

Lana

'The experience of just centering on myself for an hour is so wonderful!'

Vicki

*For narrative analysis of patient experiences, see Cassidy 1998b, Emad 1998, Gould & MacPherson 2001.

Several features of acupuncture – popularity among existing users, moderate cost, low technological demands, minimal invasiveness yet with wide medical applicability – signal why more and better use of acupuncture medicine can be viewed as likely to serve the larger society well. However, before this can happen, certain socio-cultural barriers need attention and this will best happen through carrying out more and perhaps more focused social research efforts.

What are these barriers? First, there is a straightforward deficiency of epidemiological and experiential data on acupuncture use. Since the mid 1980s, when acupuncture care began to make its presence strongly felt in English-speaking countries, there have been only a few surveys of either use or attitudes, and those that exist, despite their generally high quality, are nearly all 'snapshots' or cross-sectional studies. Second, while existing methods are good, there is room for improvement and innovation. Needed are standardised survey instruments that assess health values and the patient experience while accurately reflecting the concepts of acupuncture/East Asian medicine; currently most instruments are built on biomedical models. In future we also need more attention to gathering longitudinal data, including having core questions included in recurring national health surveys, as this would be an efficient way to monitor change in acupuncture use patterns. More subtle, yet essential, attention needs to be given to meaning, by asking the right questions in the right way, and ensuring that these respect the integrity of the medicine and the healthcare experience. Third, for socio-historical reasons, the public and biomedical perception of 'what acupuncture can do' has been narrowed to primarily emphasise the alleviation of pain in musculoskeletal complaints. But acupuncture care has a much broader clinical reach, and will serve best if its full range of applicability becomes better known. In this context, studies conducted in the UK (MacPherson et al 2006a, 2006b) report a shift toward broader use of acupuncture care. Fourth, too little effort has been spent communicating to the public, planners, and biomedical professionals the findings of new quality clinical research data on acupuncture, and the high level of professionalism of dedicated acupuncture practitioners. These barriers to the understanding of acupuncture care and its potential benefits can be addressed through appropriate social research.

WHAT ARE THE IMPORTANT QUESTIONS?

Researchers use both qualitative and quantitative approaches in doing attitudinal and epidemiological/demographic research, but the choice must be conscious and canny, for what one can glean from applying these methods differs significantly.

Because choice of method affects what questions can be answered, researchers generally agree that the first essential research step is to identify exactly what question one wants to answer and why. Thus while all research will produce *description*, including counts (frequencies, lists, statistics), among social methods only qualitative research offers *explanation* (why people chose acupuncture, how they perceive it, their reasoning, dreams, intentions and perceptions). Statistics can imply what may happen in future (*prediction*), but only if one knows both description and explanation can predictions be made with some confidence.

It may sound obvious to say: 'identify exactly what question one wants to answer', though we might wish to assume that researchers are already sensitive to this need. This is not always so. It is not unusual for questionnaire designers to take a 'shotgun' approach, asking whatever seems like it might matter, just to see by statistical manipulation what emerges afterwards as relevant. It is also not unusual for researchers to 'know' what matters and not ask their intended audience for confirmation before doing research, thus risking biased questions and statistics. Finally, some questions are subtle, even hidden from researchers: it is difficult to frame questions around topics one doesn't yet perceive (Cassidy 1994). Any methods text will develop these themes in more detail; in this short chapter we mainly sound a warning. Here, for example, is a potent 'hidden' question: when patients receive, or practitioners deliver acupuncture care, what is being delivered? Are researchers working with a reductionist definition of acupuncture, as only consisting of inserting needles into the skin at designated points? Or do they consider expectation, framing, environment, communication style, practice style and technical skill as aspects of care that will affect perceived success of outcome? How will these aspects be measured? How many of them will be measured? Consider for example just one issue: style of practice. There are many styles of acupuncture practice, such as traditional Chinese medicine (TCM), Worsley Five Element, Toyo Hari, Korean hand acupuncture, auriculotherapy, and so on. Style matters to practitioners and schools, but no current research has examined patient outcomes by practitioner practice style. Does it matter? It definitely does matter in the design of clinical trials that are concerned with 'where is an acupuncture point', 'how deep does the practitioner insert the needle' and the definition of 'sham' acupuncture! More than that, research shows that what patients and practitioners recognise as 'acupuncture' is a complex and dynamic process far broader than inserting needles, and argues that limiting assessment to needling will not assist in isolating the treatment effect, but may actively interfere with it (MacPherson et al 2006b, Paterson & Britten 2004).

Another 'hidden' question is: what is 'success of outcome'? Is it relief of symptoms, or continued use of acupuncture care, or a sense of being cared for body, mind and spirit, or increased self-efficacy, or all of these? What is 'healing'? What part does the patient–practitioner relationship play in healing? What is current public perception (or perception by other healthcare practitioners) of acupuncture?

These perceptual socio-cultural questions are listed first because they demonstrate the potential difficulty in framing appropriate research questions, and reveal the need for interview and other qualitative approaches to data gathering. In a 'best research world', answers to such questions would be gathered before, or at least alongside, quantitative description, because knowing how potential respondents perceive issues and the language they use to frame their answers, matter in designing valid survey questions. Straight quantitative questions are usually easier to frame: How many people use acupuncture care? Who are they by sex, age, health conditions, 'race', urban-rural residence, socio-economic status, insured/not, and so on (Luff & Thomas 1999)? Which conditions are commonly brought for care? Do you consider your acupuncture practitioner to be your primary care practitioner? How much do you pay at each session? How do you pay for your care? Is there parking near your practitioner's office?

Another set of questions is somewhat difficult to measure, since subtle perceptions guide experience. For example, asking 'how painful is acupuncture on a scale of 1–10?' assumes that people define or experience pain in similar ways, but they do not (Bates et al 1995, Emad 1994, Morris 1991). Comparative questions can also prove difficult to frame. Here are two to consider: 'Why do patients choose acupuncture care out

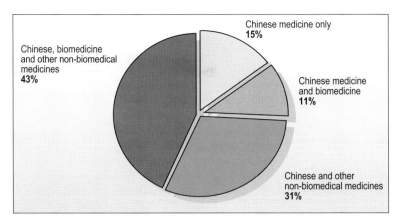

Fig 3.1   Pattern of professional healthcare used in the 3 months preceding the survey as reported by 575 Chinese medicine patients (Cassidy 1998a). (Reproduced with kind permission from Mary Ann Liebert & Co.)

of all medical options?' and 'Given the kinds of medical help you got for your condition, what role did each play in your recovery?' These questions could be reduced to Likert form and used on a quantitative survey questionnaire, but the Likert scale components should have emerged from previous interview research. In Fig. 3.1 we present an example of quantitative data derived from preceding qualitative research, namely patient reports on the patterns of professional healthcare used.

Finally, emerging from pattern of use and experiential data, there is an additional set of questions of interest, for example, 'What is changing about public perception and usage?'; 'What do we want to see change about public perception or use patterns?'; 'What approaches can change these?'; and, an important methodological issue (among many): 'How can we get "best" data from large samples?'

WHAT METHODS ARE USED TO ANSWER THESE QUESTIONS?

The potential questions are myriad; the associated methods are not (Table 3.1):

- Qualitative methods — interviews in person or by phone, observation with participation or by shadowing, written narratives, cognitive sorting tests — are best used to gather data on perception, experiences, intention, and opinion.
- Quantitative methods — surveys, oral or written — are best used to measure patterns of use.
- Qualitative methods can inform and be effectively integrated into survey formats as well as into clinical trials formats by, for example, requesting written narratives or diaries, or interviewing sub-samples of the total respondent pool.

Table 3.1 Qualitative and quantitative methods used in published studies of patterns of use and patient attitudes toward acupuncture care

Method	Description
Observation	
a) Participant observation	Researcher works alongside the healthcare practitioner, observing closely, using audio or video recordings of clinical activities and conversations, and possibly interviewing both patients and practitioner, sometimes extensively, at times separate from the clinical encounter, over a period of weeks to months. This method produces tremendous detail on perception, logic, intention, personal measures of success, and user perceptions of WHY acupuncture 'works'.
b) Shadowing	Researcher observes, usually as inconspicuously as possible, while practitioner delivers care; researcher does not help or follow up with patients, and may focus primarily on gathering medical-record data from the patient. Shadowing lasts a few hours to a few days.
Interviews	
a) In-depth	Researcher follows an open-ended protocol to interview samples of patients and/or practitioners for 60 to 90 minutes once or more times, usually to seek details on perception, logic, intention, and personal measures of success and why acupuncture 'works'. Often there is a loose topic guide to provide prompts.
b) Semi-structured	Researcher follows a pre-defined topic guide to interview patients on specific topics of particular interest to researchers; usually used in conjunction with a survey questionnaire or as part of a clinical trials/outcomes design.
c) Structured/direct questioning	Interviewer follows a strict limited question format that demands that patients respond within pre-determined parameters, such as 'How bad is your pain, on a scale of 1 to 10?' Used as part of clinical trials/outcome designs. Can be done in office, by telephone, or by computer.
Cognitive 'game' instruments	'Games' of various kinds allow respondents to reveal unconscious attitudes and beliefs, material they cannot verbalise. No cognitive tests were used in published data read for this chapter, but see Cassidy (2001).
Diaries	Participants in clinical research trials track their actions and experiences as 'daily diaries' — usually producing both quantitative data (answers to specific questions) and qualitative data (perceptual data). Diaries were not used in publications reviewed for this paper; the method is well described in Elliot (1997).

Table 3.1 (Continued)

Survey questionnaires	
a) Written in office	Respondents fill out a quantitative questionnaire in the clinic at the time of receiving care, sometimes at intake and sometimes several times during a research project. Can be computerised.
b) Mail-in	Same as above, sent out and returned by mail.
c) Telephone	Same as above, fixed interview questionnaire by telephone.
Mixed qualitative-quantitative survey questionnaires	Respondents fill out a quantitative questionnaire and then either write a narrative of their experiences as part of completing the questionnaire, or are later interviewed about their experiences. For an example of using questionnaires in qualitative interviews as a method of integrating qualitative and quantitative research, see Adamson et al (2004).
Standardised written instruments	Usually in conjunction with surveys, but sometimes in conjunction with clinical interviews, respondents complete standardised instruments designed to 'locate' their responses on a perceptual scale, e.g. of pain, general health, symptom pattern, medical values, or the like. In clinical trials, patients may fill out such instruments more than once to measure their progress during treatment. Instruments are highly sensitive to hidden agendas.
Analysis of mass survey data sets	Statistical analysis of large-scale survey data sets, such as national health statistics, to identify, e.g. patterns of use of acupuncture.
Systematic reviews	Comparative assessment of multiple published sources on the 'same' topic, to identify 'best' studies and make methodological or clinical judgements, or assess the similarities and differences in meanings obtained from qualitative studies.

Tables 3.2–3.4 provide examples of published reports using these methods. Table 3.2 focuses on qualitative methods; Table 3.3 on quantitative methods; and Table 3.4 on mixed qualitative and quantitative methods. One study from each table is discussed in more detail below.

Two potential methods are missing from current published data; both would reward use. First, at the time the earlier studies were done, data collection by computer was rare; whereas, completing survey questionnaires and standardised instruments by computer is today relatively easy, and the public is increasingly used to this approach. Second, cognitive 'games' (Cassidy 2001), such as the card sort, which allow respondents to display attitudes they did not know they held, were not used in any of the studies, even those most qualitative in nature.

Table 3.2 Examples of qualitative methods in use to study patient patterns of use and experience of acupuncture

Method type	Methods in use		
	Article example	Questions asked	Methods chosen
Observation			
a) Participant observation	Emad (1998)	How is the body experienced through encounters with acupuncture?	Participant observation, in-depth interviews with patients and practitioners in several states, rural and urban settings.
b) Shadowing	Napadow & Kaptchuk (2004)	Who uses acupuncture hospital clinics and for what conditions?	Clinic observation 18 days, two hospitals, two acupuncturists.
Interviews			
a) In-depth	Frank & Stollberg (2004)	Why do patients choose acupuncture? Do they learn about Asian medicine ideas? How do they interact with their practitioner? What do they think of their practitioner?	In-depth interviews with patients recommended by their acupuncturists to participate in study.
b) Semi-structured	So (2002)	Are treatment outcomes associated with patient's hopefulness, expectations, beliefs about the body, or patient–provider relationship?	Patient interviews before and after 3 months of acupuncture care in a clinic.
	Paterson & Britten (2004)	How do the experience and the effects of acupuncture care evolve over time?	Patient interviews three times over 6 months, patients self-referred after being told about project by their acupuncturists.
c) Structure/ direct questioning	Lin (2003)	How needle-phobic are children about acupuncture and how does this change with treatment?	Direct questioning before first treatment and after sixth/last treatment in clinic, among sick children, aged 6 to 18.

Qualitative research (Table 3.2)

Participant observation, as used by Emad (1998), is a superb method to gather data on perceptions and experiences, but it is also extremely time consuming. Interviews are more practical and have the advantage that

Table 3.3 Examples of quantitative methods in use to study patient patterns of use and experience of acupuncture

	Methods in use		
	Article example	Questions asked	Methods chosen
Survey questionnaires			
a) Written in-office	Anderson (1991)	Who seeks acupuncture care and for what? How does this compare with patient populations of other types of medical practitioners?	Written survey questionnaire completed at intake by new patients at a TCM clinic.
	Kreitler et al (1987)	What is the role of belief in pain relief with acupuncture? How much pain do people report and how much is relieved by acupuncture?	Written survey questionnaire before and two follow-ups after 4–5 acupuncture treatments of clinic patients.
	MacPherson et al (2006a)	What are the characteristics of acupuncture patients? For what main problem did they seek care?	Written survey questionnaire, cross-sectional sub-study within prospective longitudinal adverse event survey of British Acupuncture Council.
b) Mail-in questionnaires	Miller (1990)	How do recent immigrants choose between 'Eastern traditional' and 'Western modern' healthcare options?	Face-to-face interview; in-office questionnaires, mail-in questionnaires, at offices of Korean practitioners with majority of patients choosing mail-in format.
c) Telephone questionnaires	Coss et al (1998)	How aware are cancer patients about alternative therapies? What is their attitude towards them? How do patients perceive oncologists' attitudes toward alternative therapies? Should this clinic add CAM options?	Retrospective closed-question telephone survey of former patients at cancer center.
	Eisenberg et al (1998)	Who uses CAM (16 'therapies') and for what? Do they tell their MDs? What changed since the 1990 survey?	Retrospective nationally representative closed-question telephone surveys in 1990 and 1997 compared.

(*Continued*)

Table 3.3 (Continued)

Methods in use

	Article example	Questions asked	Methods chosen
Standardised written instruments			
a) With questionnaires	MacPherson et al (2003)	What are patient perceptions of practitioner empathy? Are patients enabled by acupuncture, and how? What are the perceptions of health outcomes of acupuncture care? What are the associations among these issues?	Retrospective cross-sectional study with questionnaire, with selected instruments including empathy and enablement process measures, and self-rated outcome.
b) With clinical trial	Thomas et al (2005)	What were patient beliefs about and knowledge of acupuncture before treatment? What were the expectations of acupuncture's effectiveness prior to treatment? How was the acupuncture experienced? How satisfied were the patients with their treatment? What adverse responses were experienced?	Clinical trial design using instruments like SF-36 and McGill Pain plus questions on prior expectations and beliefs in acupuncture efficacy, a standardised questionnaire on satisfaction with care received. And a patient-completed questionnaire on treatment experiences and responses.
Analysis of mass survey data set	Easthope et al (1999)	What is the incidence of acupuncture claims and what are the characteristics of patients claiming for acupuncture?	Statistical analysis of two data sets provided by Health Insurance Commission of Australia.
Systematic review	Harris & Rees (2000)	How can we rationally compare surveys of prevalence of CAM use? How is CAM to be defined? What makes a good survey?	Using formal criteria identified 'best' surveys of prevalence of CAM use in English-speaking countries.

CAM = Complementary and alternative medicine; TCM = traditional Chinese medicine.

Table 3.4 Examples of mixed qualitative and quantitative methods used to study patient patterns of use and experience of acupuncture

Method type	Methods in use		
	Article example	Questions asked	Methods chosen
Mixed survey questionnaire plus qualitative study	Cassidy (1998a, 1998b)	Who uses acupuncture care? For what purposes? What do they experience? Are they satisfied? What do they learn about Chinese medicine? How does acupuncture use relate to use of other medical care? What do they say about their experiences?	Survey questionnaire including white space to write narrative 'story' about their experiences; six clinics in five US states.
	Gould & MacPherson (2001)	Patients' reasons for seeking care and whether they experienced change, what kinds of change, and how much they attributed changes to acupuncture.	Survey questionnaires followed by semi-structured interviews with sub-sample of respondents in a clinic setting.

research can even be designed to yield high-quality longitudinal experiential data in a relatively short time. Paterson & Britten (2004) used semi-structured questionnaires (a mix of in-depth and pre-set questions) to gather longitudinal qualitative data by interviewing the same 23 patients up to three times over a period of 6 months. The resulting data meshed well with earlier cross-sectional findings as to the experiential aspects of acupuncture care, while yielding rich new data on the complexity and interactive aspects of care. These data permitted the development of a dynamic treatment model, including a critique of clinical research that focuses exclusively on the effects of needling. Patterson & Britten followed guidelines for increasing validity in qualitative research and included an unusual test of their model. This consisted of asking not just their interviewees (whose perceptions had informed development of the model), but participating acupuncturists, if the model 'made sense' and seemed to mesh with their experience. The answer was 'yes', meaning that now both patient and practitioner recognised the model as 'real' and as 'describing what I know'. Limitations, the authors noted, included difficulty recruiting to the project, which prevented theoretical sampling.

Quantitative research (Table 3.3)

Numerous surveys of 'who uses acupuncture care and for what conditions' have been published. The emerging research needs are for greater care in defining what one means when one says one is doing a 'complementary and alternative medicine' survey (Harris & Rees 2000), and for repeat surveys that seek evidence of change in use patterns. We know of three follow-up studies. Two of these, Eisenberg et al (1998) and Thomas et al (2003), compare users and providers of a range of CAM choices and explore changes over time. Since our primary interest is in acupuncture, we will focus on the work of MacPherson et al (2006a). Here the pattern-of-use study was designed as a sub-study using the same population as an acupuncture safety survey, which provided cross-sectional demographic and primary complaint data on over 9000 patients being treated by members of the British Acupuncture Council. Respondents completed a fixed-format questionnaire form. The resulting demographics were compared with general population data, to find out if acupuncture patients differed from the ordinary population, as well as with demographic data from a 1988 British survey that included acupuncture patients, to find out what had changed in the intervening years. Respondents were asked to report one 'main problem' and this was coded using an international WHO standard that is designed to allow coding of the patient's own statement, rather than requiring a biomedical diagnostic label. Our focus is on methods, not outcomes, but with regard to researchers' larger goal of understanding use and communicating to the public, it is interesting to note that this survey reports a significant drop in musculoskeletal complaints as the main reason for seeing an acupuncturist. The authors note that this indicates a 'wider case mix amongst patients than in 1988' and presumably some learning among patients that acupuncture care can serve a broad range of conditions. Limitations of the study include its cross-sectional character (comparisons were made with existing studies and required various adjustments to allow comparison), potential bias in working only with the patients of professional acupuncturists (i.e. no MD or DC acupuncturists were included), and limiting respondents to report one main clinical problem, when most seek care for multiple problems. Indeed, this may be one mechanism for the apparent widening of the indications for which patients are using acupuncture; patients first visit a practitioner with one problem and discover, through their care, that acupuncture offers solutions for coexisting conditions and problems. To date, the efforts to explore this mechanism through empirical research have been limited.

Mixed qualitative and quantitative methods (Table 3.4)

Cassidy (1998a, 1998b) offers an example of a cross-sectional mixed qualitative-quantitative study. In contrast to the present, in 1995 there were essentially no data on pattern of use or attitudes towards acupuncture care available. Even acupuncture school administrators had collected little or no data on the users of their own clinics. The goal of this study, then, was to gather first-time data on who was using acupuncture care and for what purposes, with the special proviso that the 'words of the people' were also to be gathered. The scale was to be 'nationwide' though funding was private and extremely tight.

Cassidy used a respondent-driven questionnaire research design (1994) with the perceptions of the patients — the users of acupuncture — guiding the content and phrasing of the questionnaire. To identify what mattered to patients, Cassidy began by depth interviewing a sample of 60 current and former acupuncture patients, using open-ended questions and recording the exact words used by the respondents. From this she identified not only the themes common to the respondents, but also the language in which they expressed themselves. These data were used to create a draft survey questionnaire, which included one and a half pages of 'white space', with a request to 'tell your own story'. The questionnaire was piloted first with a sample of eight professional acupuncturists, asking if the questions 'made sense' and 'were sufficient'. Next, an improved draft was piloted with a sample of acupuncture patients, who were asked whether the questions 'made sense' and 'were relevant'. Now with the questions and formatting vetted by both acupuncturists and patients (establishing 'face validity'), paper questionnaires were sent out to six 'large' acupuncture clinics in five US states to be completed by those who were willing. Returned usable questionnaires numbered 575, with 460 including a written narrative. Computer software was used to analyse both the qualitative and quantitative data. Results provided pattern-of-use data; rich knowledge of what people got out of acupuncture care; and why they were highly satisfied. Cognitive distance analysis also showed that users were not seeking something exotic ('Chinese medicine') but instead, a holistic approach to care, a finding that should be recognised as having significant implications for healthcare planners.

This early study is methodologically important because of the care taken to ensure that the questions asked were asked in ways that made sense to respondents, thus yielding trustworthy data. Such data could be used to teach in schools, to design delivery in clinics, or even provide guidance for national-level healthcare planners. It is also significant because of the unusual technique of including a large amount of 'white space' and asking respondents to 'tell their own story'. This study had the following limitations: there was insufficient funding to train project managers at locales distant to the originator locale in methods to improve response rates, so response rates were probably lower than they could have been. In addition, the project depended heavily on volunteer labour, thus unpredictable time schedules, uncertain efforts to encourage participation, and lags in returning completed questionnaires. The method also had a limited ability to reach a representative sample of acupuncture users. For example, asking respondents to 'tell their story' in this way requires significant literacy skills. In addition, most users in this survey were white, but a recent statistical analysis of US national health data suggests, in contrast, that Asian-Americans are the heaviest users of acupuncture (Burke et al 2006). O'Cathian & Thomas (2004) examine the advantages and disadvantages of using 'white space' in surveys — the advantage is in having respondents' words and 'stories' and knowing their reasoning, and the disadvantages include the time demands to analyse these data, and their mixed quality. The Cassidy survey provided cross-sectional data, and took all respondents from those just beginning through to others with years of experience. Later mixed surveys have not used the 'white space' approach, and have focused more closely on smaller samples by, for example, interviewing a sub-sample of the whole (Gould & MacPherson 2001), or doing repeat interview questionnaires to measure how attitudes change with increasing experience (Paterson & Britten 2004).

Despite the limitations noted for the research projects discussed above, data in each case were statistically valid and useful. We should remember, then, that there is no 'perfect' study — if appropriate questions are asked, good methods used, and resulting data applicable, then the study is properly defined as 'good'.

KEY AREAS THAT REMAIN AS CHALLENGES

A key challenge is defining acupuncture itself, including what practitioners actually do, the influence of 'style' of practice, and how healing emerges from the relationship of patient and practitioner. For example, if a patient sees an acupuncturist and is offered not only needling, but active listening, exercise and dietary guidance, humour in discussing child-care issues, all delivered in a room designed to calm, and with music during the treatment rest period, how much of this must be assessed in descriptive studies? How should the effects be measured? Again, if a practitioner offers a combination of styles seamlessly during treatment (e.g. TCM, Nagano style, and auriculotherapy) which, and how shall this be reported and measured?

A related challenge concerns how acupuncture medicine is to represent itself to the larger society. Currently public interest is growing, and biomedical schools are beginning to include acupuncture 'shadowing' among their requirements for graduation in both the UK and US. Realistically however, there remain considerable sociological and political barriers to overcome. One is the fact that acupuncture is widely viewed as mainly useful for accomplishing 'pain relief' especially of musculoskeletal origin. This means that many of its potential clinical strengths, as in women's reproductive health, mood issues, immune system modulation, and digestive, respiratory, neurological, and skin health, are largely ignored. We can cite historical reasons for this limited view, but even more interesting and more difficult to address are territorial issues, that is, the need some feel to protect the 'social capital' or reputation they've built up as societally recognised 'orthodox' medical specialists (Webster 1979). In settings in which only biomedical practitioners are permitted to practise acupuncture, they have few reasons to do so since their practice and their reputations are unlikely to be enhanced by such practice and there is little competition to drive its development. In other settings, a broad range of medical practitioners can and do practise acupuncture, as in the UK and US. In English-speaking countries professional acupuncturists are successful enough that their work is increasingly protected by supportive laws, and (in the US) a gradual increase in insurance coverage. But there continue to be significant barriers to 'integrative' practice, such as widespread ignorance of the many years it takes to become a practitioner of East Asian medicine, and lack of awareness of the growing body of quality research which makes the common complaint that this medicine 'lacks scientific rigor' increasingly dated. We believe these misperceptions need countering, and this in turn will require both the collection of social data on how people perceive acupuncture, and focused educational outreach efforts based on the increase in evidence. The effectiveness of such outreach also needs tracking.

We turn now to methodological challenges.

- *Most existing surveys are cross-sectional and may be dated.* We need efficient means to track changes in patterns of use and attitudes. Though some examples were noted above, in general we need to develop more avenues from which to do longitudinal studies. These could be large-scale studies of healthcare if they included acupuncture as a treatment option for all participants, and these could be funded by private charitable institutions or at the national level. Another possibility is to have questions included on national health surveys, and while these would provide pattern-of-use data only, they could usefully help chart the growth of acupuncture use. School clinics or consortia of schools could also launch longitudinal surveys.
- *Many studies use standardised instruments,* but many existing instruments are biomedical in origin, and may not accurately reflect the precepts of East Asian medicine. Ryan (1997) analyses methodological difficulties in using a biomedical standard instrument for helping patients to report 'pain' and why it didn't work among Tibetan patients. For use in clinical trials of acupuncture, Rosa Schnyer et al are developing a structured assessment instrument (Schnyer et al 2005), see Box 6.7 in Chapter 6. Equally needed are standardised instruments for use in assessing patients' (and practitioners') health values and experience of East Asian medicine. Creating such instruments is challenging but highly useful; it is a challenge we need to meet.
- *Current survey studies above a certain size should employ computerisation from the outset.* While patients and acupuncturists often still feel 'distanced' by this technology, its advantages in rapid response and analysis outweigh complaints in most cases. However,

computerisation requires appropriate support in both funding and management, and these are not insignificant costs.

- *In our urge to collect 'more' data we must not forget the power of stories!* It is 'successful care' that attracts both new users and funders, and while statistics display the reach of acupuncture care, nothing is more convincing than real people explaining in their own words what happened to them and why they are now well, especially if a sufficiency of 'stories' allows for scientific rigour in analysis. Clinical trials present real opportunities for investing in 'nested' qualitative studies of patients' and practitioners' experiences, see for example MacPherson et al (2006b). Qualitative research may take longer to gather and to analyse, but the rewards are great. Another important challenge therefore is to find creative ways to collect qualitative data even as we focus on speed and precision. Current qualitative analysis software is efficient; mixed qualitative-quantitative approaches 'work', and stories 'sell'.

Our final, and fundamental challenge: finding sufficient funding to support our research initiatives. Tables 3.2–3.4 list 18 studies published from 1987 to 2006 (several not included were epidemiological studies that took place within a single clinic). This sample may represent as much as one-half of all English-language studies of pattern of use and experience in acupuncture. In short, we are badly in need of more studies and the funding to support them, especially in the areas summarised in the above paragraphs. As researchers, and as a profession, we need to develop avenues for funding, whether they are federal or private; we are in need of 'angels'.

HOW PATIENT-BASED RESEARCH CAN TRANSLATE INTO PRACTICE

Several potential applications of patient-based research have been mentioned in the preceding paragraphs, and here we list several more, for knowing more about the users of acupuncture care has many advantages:

- Schools (both acupuncture and other medical schools) can use such data to guide students into environments or specialties that improve their success rates and serve the larger society. Schools could also use patient-based research data to modify curriculum, for example, by training students in the characteristics of holism and how these can be made to play out in healthcare delivery.
- School consortia could cooperate to seek funds and share expertise to carry out larger-scale and/or longitudinal studies of, for example, the clinical effects of differing styles of practice, or public perceptions of acupuncture in different locales, or of how healing emerges from the relationship of patient and practitioner.
- National surveys of healthcare utilisation could hereafter include questions to track patterns of use of acupuncture care, in turn

permitting tracking of the pattern of expansion of acupuncture, and providing important 'medical plurality' data to healthcare planners. Such data would also prove useful to schools and research funding agencies.

- Designers of clinical trials/outcomes studies could increasingly include 'essay' or 'diary' components, or interviewing of participant sub-samples in their design protocols, allowing them to better assess exactly what patients think is happening during their care, and what features of the care most matter to them. These data in turn could be applied in the design of intervention protocols, clinics, outreach programs, and even curriculum.
- As a healing profession, and as researchers, we need such data to help us develop effective educational outreach to inform the public, correct misconceptions, as well as to offer guidance to healthcare policy-makers and funding agencies.

SUMMARY

- There exists a wide range of good quantitative, qualitative, and mixed methods to explore questions concerning who uses acupuncture care, why and with what success. Current innovations are steadily increasing the ease and accuracy of data collection.
- Many audiences — the public, practitioners, educators, research funders, insurers, medical innovators, marketers — are interested in such data, and research can be designed to address any of these audiences.
- This chapter identifies research needs and methods, and helps readers distinguish what a particular method allows researchers to do that another might not be able to do.
- Current evidence clearly shows that users like acupuncture care and experience it as a complex holistic intervention — there is much room to develop the details of these earlier findings.
- In conclusion, the most key issue in designing quality pattern of use and experience research is to remember that we learn about meaning by asking and listening, and that our task is to ask the patients and practitioners, and pay attention to context, or, in other words, to be led not by theory or assumption, but by the emergent data itself.

ACKNOWLEDGEMENTS

Our special thanks and appreciation to Charlotte Paterson, George Lewith and Hugh MacPherson for their careful and insightful editing of the chapter. We would also like to thank those at the June 2006 Workshop who provided commentaries that improved the chapter, and the many patients and practitioners who, over the years, have generously given their time and expertise to inform us and our research.

Research resources

Bernard H R 2005 Research methods in anthropology, qualitative and quantitative approaches, 4th edn. Altamira Press, Walnut Creek, CA

Fowler F J 2001 Survey research methods, 3rd edn. Sage Publications, Newbury Park, CA

Grbich C 2007 Qualitative data analysis, an introduction. Sage Publications, Newbury Park, CA

Marshall C, Rossman G 2006 Designing qualitative research, 4th edn. Sage Publications, Newbury Park, CA

Morse J M, Field P A 1995 Qualitative research methods for health professionals. Sage Publications, Newbury Park, CA

Schutt R K 2006 Investigating the social world, the process and practice of research, 5th edn. Sage Publications, Newbury Park, CA

Sue V M, Ritter L A 2007 Conducting online surveys. Sage Publications, Newbury Park, CA

Yates S 2003 Doing social science research. Sage Publications, Newbury Park, CA

References

Adamson J, Gooberman-Hill R, Woolhead G et al 2004 'Questerviews': using questionnaires in qualitative interviews as a method of integrating qualitative and quantitative health services research. Journal of Health Services and Research Policy 9(3):139–145

Anderson R 1991 An American clinic for traditional Chinese medicine: comparisons to family medicine and chiropractic. Journal of Manipulative and Physiological Therapeutics 14(8):462–466

Bates M S, Rankin-Hill L, Sanchez-Ayendez M 1995 A cross-cultural comparison of adaptation to chronic pain among Anglo-Americans and native Puerto Ricans. Medical Anthropology 16(2):141–173

Burke A, Upchurch D M, Dye C 2006 Acupuncture use in the United States: findings from the National Health Interview Survey. Journal of Alternative and Complementary Medicine 12(7):639–648

Cassidy C M 1994 Unraveling the ball of string: reality, paradigms and the study of alternative medicine. Journal of Mind Body Health 10(1):5–31

Cassidy C M 1998a Chinese medicine users in the United States. Part I: Utilization, satisfaction, medical plurality. Journal of Alternative and Complementary Medicine 4(1):17–27

Cassidy C M 1998b Chinese medicine users in the United States. Part II: Preferred aspects of care. Journal of Alternative and Complementary Medicine 4(2):189–202

Cassidy C M 2001 Beyond numbers: qualitative research methods in oriental medicine. In: Stux G, Hammerschlag R (eds) Clinical acupuncture: scientific basis. Springer, Berlin, p 151–169

Coss R A, McGrath P, Caggiano V 1998 Alternative care. Patient choices for adjunct therapies within a cancer center. Cancer Practice 6(3):176–181

Easthope G, Gill G F, Beilby J J 1999 Acupuncture in Australian general practice: patient characteristics. Medical Journal of Australia 170(6):259–262

Eisenberg D M, Davis R B, Ettner S L et al 1998 Trends in alternative medicine use in the United States, 1990–1997: results of a follow-up national survey. Journal of the American Medical Association 280(18):1569–1575

Elliot H 1997 The use of diaries in sociological research on health experience. SociologicalResearch. Online. Available: www.socresonline.org.uk/socresonline/2/2/7.html

Emad M 1994 Does acupuncture hurt? Ethnographic evidence of shifts in psycho-biological experiences of pain. Proceedings of the Society for Acupuncture Research 2:129–140

Emad M 1998 Feeling Qi: emergent bodies and disclosive fields in American appropriations of acupuncture. Rice University, Houston

Frank R, Stollberg G 2004 Medical acupuncture in Germany: patterns of consumerism among physicians and patients. Sociology of Health and Illness 26(3):351–372

Gould A, MacPherson H 2001 Patient perspectives on outcomes after treatment with acupuncture. Journal of Alternative and Complementary Medicine 7(3):261–268

Harris P, Rees R 2000 The prevalence of complementary and alternative medicine use among the general population: a systematic review of the literature. Complementary Therapies in Medicine 8(2):88–96

Kreitler S, Kreitler H, Carasso R 1987 Cognitive orientation as predictor of pain relief following acupuncture. Pain 28(3):323–341

Lin Y-C 2003 Acupuncture and needlephobia: the pediatric patient's perspective. Medical Acupuncture 14(3):15–16

Luff D, Thomas K J 1999 Models of providing complementary therapies in primary care. Final report to Department of Health. HMSO, London

Luff D, Thomas K J 2000 Sustaining complementary therapy provision in primary care: lessons from existing services. Complementary Therapies in Medicine 8(3):173–179

MacPherson H, Mercer S W, Scullion T 2003 Empathy, enablement, and outcome: an exploratory study on acupuncture patients' perceptions. Journal of Alternative and Complementary Medicine 9(6):869–876

MacPherson H, Sinclair-Lian N, Thomas K 2006a Patients seeking care from acupuncture practitioners in the UK: A national survey. Complementary Therapies in Medicine 14(1):20–30

MacPherson H, Thorpe L, Thomas K J 2006b Beyond needling – therapeutic processes in acupuncture care: a qualitative study nested within a low back pain trial. Journal of Alternative and Complementary Medicine 12(9):873–880

Miller J K 1990 Use of traditional Korean health care by Korean immigrants to the United States. Sociology and Social Research 75(11):38–48

Morris D 1991 The culture of pain. University of California Press, Berkeley

Napadow V, Kaptchuk T J 2004 Patient characteristics for outpatient acupuncture in Beijing, China. Journal of Alternative and Complementary Medicine 10(3):565–572

O'Cathain A, Thomas K J 2004 'Any other comments?' Open questions on questionnaires – a bane or a bonus to research? BMC Medical Research Methodology 4:25

Paterson C, Britten N 2004 Acupuncture as a complex intervention: a holistic model. Journal of Alternative and Complementary Medicine 10(5):791–801

Ryan M 1997 Efficacy of the Tibetan treatment for arthritis. Social Science & Medicine 44(4):535–539

Schnyer R N, Conboy L A, Jacobson E et al 2005 Development of a Chinese medicine assessment measure: an interdisciplinary approach using the delphi method. Journal of Alternative and Complementary Medicine 11(6):1005–1013

So D W 2002 Acupuncture outcomes, expectations, patient–provider relationship, and the placebo effect: implications for health promotion. American Journal of Public Health 92(10):1662–1667

Thomas K J, Coleman P, Nicholl J P 2003 Trends in access to complementary or alternative medicines via primary care in England: 1995–2001 results from a follow-up national survey. Family Practice 20(5):575–577

Thomas K J, MacPherson H, Ratcliffe J et al 2005 Longer term clinical and economic benefits of offering acupuncture care to patients with chronic low back pain. Health Technology Assessment 9(32):iii–x, 1

Webster A J 1979 Scientific controversy and socio-cognitive metonymy: The case of acupuncture. Sociological Review Monograph 27:121–137

The safety of acupuncture

4

Hugh MacPherson, Adrian White and Alan Bensoussan

WHY ACUPUNCTURE SAFETY IS IMPORTANT

Acupuncture has generally been assumed to be a very safe modality. It can be argued that continual use over 2000 years in East Asia, involving what must be many millions of treatments, has been associated with only minimal reports of serious harm. However, it is impossible to capture in any quantitative way the level of risk from this long period of use. We have so little data on numbers of treatments, and there has been no systemic collection of data on adverse events, so it is hard to translate this long-term use and low level of reporting of adverse events into meaningful evidence.

There are several reasons why concerns about acupuncture safety have risen in the last two decades. The reasons include:

- the recent unprecedented increase in use of acupuncture in the West;
- several high-profile outbreaks of cross-infection due to acupuncture;
- the growth of evidence-based medicine; and
- the growing importance of medical ethics and human rights.

First, relatively recent increased use of acupuncture in the West has provided one stimulus for systematic research into acupuncture's safety record. The common argument has been that, given the increasingly widespread use of acupuncture, it is a public health concern that we lack knowledge about safety and effectiveness, potentially compromising public safety. Indeed, without robust data on the level of this risk, patients receiving acupuncture will be at risk to an unquantifiable extent.

Long-term and widespread use does not automatically mean that acupuncture is safe. The argument often put forward by critics of acupuncture and other complementary therapies is based on the oft-quoted nineteenth-century tradition of bloodletting. [Note: Bloodletting in traditional Chinese medicine involves minimal bleeding, unlike the large amounts of blood let by nineteenth-century doctors in the West.]

Just because doctors used bloodletting widely, genuinely believing that they were doing good, did not mean that bloodletting was safe. Therefore, it can be argued that long-term use and low levels of reporting in themselves say little about how safe acupuncture really is, and provide no context for an estimate of its safety relative to other interventions for similar conditions.

Second, these more general concerns have been fuelled by outbreaks of specific diseases that have clearly involved a cross-transmission of an infection by acupuncture. An example of this was the hepatitis B outbreak in the USA in the 1980s that was tracked down by public health officials to have been due to the use of unsterilised acupuncture needles (Kent et al 1988) (see Box 4.1).

Box 4.1   Case study of a hepatitis B outbreak (Kent et al 1988)

An investigation of an acupuncturist's practice in Rhode Island identified 35 patients who were infected with hepatitis B virus during 1984. Of 366 patients seen by the acupuncturist during 1984, tests for hepatitis B antigen identified 17 patients with hepatitis who otherwise may have gone undetected, including the acupuncturist himself. Although the practitioner ran two practices, all but one of the 35 affected patients were treated in one centre. Patients who received a greater number of acupuncture needles during their treatment course were more likely to have been infected. The investigators noted that the acupuncturist held needles by their points with ungloved hands and rubbed the needles with his fingers to test them for sharpness, both before and after inserting them. There was no evidence of a strict procedure for sterilisation.

Other well-documented hepatitis outbreaks have occurred and such incidents are obviously of great concern to the public and to the professional bodies regulating acupuncture. Such outbreaks, and their subsequent reporting, have been influential in encouraging professional bodies to rewrite their codes of practice, with autoclave sterilisation methods being replaced by single-use disposable needles. As any acupuncturist knows, there is also a risk of acupuncturists infecting themselves, especially when using an autoclave where potentially infected needles have to be handled prior to re-use. As awareness of the risks of cross-transmission grew, sterile disposable needles became the norm, a shift reinforced by the subsequent AIDS epidemic. And in the UK, there has been the added concern about the theoretical risk of transferring prions (small proteinaceous infectious particles), which are not inactivated even at very high temperatures, leading to a more stringent requirement for acupuncturists to use disposable needles (Department of Health 2006) (see Box 4.2).

Third, the growth of evidence-based medicine has resulted in a more systematic approach to measuring risk and benefit. Formulating a question, searching the literature based on key words, reviewing relevant

---

Box 4.2 The theoretical risk of transferring prions (Department of Health 2006)

In the year 1999 the Department of Health in the UK issued a warning about the theoretical risk from transmitting variant Creutzfeldt-Jakob disease (vCJD). Sometimes known as mad cow disease, or transmissible spongiform encephalopathy, over 140 cases of vCJD have occurred in the UK, seven in France and one each in Ireland, Italy, USA and Canada since 1996 (Department of Health 2006). Of great concern are the risks posed by transferring prions, which are naturally occurring proteins that can become abnormal leading to vCJD. Abnormal prions can lead to the destruction of nervous tissue especially in the brain, giving rise to a spongy appearance seen on autopsy. Because prions are unusually resistant to inactivation by high-temperature sterilisation procedures, single-use disposable needles need to be mandatory.

---

articles, synthesising and interpreting the data, and providing an informed conclusion have formed the core elements of evidence-based medicine. Researchers who have turned their attention to questions of acupuncture safety, and in reviewing the literature, have found an extraordinary range of adverse events and even deaths that have been ascribed to acupuncture. In turn the message of potential danger identified in review papers has been picked up by the popular press, see for example the article 'Can complementary medicine kill you?' in a UK men's magazine (Anon 1997). Leaving aside the question of whether all these adverse events can actually be attributed to acupuncture, it remains imperative that we acquire better evidence on safety and risk.

Fourth, advances in medical ethics and human rights have led to the need to ensure patient autonomy: patients have the right to be fully informed about possible harms of any treatment before they decide whether to receive it or not. They can only be informed if the risks are known.

In this chapter we will highlight the main strands of this research endeavour, identify the key methods of establishing the range of potential risks, set out the methods for assessing the level of these risks and identify some remaining challenges in this field. Thus we hope to provide a thorough and explicit strategy for researching acupuncture safety.

WHAT IS MEANT BY RISK?

Most research into the risks of medical treatment has been in the area of reactions to conventional drugs (Edwards & Aronson 2000), and the definitions that have been developed in that area are not necessarily relevant to the risks of acupuncture. The focus of this research has been on adverse reactions (seen from the perspective of the patient) or adverse effects (as seen from the perspective of the therapy). The primary aim is to establish their type and frequency, whether they can be attributable to the drug, whether they are avoidable, whether they are serious, and what can be learned to reduce future risk. This begs the question, 'What is an adverse event, and how is it different from an adverse effect or adverse reaction?'. It soon becomes evident that there is no single definition for all purposes. For some, the definition of an adverse event includes any event that occurred during a course of treatment whether it was actually caused by the treatment or not. For example the World Health Organisation's definition is, 'Any untoward medical occurrence that may present during treatment with a pharmaceutical product but which does not necessarily have a causal relationship with this treatment' (World Health Organisation 1992).

Adverse events can be classified in many different ways, one of which is according to the frequency with which they occur — with common adverse events being at one end of the spectrum and rare at the other. This can be helpful in that it would clearly be more of a problem if serious adverse events were common rather than rare. Another classification is according to their level of seriousness. One definition of what constitutes a 'serious' adverse event is that it 'requires hospitalization, prolongs hospitalization, is permanently disabling, or results in death' (Lazarou et al 1998). If we combine frequency and seriousness, then we have a basis for determining risk (see Table 4.1).

Criteria for assessing causality have also been developed for drug reactions (Edwards & Aronson 2000). The most important is the time course of the event: given that many drugs tend to have a short-term impact, if a person experiencing a suspected adverse reaction to the drug stops taking it, and the adverse symptoms subside, then we can have some confidence that the event can be attributed to the drug. Restarting the drug is termed a 'rechallenge'. If adverse symptoms reappear then attribution to the drug is more certain. In addition, there should be a plausible mechanism for the reaction to be attributable to the treatment.

When this approach is adapted to acupuncture, the criteria for frequency and severity have some value, though we are also faced with

Table 4.1 Table of levels of risk expressed as percentages (i.e. a 1% risk means that there is one chance in a hundred of experiencing an adverse event)

	Negligible	Minimal	>Minimal
Major complication	<0.001%	0.01%	>0.1%
Minor complication	<0.1%	0.1–10%	>10%

Adapted from BMA Ethics Science and Information Division 1993.

unique challenges, which will be addressed in more detail later in this chapter. However, we are calling attention to them here in order that the complexity of safety research is kept in mind. First, not all reactions to treatment that perhaps might be experienced as negative by patients are necessarily 'adverse' in the pharmaceutical sense of the word. Tiredness, for example, may be 'positive' in a therapeutic sense, in that it helps support a healing process, even though it might also be potentially 'negative' in terms of safety, for example if the patient were to fall asleep at the wheel of a car immediately after treatment.

It is also essential that we identify at the outset, a distinction between unavoidable and avoidable events (Yamashita et al 1999). The latter are likely to be due to inadequate practice standards, for example blood-borne infection or moxa burns to the skin. Unavoidable events may be unexpected and spontaneous reactions to routine treatment provided at acceptable standard. Avoidable events, when thoroughly investigated and reported, can lead to better training and higher practice standards.

One further classification may be of value, and that is the difference between events related directly to an active component of treatment, such as needling or moxibustion, which are sometimes known as 'direct' adverse events, and events related to the clinical judgement of the acupuncture practitioner, which are sometimes known as 'indirect' adverse events. In terms of the former, some reactions might be avoidable, such as cross-infection, and some might not, for example idiosyncratic reactions such as fainting. An example of the latter would be a missed diagnosis of a malignant condition, such that the patient's conventional treatment was delayed (Ernst 2001). In Table 4.2 we present a schema

Table 4.2 Schema for a classification of risks associated with the practice of acupuncture

Category of risk	Areas of risk	Principal types
Acupuncture	Reactions related to needling	Cross-infection Trauma Physiological responses Metal allergy Idiosyncratic reactions
Clinical judgement of the acupuncture practitioner	Commission	Incorrect treatment Advice to remove a conventional therapy Misdiagnosis leading to delayed conventional treatment
	Omission	Failure to refer Failure to explain risks

Adapted from Bensoussan & Myers 1996.

for the classification of risks, which drew on the expertise of clinical toxicologists, and emphasises the clinical judgement of the practitioner, dividing them into errors of omission and commission. Many of these issues will be revisited in later sections of this chapter where we will also identify some challenges and suggest strategies for addressing them. In the first instance however we will examine effective approaches to evaluating acupuncture safety.

METHODS OF ASSESSING ACUPUNCTURE SAFETY AND RISK

A range of methods have been used to assess the risks associated with medical interventions, some of which have been used for acupuncture studies, see Table 4.3 (World Health Organisation 1992).

Prospective studies are those that commence before the events they measure, and retrospective studies are those that collect events that have already taken place. Data may be collected by practitioners or by patients. Ideally, risk is assessed in a way that includes an incidence rate or proportion, for example, the incidence could be the number of adverse events over a period of time for a specific population, or the proportion could

Table 4.3 Commonly used and potential methods to establish risks associated with acupuncture

Method (description, comment)	Limitations
Reviews of case reports from the literature (isolated events)	(Discussed in the text following this table)
Retrospective studies, population surveys	Data unreliable and easily confounded. (For an example see below)
Prospective studies, intensive event monitoring (run for a defined period with observers specially recruited)	Limited number of observers, limited duration: both restrict generalisability. Large numbers required for rare events. (For examples see below)
Review of clinical records (either routine or purposive)	Exhaustive but expensive. For retrospective reviews, very dependent on quality of records
Case-control studies (retrospective comparison to establish causality of known adverse events)	Expensive. Difficult to establish appropriate controls
Voluntary organised reporting (systematic, e.g. Yellow Card system)	Unreliable because of under-reporting (see below)
Meta-analysis of published studies	Relies on original data, which may be heterogeneous in terms of definitions, methods, and quality

Adapted from White 2004b.

be the number of adverse events out of a total number of treatments. If there is no 'rate' (i.e. denominator) on which to base the risk, then the data will be difficult to interpret: one in ten is very different from one in a million. In the next section we will outline the different approaches to evaluating risk.

Reviews of case reports from the literature

In the earlier days of research into acupuncture safety, one of the most common approaches was to search the scientific and medical literature to find reports of cases of adverse events. Such case reports in the 1970s and 1980s often presented unusual or bizarre incidents (see Box 4.3), and demonstrated standards of practice well below those now considered acceptable. Lao et al's (2003) review supports evidence of rising standards, with their findings of a trend towards fewer reports of serious complications since 1988.

In the 1990s, researchers started systematically collecting data from the literature. A key feature of systematic literature reviews is a set of pre-defined criteria, including search words, language, searchable databases, and start and end time periods. An early example of this type of research was the study of Norheim (1996) (see Box 4.4).

In recent years there have been many literature reviews of case reports (Lao et al 2003, Rosted 1996, White 2004a), all of which have a similar methodology, though some have had variations in their specific focus, for example case reports of hepatitis (Ernst & Sherman 2003). With a few exceptions, almost all serious adverse events are associated with poor practice. An outcome from this research has been general support for the principle that only properly trained and regulated practitioners should be practising acupuncture. Some of the reviews concluded that acupuncture appeared to be relatively safe. To quote one review, 'there

---

Box 4.3 A tragic case of a do-it-yourselfer (Schiff 1965)

'The subject, an 82-year-old white Hungarian émigré, was found dead in her home by a relative. In panic, the relative called a physician who, at first sight, believed the death to be natural. However, on more detailed inspection the physician noted a sewing needle projecting from the precordial area'. It turned out that she had herself inserted an ordinary sewing needle, 1-inch long, which had pierced her heart. The author of the case report writes, 'It is impossible to know what was on the mind of a dead woman. From the condition of the heart, it can be assumed that this woman occasionally had anginal pains'.

Also, 'She was known to have practised acupuncture'. The author concluded that: 'The final diagnosis was that of cardiac tamponade due to needle puncture of the heart'.

> **Box 4.4** Literature review of case reports (Norheim 1996)
>
> Arne Norheim, a Norwegian who has been one of the pioneers of acupuncture safety research, searched Medline for the years 1981–1994 using key words 'acupuncture' and 'adverse' and 'effects'. In his search of the literature, he found 125 papers that involved 78 case reports and 193 patients. Pneumothorax was the most common organ injury, while hepatitis was the worst common infection. Among these cases, three patients were reported to have died, one with bilateral pneumothorax, another with complications from endocarditis, and the third died after a severe asthma attack. In reviewing these case reports of deaths, it was not possible to unequivocally attribute the adverse events to acupuncture. The author concluded that, 'serious adverse events are few, and acupuncture can generally be considered as a safe treatment'.

are hundreds of thousands of acupuncturists world-wide performing world-wide millions of treatments a year. From this perspective, the true incidence of serious complications could well be very low indeed' (Ernst & White 1997).

In an unusual approach, a systematic review of traumatic events by Peuker et al (1999) was accompanied by post-mortem anatomical studies. This study highlighted the risks to internal organs associated with acupuncture when practised without due care and attention. The authors stressed the risks to the heart (cardiac tamponade) and lungs (pneumothorax) when needling inappropriately, and cite incidents that have led to patient deaths (see Box 4.5). Damage to peripheral nerves, the central nervous system and blood vessels are also areas of concern discussed by the authors. To complement their literature review, human cadavers were used to establish distances between the surface of the skin and specific internal organs, so that advice about depth of needling could be provided.

There are a number of limitations associated with using case reports as evidence for safety or risks of acupuncture. Part of the problem is that case reports provide varying levels of detail. And the term 'acupuncture' covers a range of different techniques (for example, implanted needles and electro-acupuncture), which carry different types of risk. Most reports give little or no detail of precise techniques used, nor the education, experience or style of practice of the acupuncturists. Case reports tend to be of acute serious incidents, and the tone of some of these reports indicates a negative attitude to acupuncture that may have motivated the author to write the report. Therefore serious adverse events might be over-represented among case reports, while non-serious events, perhaps with a latent phase before onset, are likely to be under-represented. This is because minor reactions, such as bleeding, or local pain at the site of needling, or fainting and nausea, will be unlikely to be considered worthy of a publishable case report.

> **Box 4.5** Needling REN-17 through a hole in the sternum (Peuker et al 1999)
>
> It is possible to injure the heart when needling REN-17 perpendicularly. This is because of the little-known fact that around 5% of people have a hole in their sternum in the region of this point, known as a sternal foramen (see Fig. 4.1). Practitioners who are unaware of this may place the patient at considerable risk. There have been several reported cases and one fatality (Halvorsen et al 1995, Hasegawa et al 1991). This congenital abnormality cannot be detected by X-rays, and is usually identified by computed tomography (CT) scans. Palpation prior to acupuncture cannot detect this abnormality either, so when treating patients, this point must be needled tangentially. Peuker et al suggest that 'knowledge of normal anatomy and anatomical variations is essential for safe practice, and should be reviewed by regulatory authorities and those responsible for training courses' (Peuker et al 1999).

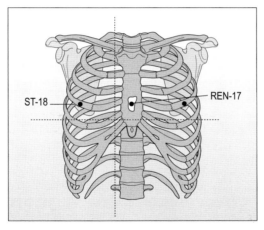

Fig 4.1   A hole on the sternum at Ren-17 is a risk factor when acupuncturists needle perpendicularly.

While case reports provide a useful background to our understanding of the type of adverse events, they tell us little about frequency, and because there is no incidence rate, they tell us little about risk. To determine frequency and therefore risk, retrospective and prospective surveys are commonly used.

Retrospective surveys

Some idea of the frequency of adverse events can come from retrospective surveys. Such surveys have tended to focus on a particular group or groups of practitioners in one location or country, and over a specified period of time. Some researchers have surveyed acupuncture practitioners (Bensoussan et al 2000), while others have surveyed general medical practitioners (not practising acupuncture) reporting on their patients' experiences (Abbot et al 1998). Retrospective surveys of patients in the general population have also provided a useful perspective (Chen et al 1990, Norheim & Fonnebo 2000, Yamashita et al 1998).

Retrospective surveys have the advantage of simplicity, requiring participants to be involved in a one-off completion of a questionnaire. A key condition is to ensure that the sample is representative of the wider population and a computer-generated random sample, with a reasonably high percentage of the sample responding, will help to minimise selection bias. The robustness of the findings will be enhanced if it can be shown that the responders are reasonably representative of the population. A good example of such a retrospective survey is that of Bensoussan et al (2000) (see Box 4.6).

There are a number of difficulties associated with retrospective surveys. Recall bias and error are potential limitations of retrospective surveys generally, whether respondents are acupuncturists, general practitioners or participants. In Bensoussan et al's survey (undertaken in 1996), the average full-time equivalent years in practice was 7.7 years, so practitioners were being asked to remember events over such a long time period it is likely that there would be some bias and error in recall, with presumably more severe events being remembered best, and trivial events forgotten. A poor response rate is a second potential problem. If such surveys involve practitioners, it is difficult to achieve more than moderate response rates (greater than 50%), as practitioners are either too busy or possibly over-sensitive about a potentially negative outcome. Both non-response bias and attrition bias may contribute to under-reporting

Box 4.6 A retrospective survey of practitioners in Australia (Bensoussan 2000)

Alan Bensoussan and his colleagues surveyed occupational health groups who provided acupuncture in three Australian states. The aim was to investigate the nature and frequency of adverse events that result from the practice of acupuncture and Chinese herbal medicine. A total of 458 (30%) of 1517 medically qualified practitioners responded to the survey, while 642 (50%) of 1278 practitioner members of non-medical associations responded. Practitioners were asked to report on adverse events that they ascribed to acupuncture since they had started in practice. More than 3000 events were reported, most commonly fainting during treatment, increased pain and nausea. Serious adverse effects included 64 reports of pneumothorax. The mean duration of practice was the full-time equivalent of 7.7 years. Bensoussan et al calculated that one adverse event occurred on average for every 633 consultations, i.e. approximately one event every 8 to 9 months of full-time practice.

by those practitioners who actually participate. A third limitation may be under-reporting, as practitioners may not want to show themselves in a bad light, nor patients their practitioners. Further research using these retrospective surveys may be useful to gain a snapshot of most commonly observed events, but have many limitations compared to prospective surveys.

Prospective surveys

Prospective surveys require participants to collect ongoing data for a specific time period. This approach reduces bias associated with poor recall, the major limitation of the retrospective approach, so can provide more accurate data. Prospective surveys can involve data collection by practitioners, by patients or by other healthcare practitioners.

This type of survey can be characterised by the recruitment of acupuncture practitioners, whether a sample through professional associations or a group in specific clinic settings, who are asked to monitor adverse events over a period of time, or covering a specific number of treatments. Standardised documentation is used with a clear description of what constitutes an adverse event. Such surveys have been undertaken in the UK with traditional acupuncturists (MacPherson et al 2001), and with doctors and physiotherapists who practise acupuncture as an adjunctive technique (White et al 2001), as well as in Japan (Yamashita et al 1999), Taiwan (Chen et al 1990) and elsewhere.

These surveys do have some limitations. For surveys in hospital clinics (Yamashita et al 1999) and teaching clinics (Yamashita et al 2001) it is only with caution that one can generalise the results beyond a specific clinical setting that may involve only a handful of practitioners. For surveys involving practitioners of professional associations, attaining a reasonable response rate is a challenge, especially as ongoing monitoring requires more of a commitment than completing a single questionnaire. For an example of such a survey, see Box 4.7.

As with retrospective surveys, prospective practitioner surveys may also tend to result in under-reporting, with attribution adding to the difficulty of interpreting the results. The quality of the data obtained will also depend to some extent on the documentation. The use of check boxes, for example, when compared to an open question, is likely to increase reporting rates.

Prospective patient surveys have the potential to overcome some of the limitations of practitioner surveys, for example such surveys may include data from patients who have negative experiences that result in discontinuing treatment. Data from patients may also be less biased because as a group they have less investment in acupuncture's reputation than practitioners for whom it is their livelihood. Patients also might be less busy than practitioners, and therefore a higher response rate might be expected from patients. In addition, patients have a lower

Box 4.7 A prospective acupuncture safety survey of reports by physicians and physiotherapists (White et al 2001)

A prospective survey was undertaken using the method of intensive event monitoring. Forms were developed for reporting minor events month by month, and for significant events as they occurred. The sample size was calculated to identify any adverse events that occurred more frequently than once in 10 000 consultations. Acupuncturists were recruited from the professional organisations of doctors and physiotherapists in the UK. Seventy-eight acupuncturists reported a total of 2178 events occurring in 31 822 consultations, an incidence of 684 per 10 000 consultations. The most common minor adverse events were bleeding (3%), needling pain (1%), and aggravation of symptoms (1%). In the case of the aggravations, resolution of symptoms followed in 70% of cases. A total of 43 significant adverse events reported, a rate of 14 per 10 000, of which none was classified as serious though 13 interfered with daily activities. One patient suffered a seizure during acupuncture. Avoidable events included forgotten patients, needles left in patients, cellulitis and moxa burns. The incidence of adverse events following acupuncture by these practitioners can be classified as minimal; some avoidable events did occur. They concluded that acupuncture in skilled hands seems to be one of the safer forms of medical intervention.

threshold for reporting adverse events. For these reasons, prospective patient surveys might be expected to provide relatively more robust evidence on acupuncture safety. A recent systematic review of prospective studies of acupuncture safety (Ernst 2001), covering a quarter of a million treatments in all, showed higher rates of adverse events when reported by patients rather than their practitioners. The authors made this point in the context of a more general one, namely that adverse event rates reported will depend on many factors; the type of acupuncture, the cultural context, the way questions are framed, how they are asked, and the definition of what constitutes an adverse event are all factors that will influence the resulting adverse event rates. Similar to other investigations, the authors 'confirm that the true incidence of serious complications is low' (Ernst 2001).

Indirect adverse events

The potential for acupuncturists to encourage their patients to continue with acupuncture rather than refer them for a medical diagnosis, thereby resulting in delayed treatment for an underlying pathology, was first addressed by Norheim (1996). In this Norwegian survey, doctors reported 10 cases of delayed doctor contact. In a more recent population survey of patients, Norheim and Fonnebo (2000) found that their data did not

> **Box 4.8** Adverse events indirectly associated with acupuncture as reported by patients in the UK (MacPherson et al 2004)
>
> In a large-scale survey of patients, the primary aim was to establish from acupuncture patients the type and frequency of adverse events they experienced and attributed to their treatment. However important secondary aims included the measurement of patient-reported adverse consequences arising from advice received about conventional/prescribed medication, or from delayed conventional diagnosis and treatment. In a postal survey of prospectively identified acupuncture patients, one in three members of the British Acupuncture Council (638) invited consecutive patients to participate. Participating patients gave baseline data and consented to direct follow-up by the researchers at 3 months. A structured questionnaire was used to collect data on perceived adverse events resulting from treatment with acupuncture. In total 9408 patients gave baseline information and consent, 6348 (67%) completed 3-month questionnaires. One hundred and ninety nine (3%) of responding patients reported receiving advice about conventional/prescribed medication, of whom six reported adverse consequences after taking this advice. Two patients reported delayed conventional treatment. These data led the authors to conclude that the risks associated with indirect adverse events are very low.

support the contention that acupuncture patients failed to seek conventional treatment for potentially serious disease. Nevertheless, other researchers (Abbot et al 1998) and reviewers of the literature (Ernst 2001) have continued to raise concerns about missed diagnoses and delayed treatment. For example, Abbott et al (1998) 'raise the possibility that a therapist's advice may be more dangerous than the therapy itself' and include 'unnecessary financial loss or disillusion with ineffective treatment' to be a potential adverse event. Inappropriate advice about prescribed conventional medication, such that the patient may be put at risk, has also been raised as a concern (Bensoussan & Myers 1996, Ernst 2001). Only more recently have these potential risks been placed in the context of the frequency and severity of occurrence in the general patient population (see Box 4.8).

CHALLENGES AND STRATEGIES

We now have some solid data on levels of risk for patients. In competent hands, acupuncture appears to be a safe modality, but some challenges remain. In this section we cover: exploring variability in patient reactions in routine care; exploring the variability that might be due to practitioner characteristics; mapping those areas where further safety data would be useful; improving definitions and documentation; exploring the impact of treatment reactions and adverse events on outcome; and monitoring safety within a clinical trial. An additional challenge, the improvement of practice in order to reduce adverse events, is discussed in the following section.

Exploring variability in patient reactions in routine care

In general it is of value to explore the patient perspective, one that has been consistently under-utilised in medical research (Vincent & Coulter 2002). It should be noted that not all 'adverse' events experienced by patients are seen as unwelcome. The concept of patient-rated 'bothersomeness' would factor in the other dimensions to the experience of acupuncture, whereby positive reactions modify the experience of the negative ones (Thomas et al 2005), so ideally, for patient-reported adverse events, we should also collect the patient's assessment of the impact. Certain research questions may be better answered using qualitative research methods, to explore attitudes to risk, bothersomeness, and association between attitudes and events. For example, is needle phobia or route to referral related to reaction rates when exploring variability between patients? Does the expectation of pain seem to be associated with more actual pain experienced at the site of needling? More generally, are there patient characteristics that would help us predict a higher likelihood of a negative reaction? Do some types of patients experience more negative reactions with acupuncture, perhaps being more prone to fainting? There is also some evidence regarding patients prescribed medication interacting with acupuncture. For example warfarin, which reduces blood clotting, is associated with an increased likelihood of bleeding, though we have little data on this. In addition, it is theoretically possible that some patients may be ideal responders in that they are neurochemically favourably disposed to treatment. In all these areas of research the patient perspective can contribute important insights, however the data are collected.

Exploring variability due to practitioner characteristics in routine care

There is some evidence to indicate that different practitioners report very different rates of adverse reactions (White et al 2001). The extent to which this is an artefact of variable approaches to reporting, or that there are real differences in the rates of reactions, is unclear. Some styles of acupuncture might also be implicated in higher rates of adverse events. Do practitioners who usually use strong stimulation techniques cause more bothersome reactions? Acupuncture practitioners may also use certain auxiliary techniques which have been associated with adverse events, but have been subjected to little research. Moxibustion, for example, has been associated with burns to the skin, although we know little about the methods of practice that have caused them, given that moxibustion can be used in a number of ways (moxa on the needle; moxa box; 'sparrow-pecking', etc.). Electro-acupuncture can be problematic, not only when poor implementation causes sudden and unexpected electric shocks, but also patients fitted with pacemakers are advised not to receive electro-acupuncture (Fujiwara et al 1980). Certain risks are attached to embedded needle techniques, particularly infection, and these have not been mapped well. Many acupuncturists practice Chinese herbal medicine, as many as 30% in one study (Sherman et al 2005), and little is known about the possible interaction of acupuncture and herbs. The use of auxiliary techniques varies considerably, but it can be expected that their addition to a practitioner's repertoire will also vary the level of risk.

An under-investigated area is the practice of discussing risks before a course of treatment, and the extent to which this discussion increases (or decreases) negative patient reaction on the basis of suggestion. Some practitioners also impose requirements before treatment, such as fasting for several hours. We have little knowledge of the importance of these areas of discussion and/or advice in reducing reactions such as fainting, or whether certain reactions such as light-headedness, fainting or tiredness may be increased as a result.

Mapping those areas where further data would be useful

Reliable data on the frequency of non-serious adverse events is now available from a number of major surveys, but data on type and frequency of serious adverse events are sparse, simply because such events are so rare. Methodologically, it is unclear how such adverse events could be monitored in as systematic and rigorous a fashion as is feasible.

When mapping adverse events in routine care, it should be noted that a high number of similar symptoms have been reported in healthy people not undergoing any treatment. Three studies monitored reports of young, fit subjects with health-related symptoms (some of which may be described as adverse or negative events) over the previous 3 days (Bandolier 2003). Levels of fatigue were reported by between 37% and 65% of subjects. Other common symptoms included nasal congestion, inability to concentrate and excessive sleepiness. Such data might indicate that surveys of acupuncture safety might have overestimated the associated adverse event rate. When conducting such surveys, it might be sensible to adjust the event rate for what might be expected without treatment.

Improving definitions and documentation

A major concern regarding the variability of reporting lies with the nature of definitions and the quality of documentation procedures. We know that the definition of an adverse event will impact on reporting, as will the documentation. For example, if reporters use checklists then we can expect higher levels of reporting for the same level of adverse events. One of the challenges is to develop better tools in this area, so that we can produce more consistent data, and a more robust evidence base.

There are arguments both for and against a voluntary scheme of reporting adverse events. For mild non-significant events, the effort involved would likely far outweigh putative benefits, especially because of the general unreliability of voluntary reporting schemes. Specifically, under-reporting is a problem, as has been found in voluntary schemes within conventional medicine. In a study involving 100 French GPs, they reported only 1 in 20 000 drug reactions (Moride et al 1997). A stronger case could perhaps be made for reporting serious adverse events in routine care, though such an approach is not without its challenges, not least the necessity of gaining the support of professional associations. The best alternative to voluntary reporting would probably be to conduct prospective studies over a limited period of time that are designed to answer specific research questions.

Exploring the impact of treatment reactions and adverse events on outcome

A further area awaiting investigation is the relationship of short-term treatment reactions and adverse events to longer-term health-related outcomes. For some time it has been thought that spontaneous aggravations of existing conditions might be a 'healing response', or Menken effect as it is known in Japan (Yamashita et al 1999). Even though the adverse event rate associated with aggravations is relatively small, around 1% to 3% (MacPherson et al 2001, 2004, White et al 2001), as yet we know little about the association with therapeutic impact.

When two treatments are compared, it is the health-related outcome that is usually sought. This is of course quite understandable, but decisions about treatment should also include some measure of the side-effect profile. There may be sufficiently large differences to impact on judgements and decisions, whether made by patients or policy-makers. Of particular interest in this context would be a fair comparison between acupuncture and non-steroidal anti-inflammatory medication for the treatment of painful conditions. However it is important to compare like with like and further research could usefully establish what a meaningful and fair comparison might be. Some preliminary research in Norway on acupuncture for low back pain has indicated that there are quite substantial differences in side effects when acupuncture is compared to non-steroidal anti-inflammatory medication for low back pain (Kittang et al 2001). In the naproxen group, gastrointestinal side effects were noted in 15/29, compared with 0/28 in the acupuncture group.

Monitoring safety within clinical trials

The advantage of collecting data within a trial is that patients agree to complete all necessary documentation. It is always good clinical practice (GCP) to prospectively monitor adverse events within a trial, and there are guidelines on GCP in conventional medical research that are helpful here. See http://www.mrc.ac.uk/pdf-ctg.pdf for the UK and http://www.fda.gov/cder/guidance/959fnl.pdf for the USA. Clinical trials involve relatively small numbers of patients, so will tell us little about serious adverse event rates, but they do provide investigators with the opportunity of conducting deeper investigations into the impact of treatment reactions and adverse events. For a good example of safety monitoring in an acupuncture trial of low back pain, see http://clinical-trials.gov/ct/show/NCT00065585?order=21. The safety monitoring protocol had two levels: adverse experiences (i.e. adverse events) and serious adverse events (regardless of attribution). Procedures for monitoring were clearly set out, which included a practitioner report on how likely the event was caused by acupuncture. For meaningful comparisons between trials, there needs to be more consistent high-quality reporting, ideally involving similar documentation. In this way more rigorous comparisons between treatments can be made.

TRANSLATING RESEARCH INTO PRACTICE

Translating research into improving practice is particularly pertinent in the area of safety. Can all this research into negative reactions and adverse events make a difference? We have seen a steady rise in the standards of acupuncture over recent decades, as evidenced by the reducing rates of serious adverse events (Lao et al 2003) and the increased quality of provision to acupuncturists of practice guidelines by professional associations.

It is the 'avoidable' risks that probably merit the most attention when it comes to strategies to improve practice. The more common avoidable adverse events include forgetting to remove the needles, forgetting the patient and moxa burns (Ernst 2001, Lao et al 2003). The forgotten needle is one such avoidable event which is often very worrisome for the patient. Being a forgotten patient can also be extremely distressing. What can be done to reduce these occurrences? In the UK, a 'systems' approach has now been adopted in principle in the National Health Service to reduce risk in conventional medical care. This approach, developed for investigating and avoiding medical accidents, entails going beyond blaming the individual practitioner and assessing and improving the systems of working. It could lead to a check list for acupuncture practice, and may be useful for individuals and organisations concerned with reducing the risk of adverse events.

Tiredness is potentially the most serious adverse event, given that driving home after treatment might place the patient at risk of a fatal accident. Research into translating this concern into a systematic approach to reducing the risk would be useful. For example, what are the patient characteristics and environmental aspects most highly associated with tiredness? Are there steps that the practitioner can take to reduce the risk, or telltale signs in the patient after treatment that warn the practitioner to pass on the concern before the patient leaves the clinic?

Some of the risks for patients are dependent on the competence of the practitioner. Acupuncturists are members of a professional association hopefully with exemplary codes of practice, but there may be reasons for differential risks between practitioners. Exploring these differences could flag areas where changes to practice and guidelines could be implemented. For example, research has identified the dangers associated with practitioners being over-confident in their own abilities (Kruger & Dunning 1999).

Professional associations have a responsibility to maintain standards in their professions and a number of approaches merit consideration here. Building a database of case reports may provide a useful starting point, and guidelines for such case reporting have been proposed for cases of pneumothorax (Peuker & Filler 2004). Further research would help establish how such case reports could raise general awareness, perhaps through publication, and possibly upgraded guidelines. The professional associations are best placed to explore how acupuncturists can best provide data on risk to patients. There are many ways of presenting risks to patients, some of which are better than others, and certain professional associations have already produced guidelines, but more rigorous research to identify the key data that should be presented may be helpful. Most importantly, professional associations are able to shift their members' attitudes, so that good practice in safety is not merely a 'requirement', but the aim of all practitioners for reasons of respect and ethics.

SUMMARY

The safety of acupuncture and its associated techniques cannot be taken for granted. The level of safety needs to be established and the risk quantified. Research to date shows that, in the hands of trained practitioners, acupuncture is a relatively safe technique and continued research will be of value in extending the evidence base. Changes to practice have resulted from research into the risks of acupuncture, and further changes can be anticipated that will make the treatment even safer.

Research resources

Rosenthal M M, Sutcliffe K M 2002 Medical error: what do we know, what do we do. Jossey-Bass, Wiley, San Francisco
Vincent C 2001 Clinical risk management. BMJ Books, London
Vincent C 2006 Patient safety. Churchill Livingstone, Edinburgh

References

Abbot N C, Hill M, Barnes J, Hourigan P, Ernst E 1998 Uncovering suspected adverse effects of complementary and alternative medicine. The International Journal of Risk and Safety in Medicine 11(2):99–106

Anon 1997 Can complementary medicine kill you? Mens' Health, UK

Bandolier 2003 Adverse non-drug reactions. Evidence based thinking about health care. 115:4

Bensoussan A, Myers S P 1996 Towards a safer choice: the practice of traditional Chinese medicine in Australia. Faculty of Health, University of Western Sydney, Sydney

Bensoussan A, Myers S P, Carlton A L 2000 Risks associated with the practice of traditional Chinese medicine: an Australian study. Archives of Family Medicine 9:1071–1078

BMA Ethics Science and Information Division 1993 Medical ethics today: its practice and philosophy. BMJ Publishing Group, London

Chen F P, Hwang S J, Lee H P et al 1990 Clinical study of syncope during acupuncture treatment. Acupuncture and Electro-therapeutics Research 15:107–119

Department of Health (UK) 2006 CJD. Department of Health, London

Edwards I R, Aronson J K 2000 Adverse drug reactions: definitions, diagnosis, and management. Lancet 356:1255–1259

Ernst E 2001 Desk top guide to complementary and alternative medicine, an evidence based approach. Harcourt, London

Ernst E, Sherman K J 2003 Is acupuncture a risk factor for hepatitis? Systematic review of epidemiological studies. Journal of Gastroenterology and Hepatology 18:1231–1236

Ernst E, White A 1997 Life-threatening adverse reactions after acupuncture? A systematic review. Pain 71:123–126

Ernst E, White A R 2001 Prospective studies of the safety of acupuncture: a systematic review. American Journal of Medicine 110:481–485

Fujiwara H, Taniguchi K, Takeuchi J et al 1980 The influence of low frequency acupuncture on a demand pacemaker. Chest 78(1):96–97

Halvorsen T B, Anda S S, Naess A B et al 1995 Fatal cardiac tamponade after acupuncture through congenital sternal foramen. Lancet 345:1175

Hasegawa J, Noguchi N, Yamasaki J et al 1991 Delayed cardiac tamponade and hemothorax induced by an acupuncture needle. Cardiology 78:58–63

Kent G P, Brondum J, Keenlyside R A et al 1988 A large outbreak of acupuncture-associated hepatitis B. American Journal of Epidemiology 127:591–598

Kittang G, Melvaer T, Baerheim A 2001 [Acupuncture versus antiphlogistics in acute low back pain in general practice]. Tidsskrift for den Norske laegeforening 121(10):1207–1210

Kruger J, Dunning D 1999 Unskilled and unaware of it: how difficulties in recognizing one's own incompetence lead to inflated self-assessments. Journal of Personality and Social Psychology 77:1121–1134

Lao L, Hamilton G R, Fu J et al 2003 Is acupuncture safe? A systematic review of case reports. Alternative Therapies in Health and Medicine 9:72–83

Lazarou J, Pomeranz B H, Corey P N 1998 Incidence of adverse drug reactions in hospitalized patients: a meta-analysis of prospective studies. Journal of the American Medical Association 279:1200–1205

MacPherson H, Thomas K, Walters S et al 2001 A prospective survey of adverse events and treatment reactions following 34,000 consultations with professional acupuncturists. Acupuncture in Medicine 19:93–102

MacPherson H, Scullion A, Thomas K J et al 2004 Patient reports of adverse events associated with acupuncture treatment: a prospective national survey. Quality and Safety in Health Care 13:349–355

Moride Y, Haramburu F, Requejo A A et al 1997 Under-reporting of adverse drug reactions in general practice. British Journal of Clinical Pharmacology 43:177–181

Norheim A J 1996 Adverse effects of acupuncture: a study of the literature for the years 1981–1994. Journal of Alternative and Complementary Medicine 2:291–297

Norheim A J, Fonnebo V 2000 A survey of acupuncture patients: results from a questionnaire among a random sample in the general population in Norway. Complementary Therapies in Medicine 8:187–192

Peuker E, Filler T 2004 Guidelines for case reports of adverse events related to acupuncture. Acupuncture in Medicine 22:29–33

Peuker E T, White A, Ernst E 1999 Traumatic complications of acupuncture. Therapists need to know human anatomy. Archives of Family Medicine 8:553–558

Rosted P 1996 Literature survey of reported adverse effects associated with acupuncture treatment. American Journal of Acupuncture 24:27–34

Sherman K J, Cherkin D C, Eisenberg D M 2005 The practice of acupuncture: who are the providers and what do they do? Annals of Family Medicine 3(2):151–158

Schiff A F 1965 A fatality due to acupuncture. Medical Times 93(6): 630–631

Thomas K J, MacPherson H, Ratcliffe J et al 2005 Longer term clinical and economic benefits of offering acupuncture care to patients with chronic low back pain. Health Technology Assessment 9(32):iii–x, 1

Vincent C A, Coulter A 2002 Patient safety: what about the patient? Quality and Safety in Health Care 11:76–80

White A 2004a A cumulative review of the range and incidence of significant adverse events associated with acupuncture. Acupuncture in Medicine 22:122–133

White A R 2004b Evidence on the safety of acupuncture, and its effectiveness in three common indications (dissertation). Peninsula Medical School, Universities of Exeter and Plymouth

White A, Hayhoe S, Hart A et al 2001 Survey of adverse events following acupuncture (SAFA): a prospective study of 32,000 consultations. Acupuncture in Medicine 19:84–92

World Health Organisation 1992 International monitoring of adverse reactions to drugs: adverse reaction terminology. WHO Collaborating Centre for International Drug Monitoring, Uppsala, Sweden

Yamashita H, Tsukayama H, Tanno Y et al 1998 Adverse events related to acupuncture. Journal of the American Medical Association 280:1563–1564

Yamashita H, Tsukayama H, Tanno Y 1999 Adverse events in acupuncture and moxibustion treatment: a six-year survey at a national clinic in Japan. Journal of Alternative and Complementary Medicine 5:229–236

Yamashita H, Tsukayama H, White A R et al 2001 Systematic review of adverse events following acupuncture: the Japanese literature. Complementary Therapies in Medicine 9:98–104

Measuring patient–centred outcomes

5

Charlotte Paterson and Rosa N. Schnyer

WHY THE EMPHASIS ON MEASURING PATIENT-CENTRED OUTCOMES?

In this chapter we argue that acupuncture should be evaluated on the basis of whether it improves people's health in ways that are important to individual patients. In order to do this we need outcome measures that are patient centred, as well as reliable and sensitive to change. Although patient-centred outcomes may include objective measures, such as weight, days off work, or mortality rates, they are more often focused on subjective health (or 'quality of life') that is measured using outcome questionnaires. An outcome questionnaire that is patient centred should encompass the aims, values and treatment effects that are prioritised by individuals, and should enable each individual to provide an unambiguous assessment of change over time (Paterson 2004). This individualised approach is in keeping with the underlying philosophy of Chinese medicine.

The reason for practising acupuncture, and for researching it, is to improve the quality of patients' lives. In clinical practice the acupuncturist does this by listening to the patients, offering treatment that attends to their needs and seeking feedback from them to direct further treatment. There is an ongoing dialogue between the practitioner's expert knowledge and the patients' individual knowledge and experience of their health and illness. However when it comes to research, the patient's perspective and subjective experience is often removed, and other 'objective' criteria are used to assess whether the treatment is helpful. For example the outcome of acupuncture for people with asthma is reduced to changes in lung function tests, or the outcome for people with depression is reduced to changes in a standard psychiatric examination. When this happens, and patient-centred outcomes are neglected, research cannot answer the question of whether and how acupuncture addresses people's health needs and improves their lives. Using such restricted outcomes runs the risk of producing false-negative results, which will be interpreted as showing acupuncture 'doesn't work'. In this chapter we do not describe the measurement of objective outcomes such as changes in blood pressure or biochemical markers. This is not because they are not important, but because their measurement is straightforward and described elsewhere. In contrast, understanding more complex and subjective treatment effects and seeking to measure them is a challenging area that is relevant not just to acupuncture, but to other holistic interventions or packages of care, including those based on conventional medicine.

Prioritising the patient's perspective does not, however, mean that other perspectives on outcome should be neglected. We recognise that a patient-centred outcome constitutes only one perspective on outcomes and that other perspectives, such as biomedically defined outcomes and outcomes based on a Chinese medicine explanatory model are also important. As we take the work forward in this area we need to investigate and understand the associations between these different perspectives on outcome. In particular situations, additional perspectives may also be important, such as that of parents and carers, or that of health service policy-makers or managers. Although in practice there may be overlap between these different standpoints, research designs should be explicit about their primary orientation and, where possible, deepen our understanding by encompassing more than a single perspective. We return to this issue of multiple perspectives later, and one integrative model is presented in Box 5.5.

In this chapter we will trace the development of outcome measures that encompass the three perspectives of biomedicine, patients, and the Chinese medicine theoretical model. We will describe how qualitative methods have been used to develop patient-centred outcome agendas and tools for research into acupuncture and Chinese medicine. This research highlights the wide range of possible treatment effects; the importance of recognising treatment as a dynamic process that will result in different effects over many months or years of treatment; the importance of individual aims and outcomes; and the particular difficulties posed by evaluating the use of acupuncture to maintain health in chronic or progressive conditions. We will start, however, with a brief section on terminology.

OUTCOME MEASURES, PSYCHOMETRICS, AND ALL THAT JAZZ

The term 'outcome measure' or 'outcome tool' encompasses all the different questionnaires and instruments that are used to measure the effects of treatment. The term 'tool', or 'instrument', is useful because it reminds us that just as an instrument like a thermometer has to be designed and tested to be accurate and reliable, so questionnaires should be designed and tested to make them valid, reliable and sensitive

> **Box 5.1** Psychometric testing (Fitzpatrick et al 1998)
>
> Eight criteria that investigators should have in mind when they select a patient-based outcome measure for use in a clinical trial.
>
> - Is the content of the instrument appropriate to the questions which the clinical trial is intended to address? (Appropriateness.)
> - Does the instrument produce results that are reproducible and internally consistent? (Reliability.)
> - Does the instrument measure what it claims to measure? (Validity.)
> - Does the instrument detect changes over time that matter to patients? (Responsiveness.)
> - How precise are the scores of the instrument? (Precision.)
> - How interpretable are the scores of the instrument? (Interpretability.)
> - Is the instrument acceptable to patients? (Acceptability.)
> - Is the instrument easy to use and to process? (Feasibility.)

to change. Developing a new outcome tool is consequently a big undertaking and, unless appropriate resources and skills are available, it is better to look for an 'off-the-shelf' model.

Outcome questionnaires, which may also be termed health-status, subjective-health, or quality-of-life measures, may be *generic* (spanning all aspects of health) or *problem specific*. The term 'psychometric testing' refers to the methods used to develop and test out an outcome questionnaire to ensure that it performs well and that it measures what we want it to measure (see Box 5.1). Traditionally these psychometric properties have been determined on the basis of quantitative statistical techniques, but more recently researchers have also started to interview respondents to discover what dimensions are of importance to them and how and why they make their responses to questionnaire items.

METHODS OF MEASURING PATIENT-CENTRED OUTCOMES

Shifting perspectives and the development of subjective health status questionnaires

Traditionally, over thousands of years, acupuncture and Chinese medicine have been researched and developed using case study methods. Although these methods include patients' symptoms and progress, they are primarily focused on the practitioners' interpretation of these changes and the practitioners' perspective. Subsequently, in the early 1970s, the advent of clinical trials in acupuncture heralded a period of biomedical dominance in research methods, including outcome measurement. In the world of clinical trials, acupuncture needling has often been investigated in just the same way as a drug, and outcomes were chosen according to medical diagnosis and biomedical perceptions. Trial design demanded a single primary outcome measure and initially priority was given to objective scientific measures, such as blood pressure and biochemical markers.

However many health problems, such as pain or anxiety, can only be evaluated by subjective states. The development of subjective health status questionnaires, and their increasing use in the evaluation of people's response to treatment, gives patients a voice in the measuring process. This is especially important for people with chronic disease for whom treatment rarely aims at cure, and where such aims as improvement in well-being, function and 'quality of life' may mean different things to different people. These considerations are also particularly relevant to acupuncture, because the individualised nature of the treatment focuses on the concerns of that individual rather than on standard outcomes for any one diagnosis or condition. The term 'subjective health' also implies that patients, rather than health professionals or researchers, measure their own function and feelings. This has become the norm since research with cancer patients (Slevin et al 1988) and with outpatients (Hall et al 1976, Orth-Gomer et al 1979) showed that doctors, carers and patients will make different assessments of both the outcome of specific therapies and of general 'quality of life'.

In the last 10 years there has been an explosion of interest in developing and using such subjective health questionnaires in research and clinical practice. However, surprisingly little is known about the extent to which these subjective health questionnaires actually do encompass the aims, values and benefits prioritised by patients (Carr & Higginson 2001, Gill & Feinstein 1994). Most of them were developed on the basis of the knowledge of medical experts and the literature, rather than from patients themselves. The recent move towards using qualitative methods in the development of questionnaires is a big step forward (McColl et al 2003) but many of the standard subjective health measures, such as the SF-36 (Garratt et al 1993) were not developed in this way. Consequently although patients are required to respond to the questions, the questions themselves may not prioritise the issues that are important to patients. In this respect many subjective measures are not properly patient centred.

One strategy to make outcome measures more patient centred has been the development of individualised outcome tools. These individualised measures require respondents to identify the main problem and the ways in which it affects their lives, before scoring these items for severity. In this respect they differ from other subjective health measures where the questionnaire items are already defined and the patient is only asked to score the severity. (See Box 5.2 for some examples of individualised questionnaires.) All these individualised questionnaires are interviewer administered, at least on the first occasion, and only the Measure Yourself Medical Outcome Profile (MYMOP) has been developed and validated for acupuncture patients.

> **Box 5.2** Individualised outcome measures (Chapman et al 2001, Guyatt et al 1987, Hickey et al 1996, Paterson 1996, Paterson & Britten 2000, 2003, Ruta et al 1999, Tugwell et al 1987)
>
> - The Schedule for the Evaluation of Individual Quality of Life (SEIQoL) (Hickey et al 1996) and the Patient-Generated Index (PGI) (Ruta et al 1999) both involve a three-stage process in which the respondents are required to nominate those aspects of life which they feel are most important, to rate how badly affected they are in each of these areas, and to value improvements in each area. SEIQoL encompasses all aspects of life, whereas the PGI is focused on health. Their main disadvantage remains their length and complexity.
> - Disease-specific individualised measures include MACTAR, a measure of functional impairment in rheumatoid arthritis (Tugwell et al 1987), and a number of questionnaires which include individualised sections within a pre-set questionnaire, such as that developed for people with chronic lung disease (Guyatt et al 1987).
> - MYMOP is a brief problem-specific questionnaire that has been shown to be reliable and highly responsive amongst general and complementary practitioner patients and subsequently has been used in a number of other evaluations (Chapman et al 2001, Paterson 1996). Two qualitative evaluations in acupuncture patients have demonstrated that although it enables most individuals to specify and measure changes in what is most important to them it fails to encompass some of the more subtle and longer-term changes associated with acupuncture treatment, such as changes in personal and social identity (Paterson & Britten 2000, 2003). It may be supplemented with other questionnaires (see Box 5.4).

Despite these attempts to make outcome measures more patient cen-tred, it remains the case that these questionnaires are generally developed in order to evaluate biomedical interventions, such as a new drug. Consequently they do not necessarily include, or prioritise, all the effects of complex and holistic interventions such as acupuncture. Whilst many acupuncture patients do value changes in presenting symptoms and bio-medically defined functions, these changes are often only one aspect of the total effect of acupuncture. Unless the whole range of patient-centred outcomes is measured, the unique contribution made by acupuncture and other holistic interventions may not be fully evaluated. In the next section we will describe some of the research that has sought to understand and categorise some of the other treatment effects perceived by people receiv-ing acupuncture for long-term conditions. These wider, 'whole-person' changes are likely to be experienced by patients receiving other complex interventions for long-term health problems, and in this respect acupunc-ture research may be useful to researchers in other disciplines.

What treatment effects do acupuncture patients experience and value?

In order to make outcome measures more relevant to evaluating the full effects of acupuncture and Chinese medicine, we need to understand in more detail what treatment effects are experienced and valued by acupuncture patients. Traditionally medical research has chosen outcome measures according to the disease that is being treated. However, from the perspective of acupuncture practitioners there are additional treatment effects from acupuncture treatment that may be experienced by patients with any chronic illness. These additional, whole-person effects relate to the holistic perspective of acupuncture, and the underlying Chinese medicine therapeutic theory. A number of qualitative studies have sought to explore the patient's perspective on treatment effects and to investigate whether these postulated whole-person effects of acupuncture are evident to the person being treated.

In 1995 Cassidy analysed both structured questionnaire responses and 'handwritten stories' from 460 users of acupuncture/Chinese medicine in several centres in the USA (Cassidy 1998). These respondents experienced and valued acupuncture as holistic care. In addition to valuing relief of presenting complaints, these users described other 'expanded effects of care', which were categorised as improvements in *physiological coping* (such as increases in energy, increases in relaxation and calmness, reduction in reliance on prescription drugs, reduction in the frequency of 'colds', and quicker healing, as from surgery) and improvements in *psychosocial coping* (such as increases in self-awareness, an increased sense of wholeness, balance, centredness, well-being, increases in self-efficacy and all-round changes in lives). In addition respondents reported enjoying a close relationship with their practitioner, learning new things, and feeling more able to guide their own lives and care for themselves.

A few years later a smaller study in York in the UK, which combined a similar questionnaire with interviews with 11 long-term acupuncture patients, came to comparable conclusions (Gould & MacPherson 2001). Questionnaire responses indicated that 75% of respondents had noticed changes in physical symptoms, 67% in emotional and mental symptoms, 54% in inner life changes (outlook and attitude to health), 40% in lifestyle behaviour and 27% had experienced major life changes. Nearly half the patients had changed their focus of acupuncture treatment over time, often to one of general health and well-being.

Building on the results of these two earlier studies, a longitudinal study in 2001 included both private and NHS-funded patients, and interviewed a consecutive sample of 23 people with chronic illness, who were having acupuncture for the first time (Paterson & Britten 2003, 2004). Each person was interviewed three times over 6 months. The analysis, using a method based on grounded theory, sought to describe the treatment effects in more conceptual terms and to describe their emergence over time. People described their experience of acupuncture in terms of the acupuncturist's diagnostic and needling skills; the therapeutic relationship;

and a new understanding of the body and self as a whole being. All three of these components were imbued with holistic ideology. Treatment effects were perceived as changes in symptoms and medication; changes in energy and relaxation; and changes in self-concept (self-awareness, self-confidence, self-efficacy, self-responsibility and self-help). This qualitative study, and others like it, was also used to develop a set of outcome questionnaires that were capable of encompassing the whole range of perceived treatment effects. A summary of a vignette from one of these studies is provided in Box 5.3. It demonstrates the outcomes that were important to a patient, and those identified by her acupuncturist. The outcomes were complex and emerged over time.

Two other qualitative studies that explored the experience of patients with chronic cystitis (Alraek & Baerheim 2001) and side effects from breast cancer treatment (Walker et al 2004) also reported benefits wider than symptomatic improvement. These included more energy and relaxation, improved coping, and valuing the process of treatment and the therapeutic relationship.

In summary this portfolio of studies confirms the existence of 'whole-person' treatment effects that include physical, emotional and social components, and also highlights the importance of the process of care

Box 5.3   A qualitative vignette

Jenny was constantly exhausted, panicky, and not sleeping. She had taken antidepressants in the past but thought that they had suppressed things rather than helped her to make changes for herself and sort out what was really going on in her life. Jenny enjoyed her acupuncture because it gave her the opportunity to talk about everything that was going on in her life and it treated her holistically. The ideas of the elements and balance made 'poetic sense' to her and she learnt a number of self-help strategies such as meditation. After the first acupuncture treatment she felt relaxed and her sleep improved, but this improvement was short-lived. Gradually the effects lasted longer and after 10 weeks of treatment she was sleeping better and feeling really up-beat. She had a week off work and was 'able to give myself some space, to leave the washing up and sit and read the paper, and to start to remember what it feels like to be who I am'. Her acupuncturist Belinda noted that 'she's become more relaxed, more confident and taking action on her issues. Her eyes are more sparkly, her face is more animated and she does talk about the future'. Belinda's diagnosis and treatment strategy had remained constant and it guided both her needling and the strategies she used to promote and reinforce cognitive changes. She was treating Spleen deficiency, which she thought was largely a result of Jenny being brought up with worry and anxiety, and the associated effects on the Kidney and the Shen, or spirit. Clinically, Belinda was pleased with Jenny's progress and aimed to continue monthly treatments in order to maintain health and reinforce Jenny's new insights and cognitive changes.

and the therapeutic relationship. One challenge for the future is to synthesise these results more coherently and at a more conceptual level and to relate them to similar studies of other holistic interventions (Andrews 2002, Luff & Thomas 2000, Pawluch et al 2000, Verhoef et al 2005b).

The development of outcome tools for acupuncture and holistic therapies

Developing outcome tools that are specifically designed for measuring the spectrum of effects of acupuncture is being pursued from a number of different perspectives. These include patient-centred perspectives, building on the knowledge outlined in the previous section; practitioner perspectives, building on the theory base of Chinese medicine; and the wider perspective of holistic care.

PATIENT-CENTRED PERSPECTIVES

One programme of work on patient-centred outcome questionnaires for acupuncture has been integral to some of the qualitative work outlined above. Starting with the development and validation of the MYMOP questionnaire (see Box 5.2) this programme aims to develop a set of patient-centred questionnaires that encompass the changes in symptoms and medication; energy and relaxation; and self-concept (self-awareness, self-confidence and self-responsibility). A series of studies has tested out a number of generic questionnaires (Paterson 1996) and has also focused on methods of measuring changes in medication (Paterson et al 2003), well-being, and self-concept (Paterson 2006). This work has resulted in a set of patient-centred outcome tools for acupuncture and Chinese medicine (SPOT-ACM), which is currently being validated as a set in a quantitative study. The questionnaires that make up this set are listed in Box 5.4.

Box 5.4 A set of patient-centred outcome tools for acupuncture and Chinese medicine (SPOT-ACM)

A set of questionnaires to measure changes in: symptoms and medication; energy and relaxation; and changes in self-concept (self-awareness, self-confidence, self-responsibility and self-help).

- Measure Yourself Medical Outcome Profile with additional open question (MYMOP-qual) (Paterson & Britten 2000).
- Medication Change Questionnaire (Paterson et al 2004).
- Wellbeing questionnaire (W-BQ12) (Bradley 2000, Paterson 2006).
- Patient Enablement Index (PEI) (Howie et al 1998, Paterson 2006).
- (For economic evaluations) SF-6D (Brazier et al 2002) or EQ-5D (Brooks 1996).
- (Optional) problem-specific questionnaire.

PRACTITIONER PERSPECTIVES

Researchers in Hong Kong and China have worked from the perspective of the principles of diagnosis and practice in Chinese medicine to develop a Chinese quality of life instrument (ChQoL) (Leung et al 2005). The questionnaire has been developed and tested according to standard psychometric procedures and has been shown to have internal consistency, construct validity and good reproducibility. Its responsiveness to change remains to be demonstrated. It is available in Chinese, with a 'tentative' English translation, and consists of 50 items each scored on a five-point scale. There are three domains, each with four or five facets: the Physical Form domain (complexion, sleep, stamina, appetite and digestion, climate adjustment); Spirit domain (consciousness, thinking, spirit of eye, verbal expression); and Emotion domain (joy, anger, depressed mood, fear).

THE WIDER PERSPECTIVE OF HOLISTIC CARE

A number of other researchers have worked from the perspective of measuring holistic or integrative care. In as much as acupuncture is likely to form a part of truly integrative care packages, this emergent body of work is important. A whole systems approach to evaluating integrative care promotes combining qualitative and quantitative methods and developing tools that relate to the emphasis on wellness and healing of the whole person (Bell et al 2002, Mulkins & Verhoef 2006, Ritenbaugh et al 2003). In addition to objective parameters, symptoms, and well-being/quality of life, these authors seek to encompass dimensions such as: movement towards wholeness; personal transformation; enhanced relationships or feeling connected; 'unstuckness'; goal attainment; satisfaction; and enablement. More research is needed to evaluate to what extent these dimensions can be measured by validated questionnaires, such as those listed in Box 5.4.

There are a number of outcome tools that focus on holism that are still at an early stage of development. For example, the Arizona Integrative Outcomes Scale is a single VAS scale which assesses self-rated global sense of spiritual, social, mental, emotional and physical well-being, and there is some evidence of validity and responsiveness to change (Bell et al 2004). Another questionnaire, the Holistic Practice Questionnaire (Long et al 2000), has items covering health and healing, the user–practitioner relationship and user beliefs and expectations. The same researcher (Long) has also piloted a 'You and your Therapy' questionnaire that has 10 items covering changes in well-being, self-confidence and self-efficacy, relationships and presenting problem. Neither of these questionnaires is yet available in a validated form. Finally there are questionnaires that focus on the process, rather than the outcome of care, such as the CARE questionnaire that measures empathy (Mercer

2002) and has been used in acupuncture research (MacPherson et al 2003, Price et al 1996).

CHALLENGES AND POTENTIAL APPROACHES

We have illustrated the considerable body of work that now exists about the range of outcomes that are important to patients and practitioners and how they should be measured. However this emergent work is still not widely appreciated and it requires more synthesis and dissemination, so that it can be used in future evaluations of acupuncture and thereby developed further. In addition there are a number of challenges, both conceptual and practical, that require a multidisciplinary approach and innovative solutions. All of this work is urgent, as sensitive and appropriate outcome measurement is a prerequisite for high-quality evaluation of acupuncture, whether this uses descriptive or experimental designs.

Synthesising current evidence

The studies described in the section entitled 'What treatment effects do acupuncture patients experience and value?' that have investigated the outcomes experienced and valued by acupuncture patients, appear to report similar results. However the authors have each described the outcomes using different categories and terminology. This work could be moved forward by carrying out a high-quality synthesis of the findings. One approach to synthesising the results of qualitative studies is the meta-ethnographic method. This method has been shown to result in a higher degree of insight and conceptual development than is likely to be achieved by a narrative literature review (Campbell et al 2003). The synthesised categories or dimensions of patient-centred outcomes which such a study would aim to produce, would bring clarity to the development of appropriate outcome measures. They would also facilitate the construction of frameworks or models that link patient-centred outcomes with outcomes from a biomedical or East Asian medicine perspective.

Clarity on the dimensions of the outcomes of acupuncture and Chinese medicine would also promote work on the extent to which these are similar or different from outcomes of other holistic therapies, such as naturopathy and homeopathy, and to integrative packages of care. In addition to carrying out more primary research in this area, a further synthesis could be attempted between the acupuncture outcome studies and those studies describing other CAM/integrative outcomes, of which these are only a selection (Long 2003, Miller et al 2003).

Synthesising current evidence will also help identify the gaps where more research is required. For example, little work has been done on whether different outcomes are important for different socioeconomic and cultural groups. Another area where new research and thinking is required is on how to evaluate treatment effects valued by people with long-term progressive conditions. Here a desire for symptom relief may be matched by an appreciation of the process of care, including support, and hope, and slowing of the rate of deterioration of function and well-being. A third relatively neglected area is conceptualising and measuring acupuncture outcomes related to health maintenance and health promotion, which is a particular challenge when it is in the context of a chronic illness: so-called 'health within illness' (Lindsey 1996).

Incorporating patient-centred outcomes in clinical trials and economic studies

If we are postulating that acupuncture outcomes are individualised and wide ranging, this raises problems in trial research where only one or two predetermined primary outcomes are required. If, for example, the set of outcome questionnaires listed in Box 5.4 as SPOT-ACM, are all required in order to encompass the outcomes that are important to all the individuals in the trial, then it makes no sense to choose just one of them as a primary outcome measure. There are various approaches to this problem. It may be possible to produce some summary measure from such a set of questionnaires, or it may be preferable to use methods such as participant-centred analysis (Aickin 2003). We need to develop methods which are consistent with the aims and philosophical basis of acupuncture, and are also acceptable to evidence-based medicine experts that work within the biomedical tradition.

Economic studies pose extra problems when researching therapies such as acupuncture that promote individualised, wide-ranging, and long-term changes in health. Classic cost-effectiveness studies use utility outcome measures such as SF-6D or EuroQol (see Box 5.4) which do not encompass outcome dimensions such as changes in self-concept or coherence and are therefore likely to underestimate the cost-effectiveness of acupuncture (and other interventions that are associated with more than symptomatic and functional change). Such studies may also fail to measure the full impact of these wider changes because the changes may take place over an extended period of time and may affect health costs for many years in the future. There is mounting evidence that the relative benefits of acupuncture may increase over 1 or 2 years of follow-up (Ratcliffe et al 2006, Witt et al 2006, Wonderling et al 2004) and economic modelling strategies may be required to assess the economic effect of such changes over 10 or 20 years. It has also been suggested that the use of cost-consequence studies (where all the costs and the outcomes are measured and presented out in a table), rather than cost-effectiveness studies, may allow for a wider variety of outcomes and be more useful for decision-makers (Coast 2004).

Acupuncture as a complex intervention or whole system: relationships between outcome and process 'components'

This chapter has taken a conventional approach to the dimensions of *outcomes*, largely defining them as changes that persist beyond the consultation (such as reduced pain, more energy, better self-esteem etc.) and as separate to the valued aspects of the *process* of care (such as being recognised, supported, touched, experiencing empathy and enablement and making new meaning). This categorisation into process and outcome, whilst helpful in the context of developing outcome measures for use in clinical trials, does not mirror the interview data in the qualitative studies quoted above, in which patients talked of benefits in ways that didn't distinguish process and outcome. Consequently it is important to understand the links and feedback loops between different aspects of process and outcome, and to improve on early models of such interactions. One such model has highlighted, in addition to 'diagnostic and needling skills', the process factors of the 'therapeutic relationship' and 'new holistic understandings' (Paterson & Britten 2004). To this may be added the physical body experiences/embodied experience of acupuncture and the practitioner's intention, both of which are central to the Chinese medicine explanatory model.

Widening the focus to understand the relationship between the process factors and outcome may be particularly important for research that aims to improve the practice of acupuncture. An example of such research is the excellent work by Mercer and colleagues, which has measured empathy with the CARE questionnaire, and investigated linkages between empathy, enablement and clinical outcomes (MacPherson et al 2003, Mercer 2002, Price et al 1996). In considering aspects of outcome and process, researchers must guard against making implicit judgements about certain aspects of outcome, such as improved function, being more important than aspects of process, such as 'feeling heard'. Further research is required to understand how different patient populations value these different factors. Many of these issues are not specific to acupuncture, but may be an area where acupuncture research will make important contributions to methods of researching complex interventions (Campbell et al 2000) and whole systems research (Verhoef et al 2005a).

Integrating multiple perspectives on outcome

In this chapter we have argued that acupuncture should be evaluated on the basis of whether it improves people's health in ways that are important to individual patients. We have emphasised patient-centred outcomes and an individualised approach because this is in keeping with the underlying philosophy of East Asian medicine, but we have also acknowledged the importance of other perspectives on outcome. Box 5.5, a four-dimensional approach to the study of East Asian medicine,

---

Box 5.5 A four-dimensional approach to the study of East Asian medicine

1. An analysis of the complex intervention intact, which captures the impact of the intervention on the person as a whole system, and the short- and long-term benefit of the intervention. Outcome measures would take a patient-centred perspective and might include a range of subjective health questionnaires, individualised questionnaires and qualitative methods.
2. An analysis of the components of the intervention to capture the treatment effects as:
   a. changes in endogenous biological processes in specific subsystems and;
   b. changes in affective states and neuropsychological functioning (memory and cognition).
   Outcome measures might include conventional biomarkers, biomechanical evaluations and standardised questionnaires of psychological states or traits.
3. A *Qi*-based analysis to validate the East Asian medicine framework and correlate East Asian medicine constructs of illness and health with both biomedical and whole system concepts. Outcome measures would take a *Qi*-based perspective and might include questionnaires developed on that basis.
4. A healthcare utilisation analysis that evaluates the social and economic impact of the integration of East Asian medicine into the customary healthcare for particular patients or patient groups. Outcome measures might include health utility scales such as EuroQol, changes in healthcare utilisation such as conventional medication and hospital-based costs, and societal costs such as days off work.

---

illustrates how multiple perspectives may be integrated into a research model. Each approach would involve measuring outcomes from a different perspective, and more than one approach could be included in any one project.

SUMMARY

Measuring outcomes from the patient's perspective is especially important in acupuncture research, because acupuncture is an individualised and participative therapy which can engender broader changes beyond a single condition. Prioritising the patient's perspective does not, however, mean that other perspectives on outcome should be neglected. Patient-centred outcomes can be part of a multivariate set of outcomes that include biomedically defined outcomes, outcomes based on an East Asian Medicine theoretical model, and health economic measures. The substantial body of knowledge on the range of treatment effects experienced and valued by people receiving acupuncture is largely the result of qualitative and mixed method studies. This work forms the basis of a range of outcome questionnaires that are currently being developed or validated for use in research into acupuncture and other holistic therapies. Synthesis of the qualitative research findings would provide an even firmer basis for the further development of appropriate outcome questionnaires and for their use within the context of clinical trials. It would also facilitate comparisons between the range of outcomes that are experienced with acupuncture and those experienced with other holistic therapies and integrative packages of care. Evaluating aspects of the process of care alongside more sustainable outcomes helps our understanding of the complexity of the acupuncture consultation, feeding into both research trial design and improving the teaching and practice of acupuncture.

Research resources

Bowling A 2001 Measuring disease: a review of disease-specific quality of life measurement scales, 2nd edn. Open University Press, Buckingham

Bowling A 2005 Measuring health: a review of quality of life measurement scales, 3rd edn. Open University Press, Buckingham

Canadian Interdisciplinary Network for Complementary & Alternative Medicine Research. [Online] Available: www.incamresearch.ca

Fitzpatrick R, Davey C, Buxton M J et al 1998 Evaluating patient-based outcome measures for use in clinical trials. 2(14) Health Technology Assessment [Online] Available: http://www.ncchta.org

Measure Yourself Medical Outcome Profile (MYMOP) [Online] Available: www.hsrc.ac.uk/mymop

Streiner D L, Norman G R 2003 Health measurement scales. A practical guide to their development, 3rd edn. Oxford University Press, New York

References

Aickin M 2003 Participant-centered analysis in complementary and alternative medicine comparative trials. Journal of Alternative and Complementary Medicine 9(6):949–957

Alraek T, Baerheim A 2001 'An empty and happy feeling in the bladder...': health changes experienced by women after acupuncture for recurrent cystitis. Complementary Therapies in Medicine 9:219–223

Andrews G J 2002 Private complementary medicine and older people: service use and empowerment. Ageing and Society 22(3):343–368

Bell I R, Caspi O, Schwartz G E R et al 2002 Integrative medicine and systemic outcomes research. Archives of Internal Medicine 162:133–140

Bell I R, Cunningham V, Caspi O et al 2004 Development and validation of a new global well-being outcomes rating scale for integrative medicine research. BMC Complementary and Alternative Medicine 4(1) [Online] Available: http://www.biomedcentral.com/1472-6882/4/1

Bradley C 2000 The 12-item well-being questionnaire. Origins, current stage of development, and availability. Diabetes Care 23:875

Brazier J, Roberts J, Deverill M 2002 The estimation of a preference based measure of health from the SF-36. Journal of Health Economics 21:271–292

Brooks R 1996 The EuroQol group. EuroQol: the current state of play. Health Policy 37:53–72

Campbell M, Fitzpatrick R, Haines A et al 2000 Framework for design and evaluation of complex interventions to improve health. British Medical Journal 321:694–696

Campbell R, Pound P, Pope C et al 2003 Evaluating meta-ethnography: a synthesis of qualitative research on lay experiences of diabetes and diabetes care. Social Science & Medicine 55(4):671–684

Carr A J, Higginson I J 2001 Are quality of life measures patient centred? British Medical Journal 322:1357–1360

Cassidy C 1998 Chinese medicine users in the United States. Part II: preferred aspects of care. Journal of Alternative and Complementary Medicine 4(2):189–202

Chapman R, Norton R, Paterson C 2001 A descriptive outcome study of 291 acupuncture patients. The European Journal of Oriental Medicine September:48–53

Coast J 2004 Is economic evaluation in touch with society's health values? British Medical Journal 329:1233–1236

Fitzpatrick R, Davey C, Buxton MJ et al 1998 Evaluating patient-based outcome measures for use in clinical trials. 2(14) Health Technology Assessment [Online] Available: http://www.ncchta.org

Garratt A, Ruta D, Abdulla M I 1993 The SF-36 health survey questionnaire: an outcome measure suitable for routine use in the NHS? British Medical Journal 306:1440–1444

Gill T M, Feinstein A R 1994 A critical appraisal of the quality of quality-of-life measurements. Journal of the American Medical Association 272:619–626

Gould A, MacPherson H 2001 Patient perspectives on outcomes after treatment with acupuncture. Journal of Alternative and Complementary Medicine 7:261–268

Guyatt G H, Berman L B, Townsend M et al 1987 A measure of quality of life for clinical trials in chronic lung disease. Thorax 42:773–778

Hall R, Horrocks J C, Clamp S E 1976 Observer variation in assessment of results of surgery for peptic ulceration. British Medical Journal 1: 814–816

Hickey A, Bury G, O'Boyle C A et al 1996 A new short form individual quality of life measure (SEIQoL-DW): application in a cohort of individuals with HIV/AIDS. British Medical Journal 313:29–33

Howie J G R, Heaney D J, Maxwell M et al 1998 A comparison of the Patient Enablement Instrument (PEI) against two established satisfaction scales as an outcome measure of primary care consultations. Family Practice 15:165–171

Leung K, Liu F, Zhao L et al 2005 Development and validation of the Chinese quality of life instrument. Health and Quality of Life Outcomes 3:26

Lindsey E 1996 Health within illness: experiences of chronically ill/disabled people. Journal of Advanced Nursing 24:465–472

Long A F 2003 Outcome measurement in complementary and alternative medicine: unpicking the effects. Journal of Alternative and Complementary Medicine 8(6):777–786

Long A F, Mercer G, Hughes K 2000 Developing a tool to measure holistic practice: a missing dimension in outcomes measurement within complementary therapies. Complementary Therapies in Medicine 8:26–31

Luff D, Thomas K J 2000 'Getting somewhere', feeling cared for: patients' perspectives on complementary therapies in the NHS. Complementary Therapies in Medicine 8:253–259

MacPherson H, Mercer S W, Scullion T 2003 Empathy, enablement and outcome: an exploratory study on acupuncture patients' perceptions. Journal of Alternative and Complementary Medicine 9(6):869–876

McColl E, Meadows K, Barofsky I 2003 Cognitive aspects of survey methodology and quality of life assessment. Quality of Life Research 12:217–218

Mercer S W 2002 Empathy and quality of care. British Journal of General Practice 52(suppl):S9–S12

Miller W L, Crabtree B F, Duffy M B et al 2003 Research guidelines for assessing the impact of healing relationships in clinical medicine. Alternative Therapies in Health & Medicine 9(suppl 3):80A–95A

Mulkins A, Verhoef M 2006 Supporting the transformative process: experiences of cancer patients receiving integrative care. Integrative Cancer Therapies 3(3):230–237

Orth-Gomer K, Britton M, Rehnqvist N 1979 Quality of care in an outpatient department: the patients' view. Social Science & Medicine 13A:347–350

Paterson C 1996 Measuring outcome in primary care: a patient-generated measure, MYMOP, compared to the SF-36 health survey. British Medical Journal 312:1016–1020 Available: http://www.hsrc.ac.uk/mymop

Paterson C 2004 Seeking the patient's perspective: a qualitative assessment of EurQol, COOP-WONCA charts and MYMOP. Quality of Life Research 13:871–881

Paterson C 2006 Measuring changes in self-concept: a qualitative evaluation of outcome questionnaires in people having acupuncture for their chronic health problems. BMC Complementary and Alternative Medicine 6:7

Paterson C, Britten N 2000 In pursuit of patient-centred outcomes: a qualitative evaluation of MYMOP, Measure Yourself Medical Outcome Profile. Journal of Health Services Research Policy 5:27–36

Paterson C, Britten N 2003 Acupuncture for people with chronic illness: combining qualitative and quantitative outcome assessment. Journal of Alternative and Complementary Medicine 5(9):671–681

Paterson C, Britten N 2004 Acupuncture as a complex intervention: a holistic model. Journal of Alternative and Complementary Medicine 10:791–801

Paterson C, Symons L, Britten N 2003 Medication change as an outcome: developing the Medication Change Questionnaire. FACT Focus on Alternative and Complementary Therapies 8(4):526

Paterson C, Symons L, Britten N et al 2004 Developing the medication change questionnaire. Journal of Clinical Pharmacy and Therapeutics 29:339–349

Pawluch D, Cain R, Gillett J 2000 Lay constructions of HIV and complementary therapy use. Social Science & Medicine 51:251–264

Price S, Mercer S W, MacPherson H 1996 Practitioner empathy, patient enablement and health outcomes: a prospective study of acupuncture patients. Patient Education and Counseling 63:239–245

Ratcliffe J, Thomas K J, MacPherson H et al 2006 A randomised controlled trial of acupuncture care for persistent low back pain: cost effectiveness analysis. British Medical Journal 333:626–629

Ritenbaugh C, Verhoef M J, Fleishman S et al 2003 Whole systems research: a discipline for studying complementary and alternative medicine. Alternative Therapies in Health & Medicine 9(4):32–36

Ruta D, Garratt A, Russell I T 1999 Patient centred assessment of quality of life for patients with four common conditions. Quality in Health Care 8:22–29

Slevin M L, Plant H, Lynch D et al 1988 Who should measure quality of life, the doctor or the patient? British Journal of Cancer 57:109–112

Tugwell P, Bombardier C, Buchanan W W et al 1987 The MACTAR Patient Preference Disability Questionnaire – an individualised, functional priority approach for assessing improvement in physical disability in clinical trials in rheumatoid arthritis. Journal of Rheumatology 14:446–451

Verhoef M J, Lewith G, Ritenbaugh C et al 2005a Complementary and alternative medicine whole systems research: beyond identification of inadequacies of the RCT. Complementary Therapies in Medicine 13:206–212

Verhoef M J, Mulkins A, Boon H 2005b Integrative health care: how can we determine whether patients benefit? Journal of Alternative and Complementary Medicine 11(suppl 1):S-57–S-65

Walker G, de Valois B, Young T et al 2004 The experience of receiving traditional Chinese acupuncture. The European Journal of Oriental Medicine 4(5):59–65

Witt C, Liecker B, Linde K 2006 Pragmatic randomized trial evaluating the clinical and economic effectiveness of acupuncture for chronic low back pain. American Journal of Epidemiology 164:487–496

Wonderling D, Vickers A J, Grieve R et al 2004 Cost effectiveness analysis of a randomised trial of acupuncture for chronic headache in primary care. British Medical Journal 328:747

Exploring treatment effects: studies without control groups

6

Adrian White, Peter Wayne and Hugh MacPherson

INTRODUCTION

This chapter is the first in a series of three which look at the ways in which we can investigate the 'effectiveness' of treatment with acupuncture. By the term 'effectiveness', in this context, we mean the health benefits that patients experience after acupuncture treatment. This chapter describes the first steps in this process, namely the various types of research study that are uncontrolled, and known as 'non-experimental'. Studies without control groups describe the effects of acupuncture in normal clinical practice, and are non-experimental: there is no attempt to interfere with normal practice, or to compare the effect of acupuncture with anything else. First, we should briefly revisit the reasoning behind different types of study design, and the conclusions that we can make from different types of study.

A useful distinction can be made between a clinician's way of thinking, and a scientist's way of thinking, which are often quite different. An acupuncturist is often surrounded by grateful patients every day, and neither patient nor practitioner has any difficulty in accepting that acupuncture is an effective treatment. But, to a scientist, the reports of grateful patients are not, in themselves, proof that acupuncture is itself effective: the patients could, in theory, have improved spontaneously — many medical conditions fluctuate quite dramatically, and patients may seek acupuncture treatment at the time when they have their worst symptoms so will inevitably improve whatever treatment they have (what scientists would call 'regression to the mean' or natural history of course of a disease). In theory, they might not have been helped by acupuncture at all. It is tempting to argue that finding more and more reports is stronger evidence — in other words, that describing 100 patients who have improved with acupuncture is evidence that it must be effective. Unfortunately not: the scientist argues that all of them could have started treatment at a time of worst symptoms, so they would all have inevitably improved (even without treatment).

A scientist might also want to find out about the effectiveness of different components of the acupuncture treatment — the consultation, the diagnosis, the interaction with the therapist, the points needled, the needle stimulation and so on. The clinician is much less likely to worry about 'which part worked', as long as the patient is better. Acupuncturists should be reassured that scientists are not picking on them alone in asking this kind of question! It is simply the way that scientific enquiry takes place, and it is one particular way to investigate the natural world and establish our 'knowledge' of it.

Clinicians should not be surprised or offended when scientists describe them as 'biased' in favour of acupuncture. In truth, everyone in the world holds beliefs and expectations about many things, and everyone is in that sense 'biased' including medical scientists (Kaptchuk 2003). The problem with bias is that it can affect the way we make up our mind about these things: to take a simple example, acupuncturists might only remember and record the successes they have had with their treatment, and not the failures. This is known as 'selection bias'. However many clinicians might protest their innocence and integrity, the only way to convince a scientist is to organise things so that it is patently clear that every patient treated has been included, which usually means having someone else involved. This is the essence of rigorous research — it is research that attempts to identify and eliminate every way in which the result could be influenced by bias. Nobody is saying that it's wrong or dishonest to be biased: what is wrong is to draw conclusions about the effectiveness of treatment when the result could have been due to bias. This is the essence of the scientific method, which is recognised as a particularly powerful way of developing knowledge and understanding about the world.

We can build up evidence about the effectiveness of acupuncture from a series of studies, as summarised in Box 6.1. Clearly, anyone who is assessing the evidence should not accept it without considering whether it is biased. In this chapter we will be discussing a range of studies from initial observations, where attribution can be expected to be weak, through to pilot studies which help inform full-scale studies where attribution can be expected to be strong. In practice, evidence builds up piecemeal. It is worth noting that it is usually the practitioner that starts the whole process off with an observation; researchers then become increasingly involved with progression along the pathway.

The non-experimental studies that we describe here, i.e. the first three methods in Box 6.1, are important 1) because they add to the body of evidence and 2) because they point the way for other studies

> **Box 6.1**   Pathways for building an evidence base of treatment effects
>
> 1. Case report: clinical observation of an outcome in one patient given acupuncture: anecdote or case report.
> 2. Case series: repeated observations to confirm that there is an association between acupuncture and improvement. This also may help establish whether particular patients or treatments are associated with a good (or poor) outcome.
> 3. Qualitative study: an investigation of the experience of the acupuncture consultation, from perspectives of patient or acupuncturist. This can provide information on perceptions of patients, acceptability of treatment, factors associated with satisfaction, etc., all of which can help in making other studies more valid.
> 4. Controlled trial: a comparison between a group that receives acupuncture and a control group that receives usual care, some other treatment, or sham acupuncture. This is an experiment to test whether patients' improvement is really due to the acupuncture (see Chapters 7 and 8).

that will hopefully provide more conclusive evidence. High-quality, non-experimental studies should form the foundation and basis for more definitive 'experimental' studies.

Researchers cannot design a study 'out of the blue', they need to build on the experience and results of previous studies. So the need for good quality in all research cannot be emphasised too strongly, and means: 1) thinking carefully and critically about every aspect of the study, and discussing it with colleagues; 2) writing a protocol that will guide the study; 3) being clear and consistent in applying the protocol; and 4) reporting the study fully so that readers can know exactly what has been done and can replicate it if necessary.

All studies, including non-experimental studies, should be published in a journal where they can be accessed by other acupuncturists and researchers. This is not just a sign of good quality, but also an obligation to the participants who have contributed to the study, and to the acupuncture community as a contribution to the advance in knowledge. It is particularly important to report any mistakes that have been made, so that lessons can be learned by other people and precious time and resources can be saved.

One final introductory point might be helpful to readers who will be evaluating other people's studies and possibly planning their own. A triad of components is fundamental to any study:

- Patients: who were they, and why this group?
- Intervention: what precisely did the treatment consist of, and why?
- Measurement: how were changes in patients' conditions measured?

In addition, researchers will be interested in a fourth aspect of any study:

● Methods and procedures: how was the study actually performed, i.e. how was it developed, how were patients recruited and treated, and how were findings analysed?

The chapter starts by describing different types of non-experimental studies in general that have contributed to the evidence base of acupuncture, giving some examples, and then illustrates some 'pilot' studies that have explored particular questions that have arisen in the planning of a subsequent experimental study.

DESCRIPTION OF SOME NON-EXPERIMENTAL RESEARCH METHODS

The simplest project, and one that readers may not at first glance regard as a research project at all, is a *case report*. This is simply a description of a patient, the treatment he or she received, and the outcome, as described in Box 6.2. Usually, a chronological framework is used to describe a case history, i.e. presentation, examination findings, treatment given and the outcome. This is followed by a discussion which puts the case into context, for example describing other similar cases that have been published before. It might also describe the possible mechanism if that is relevant, and then summarise the learning point or any other reason why the author has gone to the trouble of writing the case report. Case reports can be very live and powerful because they are so full of personal detail, and can be used for illustrating points of diagnosis or treatment. It should be noted that the case study has had a central role in the development of the knowledge base of traditional Chinese medicine (Cullen 2001).

Box 6.2 A case report of a golfer with 'the yips' treated by acupuncture (Rosted 2005)

Rosted (2005) reported treating a patient with 'the yips', the nervous twitch suffered by golfers as they try to putt the ball, which often destroys a good round of golf. Rosted described the patient's background and occupation, how the condition had developed over about 2 years the acupuncture approach, and its (highly beneficial) effects which continued at follow-up 24 months later. In the discussion, Rosted gave more details of the background of the condition, and how other treatments are often unsatisfactory. Although of course this patient's response to treatment could be the result of expectation, it was sufficiently dramatic to encourage Rosted to plan a formal prospective case series, offering the treatment to members of local golf clubs at no cost, and planning the treatment and measurement schedules that he would use (Rosted 2005).

The events described in a case report could, of course, be unique to that patient and possibly due to other events in the patient's life that nobody recognises. Much more powerful evidence is a description of the same kind of outcome occurring repeatedly in similar patients. A *case series* is a description of patients (usually consecutive patients), who have a particular disorder and are treated in a similar manner, and their outcome after treatment. A rigorous case series should include all patients, not just those who responded (that would be selection bias), and should describe the assessment of symptoms both before and after treatment, as described in Chapter 5.

A case series illustrates an important general point — that by planning ahead, information can be collected that is comprehensive, and then checked for accuracy and missing data. This is the strength of a *prospective* study, and is greatly superior to collecting information by looking through the clinical records, or by asking the patient to try to remember — which are both *retrospective* methods (White & Ernst 2001). For example, it is much better to ask patients to score their pain on a scale before treatment and then again at the end (prospective), than to ask them after treatment to try to estimate their improvement (retrospective). Of course there are occasions when information can only be collected retrospectively, such as history preceding onset of musculoskeletal pain.

A *qualitative* study is a different kind of investigation, but is briefly described here because of its important contribution to knowledge about acupuncture. In contrast to the other studies in this section which are quantitative — they measure treatment effectiveness in numbers such as scores or ratings — a qualitative investigation explores treatment, perhaps using the patient's or the practitioner's own words or observing the process of treatment. The qualitative researcher is interested in the processes and experiences around treatment, such as what were the patients' expectations of treatment and their feelings afterwards. While studies of this kind are not usually regarded as strictly 'evidence of an effect', nevertheless they play a vital role in understanding acupuncture more deeply and guiding the design of other studies so that they reflect real events more accurately and measure the things that patients feel are important. Examples are given in Chapters 3 and 5 of qualitative studies that provided valuable information on the range of changes that patients noticed after treatment with acupuncture.

Returning to quantitative studies, the reader should be acquainted with the term 'cohort study', which is often confused with 'case series'. In a cohort study a group of people are identified who have something in common — for example, a new diagnosis of hepatitis C — and followed over time to see the outcome, without any treatment or other intervention. The term is not often appropriate for studying the outcome of treatment, for which 'case series' is usually correct. However, the term 'cohort' is often used incorrectly, including the title of our example in Box 6.3!

'Audit' is a word which has been used in different ways. The original use of the word 'audit' (derived from *audire* = to hear) was to describe

> **Box 6.3** A cohort series of patients with neck pain attending a hospital clinic (Blossfeldt 2004)
>
> Blossfeldt, working in a hospital-based pain clinic, was able to collect 172 patients with neck pain over a 6.5-year period. He arranged to follow them up prospectively, measuring pain at the beginning of treatment, and then a rating of improvement at the end of treatment, and 6 and 12 months later. Successful treatment was judged to be an improvement of at least 50% reduction in pain. Altogether 153 patients were evaluated, and 68% had a successful outcome at the end of treatment. Forty-nine per cent of those who completed treatment had maintained the benefit after 6 months, and 40% at 1 year. As might be expected in these patients with rather severe symptoms, the success rate was higher in patients with a short duration of pain (Blossfeldt 2004).

> **Box 6.4** An audit of outcomes in a single clinic (Grabowska et al 2003)
>
> An audit was carried out between May 1999 and April 2000 at a university-based acupuncture clinic. Two acupuncturists saw a total of 69 clients of whom three-quarters were female; just over a third were less than 29 years of age; two-thirds were below the age of 40; 67% of clients were Caucasian; a third smoked; and three-quarters currently consumed some alcohol. Most had no experience of using complementary and alternative medicine (CAM), therefore the service provided their first access to CAM. Of those attending a follow-up appointment, 43 (80%) reported feeling better, 10 the same, and 1 worse. No side effects were reported by 50 (73%) clients, but 4 reported minor side effects (1 bruising and 3 drowsiness). The process of carrying out the audit provided the opportunity for the practitioners to reflect on their clinical practice and improve service delivery (Grabowska et al 2003).

a financial investigation of a business, by examining the cash records and asking probing questions to decide whether the accounts were an honest record. This idea of *quality* is usually present in an audit. In a health context, the word is mainly used in a similar sense, to check whether clinical practice meets certain, agreed standards such as sending letters to referring physicians, or reporting of side effects (White 2004). If there are any shortcomings, these are then put right in an 'audit cycle' in which changes are put in place and another audit conducted after an agreed time. The term 'audit' is also used in a slightly different sense by some authors to describe a study in which they have measured (usually retrospectively) the outcomes on all patients attending a particular clinic. Their aim usually is not to measure whether the care has been of high quality, but to measure the outcome of patients (see Box 6.4 for an example).

Note the difference between a case series, a cohort and an audit: a case series includes patients with a particular condition who have a particular

> **Box 6.5** A cross-sectional survey of patients with their retrospective assessment of outcome (MacPherson et al 2003)
>
> An exploratory, retrospective survey of acupuncture patients' perceptions of practitioner empathy, patient enablement, and health outcome was conducted to investigate the associations between them. Questionnaires were distributed to 192 patients randomly selected from a population of 6348 who, several months previously, had participated in a survey of acupuncture safety, and had agreed to be contacted again. The main measures included patients' perceptions of their practitioners' empathy using the Consultation and Relational Empathy Measure, the Patient Enablement Instrument, and the Glasgow Homeopathic Hospital Outcome Scale (measuring change in main complaint and well-being). A total of 143 (74%) patients responded (27% men and 73% women) with an average age of 51 years. The majority of patients (71%) were in the middle of an ongoing course of treatment at the time of completing the questionnaires for this study. Patients' enablement was found to be significantly positively correlated with perception of their practitioners' empathy. Enablement in turn was strongly positively correlated with the outcome of both the main complaint and improved well-being (MacPherson et al 2003).

intervention; a cohort identifies patients with a particular condition or 'exposure' to some risk, from some database; and an audit generally includes patients who attend a particular clinic, and aims to improve some aspect of care.

Sometimes, 'surveys' are used to explore certain aspects of acupuncture treatment, but have an inherent weakness: surveys rely on people responding to a request for information, and there will usually be a proportion of people who do not respond. Those who do respond are likely to be biased in some way, for example by having a good effect of treatment, which can limit the conclusions that can be drawn. A 'cross-sectional' survey of patients or of clinics, for example, collects data from responders on one occasion, as shown in Box 6.5. In contrast, a 'longitudinal' survey collects data on more than one occasion, and therefore can start to investigate how much the different factors might have contributed to a particular outcome.

PILOT STUDIES, AND OTHER TYPES OF PRELIMINARY STUDY

A 'pilot study' is any study that is specifically designed as a forerunner of a more definitive study, for example a randomised controlled trial (RCT), to help develop and design it. Often, pilot studies mainly address the *feasibility* of the RCT, and so sometimes pilot studies are given the generic name 'feasibility studies'. Feasibility includes every aspect of the question: 'The way we have planned this trial, will it work out?'.

The most common reason that trials do not work out is that they fail to recruit enough patients: either the patients don't exist where you hoped to find them, or they have features which exclude them from the study, or they just do not want to join in. It is highly advisable to run a pilot study just to test the question of whether recruitment will be adequate. Many other problems can arise during a trial that might have been anticipated with a pilot study: participants may not be satisfied to be allocated to the control therapy so they drop out; they find they cannot attend every week for acupuncture treatment; they cannot answer the questionnaires, or perhaps move away from the district so cannot be contacted for follow-up.

A pilot study can also be used to test the feasibility of various procedures that make up the study: the details of recruitment, enrolment, and baseline evaluation of each participant, the roles of the various research staff such as coordinator or nurse, the processes of treatment and the control intervention, and the success of blinding. In the latter case the pilot study would need a control group, but it is not really experimental and will not produce definitive results in the way that the main RCT will.

Another piece of information that a pilot study may be designed to provide is the size of the treatment effect and its variability between patients. This important information is needed to calculate the number of participants that will be needed for the main study – the 'sample size calculation' – which is beyond the scope of this chapter. The information that is needed is the average change in symptoms after treatment, and the variability of that change between different patients. If this information is not already available from published case series, then the pilot study needs to be designed large enough to provide it.

In practice, of course, a pilot study will often be designed to explore several of these issues at once. For example, in one study described in Box 6.6, the researchers wanted to know whether the acupuncture treatment would be acceptable to patients and healthcare staff in the context of a hospital ward, and what was the size of the expected effect.

One big unknown in many published acupuncture studies is whether the acupuncture treatment that was given really was the best treatment for the patients. There is no point in testing an acupuncture treatment unless it is the best possible treatment for the particular group of patients. The fact that we often don't know what works best probably undermines the value of the present body of acupuncture research more than any other factor. Part of the difficulty arises from the differences in making reliable diagnosis, and a method of standardising the collection of information from patients is described in Box 6.7.

Another way of tackling the problem is by comparing the different techniques in similar patients, and one good example is shown in Box 6.8. Note that this is technically an experimental study, but is included in this chapter because of its exploratory role in acupuncture research.

Box 6.6 Establishing the acceptability of acupuncture in a new context (Vickers et al 2006)

Vickers and colleagues undertook a pilot study of acupuncture for postoperative pain after thoracotomy – a surgical procedure which is notorious for generating post-operative pain in the chest wall, which becomes a serious chronic problem in about 5% of patients. Before surgery, semi-permanent needles were inserted at points BL12 to BL19 and the point Wei Guan Xia Shu, and covered with the same occlusive dressing as was covering the indwelling epidural catheter. Additional needles were placed in ST36 and Shenmen ear point. The specific aims of the pilot study were to determine whether it was feasible to place needles so close to the surgical field, whether at least 75% of the patients found it acceptable and returned pain scores up to 30 days post-operatively, whether there were any side effects, what was the best outcome and time point, and to provide data for sample size calculations. The needles were replaced 3 or 4 days later, and removed after about 3 weeks. The needles were counted at various stages to see how well they were retained in the skin. In addition, the study provided data on the rate of patient accrual into the study. The pilot showed that the acupuncture was feasible and acceptable and the body pain index score showed the least variability and was therefore best for the main study. In addition, the authors calculated that the main study which would require 140 patients to show a difference between groups in numbers of patients with moderate or severe pain of 20% (Vickers et al 2006).

Box 6.7 Development of a Chinese medicine diagnostic assessment instrument – a Delphi study (Schnyer et al 2005)

Diagnosis in traditional Chinese medicine uses information from the context and qualitative nature of a patient's illness. These researchers wanted to standardise the process of collecting and using this information, to potentially improve the reliability of diagnosis in clinical trials of acupuncture. The questionnaire needed to be consistent with accepted Chinese medicine diagnostic categories and to include the full range of each concept's meaning. A panel of TCM expert clinicians was convened and their responses were organised using the Delphi process – an iterative, anonymous, idea-generating and consensus-building process. Over three rounds of iteration, the TEAMSI-TCM (Traditional East Asian Medicine Structured Interview, TCM version) was developed. This was specifically designed to assess women, with a focus on gynaecological conditions; with modifications it can be adapted for use with other populations and conditions. TEAMSI-TCM is a prescriptive instrument that guides clinicians to use the proper indicators, combine them in a systematic manner, and generate conclusions. In conjunction with treatment manualisation and training it may serve to increase inter-rater reliability and inter-trial reproducibility in Chinese medicine clinical trials (Schnyer et al 2005).

Box 6.8 A study to explore variations in acupuncture techniques and outcome (Harris et al 2005)

Harris and colleagues (2005) conducted one of the few pilot studies that explored factors to do with acupuncture process: the objective of this study was to investigate whether variations in acupuncture treatment such as needle placement, needle stimulation, and treatment frequency were important factors in treatment. The authors recruited 114 patients with a diagnosis of fibromyalgia. They compared traditional acupuncture sites with non-sites, stimulation with no stimulation, and treatment given once, twice and three times a week. They measured pain, fatigue and physical function. They actually found no differences in outcome: 25–35% of subjects had a clinically significant decrease in pain, but this was not dependent upon needle stimulation or location. They did observe an effect of frequency of treatment, with three sessions weekly providing more relief of pain than sessions once weekly. Among treatment responders, improvements in pain, fatigue, and physical function were highly co-dependent (Harris et al 2005).

Box 6.9 Testing blinding procedures in a pilot study

In planning a definitive trial of Western medical acupuncture for tension-type headache, acupuncture treatment with brief needling of trigger and segmental points was to be compared with a sham treatment that ideally should feel to patients the same as acupuncture, but have no effect. This sham was initially based on that previously used successfully by Lao et al (1994), namely a plastic guide tube tapped over a bony prominence somewhere near the acupuncture point. During the pilot study, it was discovered that placing a cocktail stick (or tooth-pick) in the tube seemed more manageable and realistic. In addition, the study was designed to involve minimal interaction between the patient and the practitioner, to reduce the impact of unintentional influence: the patients would interact as they normally would with the nurse — who remained blinded throughout — discussing the treatment and the outcome with her but not with the practitioner. These procedures were tested in a pilot study, which also explored the use of the daily diary as an outcome measure. Minor changes were made to the order in which the headache diary questions were presented, which led to a much smaller amount of missing data on medication in the subsequent study (White et al 1996).

For studies where it is planned to use a sham treatment in order to blind patients, the sham procedure itself may need to be explored in a pilot study as well as the success of blinding. One such pilot study is described in Box 6.9.

Another area that might need piloting is in the area of what outcomes should be assessed (for example, pain, stiffness, disability), and

Box 6.10 A step-wise structuring of pilot studies that builds towards a full-scale efficacy trial (Lao & Berman 2005)

Berman and colleagues conducted a series of three studies of progressively rigorous design in a step-wise programme to determine the effectiveness of acupuncture for treating knee pain. First, they recruited and treated a series of 12 patients with standardised acupuncture twice a week for 8 weeks (Berman et al 1995). They measured the WOMAC and Lequesne scores at baseline, 4, 8 and 12 weeks, and various other measures like timed 50-foot walk and global assessment of change. This pilot study identified sufficiently worthwhile effects to justify further studies. Second, they conducted an RCT with 73 patients to compare acupuncture with usual care control group (offering the control group acupuncture after 12 weeks) (Berman et al 1999). The results and experience of this study allowed the research team to win a large NCCAM grant to undertake a definitive RCT in which acupuncture was compared with a novel sham acupuncture and an education control in 570 patients (Berman et al 2004). This study revealed a significant effect of acupuncture and is considered a landmark in acupuncture research (Lao & Berman 2005).

how they should be measured. In conventional medicine, appropriate outcome measures have been established and validated for many different conditions. In principle, studies in acupuncture researchers should first consider the conventional outcomes, so that their results can be compared with the effects of other treatments. Typically, large rigorous trials will use one or two measures of the main symptom or symptoms, together with a functional measure particularly for musculoskeletal or neurological disorders, and a quality-of-life measure. It may be necessary to investigate, in a pilot study, how well the effects of acupuncture treatment can be measured by these various conventional instruments. Researchers have often expressed concern that the effects of acupuncture are too broad to be truly captured by conventional measures, and there has also been more widespread use of patient-centred outcome measures such as MYMOP, as discussed in Chapter 5.

Finally, it may be instructive to describe an example of how one research group exploring acupuncture for osteoarthritis of the knee progressed step-wise from a case series, through a non-randomised controlled trial to a definitive RCT (see Box 6.10). Each step involved higher levels of rigour, and built on the experience and knowledge gained in previous steps.

CHALLENGES AND POTENTIAL APPROACHES

A major challenge in the field of acupuncture research is that we need more data derived from clinical acupuncture practice. We need more information on every aspect of acupuncture patients and acupuncture treatments in order to design better studies that truly reflect real practice. Therefore, all acupuncture practitioners are to be encouraged to routinely collect data prospectively and systematically on all their patients, and to write them up as publishable reports. Although this may seem daunting to someone who has never done it before, help is often available from others who have some experience of research. Most good research is the product of collaboration between teams of people with different areas of expertise.

We shall use the four headings that we set out in the Introduction for further detailed discussion in this section.

Patients

There remains a considerable need for more information on what factors predict patients' outcome: who will have a good response, and who will have a poor response from acupuncture – not just the duration of symptoms, but also the precise clinical condition. For example, are there subgroups of patients with shoulder pain that respond better than most? Do otherwise fit patients who suffer a sports injury respond better than the slightly older patient with a diagnosis of arthritis? What types of back pain respond best to acupuncture: with or without leg pain or with or without history of acute strain? How does a claim for compensation influence the response to acupuncture for whiplash injury? Information on all these questions can be provided by carefully conducted, prospective case series. This will help for example when planning a trial, to know whether to recruit only a subgroup of patients with a specific condition on the basis that preliminary studies show better effects.

Descriptive qualitative studies can be used to explore the patient's perspective on treatment and services. For example knowing the needs of patients within a palliative care can help plan how best to deliver the service. Similar research could be used to enhance a pain service or a private practice.

Interventions and comparison interventions

There remains a great need for more information about diagnosis and treatment in traditional Chinese acupuncture. We have described one method of standardising the approach to diagnosis and treatment, but more experience is required in the use of standardised methods in different settings and with graduates of different schools. The wide range of different approaches to acupuncture treatment should be explored, looking for common features and understanding differences, and exploring the effectiveness of different approaches in different kinds of patient and different kinds of condition. We also need to understand more about individual preferences for particular treatment approaches, for example how these preferences develop, how they evolve over time, and what processes influence change or resistance to change.

Acupuncture can be seen as a complex intervention: if we are to conduct accurate and meaningful definitive studies into acupuncture, we shall need more information on every possible aspect that might influence the outcome of treatment. This could include the peculiarities of a therapeutic relationship with an acupuncturist compared with other therapists, specific expectations of acupuncture in the patient and the therapist, physiological effects of needle insertion at off-point locations, wrong-point locations and correct-point locations, and the effects of different stimulation techniques and different schedules of treatment. The whole exploration of this area will start with careful descriptions and consensus views, progressing through exploratory studies to formulate hypotheses that can be tested.

One of acupuncture's strengths — its application in a wide variety of clinical conditions — is also a challenge: how should the methods of diagnosis and treatment be adapted for treating different conditions?

The reason that it is so difficult to develop a truly inactive control intervention against which to test acupuncture is that we are still fundamentally ignorant of the mechanisms of acupuncture. Until this has been resolved, studies could usefully explore the impact of various interventions that have been used as controls, both those that penetrate the skin and those that do not. By 'impact' we mean not only the effect on the condition itself, but whether it matches patients' beliefs and expectations of acupuncture.

Outcome measures

Detailed exploration of relevant outcome measures is covered in Chapter 5 of this book. In addition, economic evaluation of acupuncture will become increasingly important as part of the evidence base for acupuncture, and studies can usefully explore the background to the costs and benefits of acupuncture treatment.

Procedures

One of the greatest problems facing clinical trials of acupuncture historically has been the determination of the sample size. Large case series that accurately measure and report changes in the appropriate outcome measures could provide valuable information for researchers.

When this information, for example on the standard deviation of the measure, is not available from large observational studies, it may be necessary to try to gain this information from a pilot study. However, it is not clear how big the pilot study needs to be. One commonly cited rule of thumb is that 30 patients is sufficient to estimate the standard deviation, but one paper concludes that this is likely to be far too small when the treatment effects are not very large (Browne 1995).

It would be valuable to investigate what particular features might attract potential participants to an acupuncture study, and what features might make them less likely to volunteer or continue to participate. Following on from this, it might be worth investigating what the specific barriers to recruitment to acupuncture trials might be, and the extent that these could be overcome.

TRANSLATING RESEARCH INTO CLINICAL PRACTICE

The information provided in uncontrolled studies may be relevant to acupuncturists and to those who are responsible for providing acupuncture services. It builds on what practitioners were taught as students and continue to learn in discussion with colleagues, to form a knowledge base on how to best advise and treat patients with different conditions. If a case series shows that patients with chronic neck pain are less likely to respond to acupuncture than those with a short history for example, a practitioner could enhance his management of neck pain by not persisting too long in a course of treatment, when early success has not occurred.

The findings of these uncontrolled studies do provide some level of evidence base for clinical decision-making in clinical practice. For example, a case series might be used to provide some evidence on which to base a decision to provide acupuncture for patients with diabetic neuropathy in a clinic that is enthusiastic. However, this type of study cannot establish causality (meaning: 'acupuncture caused this improvement') so is unlikely to influence spending of major resources in making policy changes.

SUMMARY

Investigation of the effectiveness of acupuncture is a multi-faceted and progressive exercise that ideally involves conducting a range of studies from non-experimental through to experimental studies. Non-experimental studies can explore patient and practitioner experiences, the dimensions to diagnosis and treatment, and the impact of these on outcome. These preliminary steps in this process are of crucial importance in providing information on which relevant and definitive trials can be based. Whereas non-experimental studies are, by definition, of less rigour than carefully designed experimental studies, nevertheless they should be conducted with high regard for quality. This involves careful and critical design with input from others with special knowledge and skills, following a precise study protocol and careful reporting of the study including any aspects that were unsuccessful.

Case reports are the fundamental building blocks of all research; they are followed by case series that an observed effect is consistent and repeatable. Qualitative studies add important depth of information about acupuncture without which clinical trials may be irrelevant. There is such variety and complexity in acupuncture treatment — the individual patients, the range of conditions treated, and the different aspects of diagnosis and treatment — that it has proved extremely difficult so far to design studies that all acupuncturists can accept as truly reflecting practice. Any information that throws light on even the smallest corner of this huge challenge is to be welcomed.

Research resources

Altman D G 1991 Practical statistics for medical research. Chapman & Hall, London

Lewith G, Jonas W B, Walach H (eds) 2002 Clinical research in complementary therapies. Churchill Livingstone, Edinburgh

Sim J, Wright C 2000 Research in health care: concepts, designs and methods. Stanley Thornes (Publishers) Ltd, Cheltenham

Vincent C, Furnham A 1997 Complementary medicine. A research perspective. Wiley, Chichester

The following journal articles, part of a major series on research methods, are particularly relevant to this chapter:

Grimes D A, Schulz K F 2002a An overview of clinical research: the lay of the land. Lancet 359(9300):57–61

Grimes D A, Schulz K F 2002b Descriptive studies: what they can and cannot do. Lancet 359(9301):145–149

Grimes D A, Schulz K F 2002c Bias and causal associations in observational research. Lancet 359(9302):248–252

Grimes D A, Schulz K F 2002d Cohort studies: marching towards outcomes. Lancet 359(9303):341–345

Schulz K F, Grimes D A 2002e Case-control studies: research in reverse. Lancet 359(9304):431–434

References

Berman B, Lao L, Greene M et al 1995 Efficacy of traditional Chinese acupuncture in the treatment of symptomatic knee osteoarthritis: a pilot study. Osteoarthritis Cartilage 3:139–142

Berman B M, Singh B B, Lao L et al 1999 A randomized trial of acupuncture as an adjunctive therapy in osteoarthritis of the knee. Rheumatology (Oxford) 38(4):346–354

Berman B M, Lao L, Langenberg P et al 2004 Effectiveness of acupuncture as adjunctive therapy in osteoarthritis of the knee: a randomized, controlled trial. Annals of Internal Medicine 141(12):901–910

Blossfeldt P 2004 Acupuncture for chronic neck pain — a cohort study in an NHS pain clinic. Acupuncture in Medicine 22(3):146–151

Browne R H 1995 On the use of a pilot sample for sample-size determination. Statistics in Medicine 14(17):1933–1940

Cullen C 2001 Yi'an (case statements) — the origins of a genre of Chinese medical literature. In: Hsu E (ed.) Innovation in Chinese Medicine. Cambridge University Press, Cambridge

Grabowska C, Squire C, MacRae E et al 2003 Provision of acupuncture in a university health centre — a clinical audit. Complementary Therapies in Nursing and Midwifery 9(1):14–19

Harris R E, Tian X, Williams D A et al 2005 Treatment of fibromyalgia with formula acupuncture: investigation of needle placement, needle stimulation, and treatment frequency. Journal of Alternative and Complementary Medicine 11(4):663–671

Kaptchuk T J 2003 Effect of interpretive bias on research evidence. British Medical Journal 326(7404):1453–1455

Lao L, Berman B 2005 Evaluating the effects of acupuncture on knee osteoarthritis: a stepwise approach to research, University of Maryland experience. American Journal of Traditional Chinese Medicine 6(1):5–12

Lao L, Bergman S, Anderson R et al 1994 The effect of acupuncture on post-operative pain. Acupuncture in Medicine 12:13–17

MacPherson H, Mercer SW, Scullion T et al 2003 Empathy, enablement, and outcome: an exploratory study on acupuncture patients' perceptions. Journal of Alternative and Complementary Medicine 9(6):869–876

Rosted P 2005 Acupuncture for treatment of the yips? — a case report. Acupuncture in Medicine 23(4):188–189

Schnyer R N, Conboy L A, Jacobson E et al 2005 Development of a Chinese medicine assessment measure: an interdisciplinary approach using the Delphi method. Journal of Alternative and Complementary Medicine 11(6):1005–1013

Vickers A J, Rusch V W, Malhotra V T et al 2006 Acupuncture is a feasible treatment for post-thoracotomy pain: results of a prospective pilot trial. BMC Anesthesiology 6(1):5

White A 2004 Writing case reports — author guidelines for acupuncture in medicine. Acupuncture in Medicine 22(2):83–86

White A, Ernst E 2001 The case for uncontrolled clinical trials: a starting point for the evidence base for CAM. Complementary Therapies in Medicine 9(2):111–116

White A R, Eddleston C, Hardie R et al 1996 A pilot study of acupuncture for tension headache, using a novel placebo. Acupuncture in Medicine 14:11–15

Comparing treatment effects of acupuncture and other types of healthcare

Karen Sherman, Klaus Linde and Adrian White

INTRODUCTION

In this chapter and the next, we shall discuss the use of clinical trials to evaluate whether or not acupuncture 'works', that is, is more effective than a reasonable comparison. This chapter shall discuss studies that compare acupuncture to other bona fide therapies (or as adjunctive treatments to biomedical care) while the next shall discuss studies of acupuncture compared to 'sham' or mock treatments, which generally test one 'component' of a typical acupuncture treatment. We will first describe the importance of conducting clinical trials of a therapy that has been in use for thousands of years. After that, we will describe some of the challenges of using standard frameworks of research geared toward evaluating single therapies as well as the dangers of deviating from such frameworks. Then, we will introduce the reader to the main types of clinical trial designs and finally, we will focus on the designs that have been used to compare acupuncture with other therapies.

Like most complementary and alternative medical (CAM) therapies, acupuncture is a therapy that was already in widespread use before research on CAM therapies was popular. Over the centuries, medicine has had a history of using ineffective treatments, some of which were harmful and some of which only appeared successful because the conditions they 'treated' were self-limiting and got better over time regardless of treatment. Since the 1970s, medicine has been steadily adopting a more evidence-based approach, and so if the aim is to better integrate acupuncture in healthcare, then studies evaluating the therapeutic effects of acupuncture are necessary.

The most powerful types of studies for inferring that a treatment 'works' are clinical trials, which are experiments wherein patients are given treatments assigned by the researchers. Randomised controlled clinical trials are currently considered the 'gold standard' for evaluating the effects of a medical intervention. As we shall see in the section entitled 'A field guide to cataloguing clinical trials', there are actually different types of randomised controlled clinical trials that can be undertaken, depending on the precise question being asked and the details of the trial design.

Extensive debates about the most critical type of evidence required to support the integration of complementary medicine into conventional care have been ongoing since at least the 1990s (Levin et al 1997, Vickers et al 1997). People involved in these debates often start from different positions: some are more interested in a theoretical or 'purist' approach, others in practical issues such as acupuncture's place in healthcare.

In Europe and North America, the usual model for evaluating new medical therapies is based on the testing of new pharmacological agents. New medications are introduced into practice once they have passed regulatory hurdles and have been deemed 'safe and effective' at recommended doses, frequently in placebo-controlled double-blind clinical trials where neither the patient nor the doctor knows who got the active medication. Such studies attempt to assess the effect of the 'active ingredient' of a particular medication under tightly controlled circumstances (Bombardier & Maetzel 1999). They are considered essential in demonstrating that a medication actually has a therapeutic effect. Of course, not all therapies included under the label of conventional medicine have been evaluated using these designs. Surgical procedures, psychotherapy and some complex interventions such as physical therapy are much more difficult to study in the context of a double-blind 'placebo-controlled' trial for reasons of ethics, logistical complexity and conceptual challenges.

Unfortunately, approval of a medication by a regulatory body does not tell us how well the medication will perform compared to other available therapies or whether the results would extend to individuals who are dissimilar to those who were studied (e.g. those with differing socioeconomic status, more (or less) severe disease or co-existing medical conditions). Answers to these critical and practical questions typically require further trials that compare two or more therapies to each other in a broadly defined patient population.

Some authors have proposed that, when evaluating acupuncture, the more practically oriented trials evaluating the entire package of care should be conducted first and followed by trials to evaluate the effects of specific components of acupuncture (Fønnebø et al 2007). The reason for this unusual recommendation reflects several differences between complex CAM treatments such as acupuncture and conventional biomedicine. Firstly, a course of acupuncture, when practised within the context of a traditionally based system of medicine, typically includes more than needling and traditionally may include moxibustion, tuina, Chinese herbal medicine, exercise and nutritional information. Thus, trials of a single component, most typically needling, would fail to incorporate a number of important therapeutic ingredients. Acupuncture practised in a conventional medical setting often involves needling therapy alone, though physical therapists may use manual therapies alongside needling. Secondly, acupuncture is commonly customised to the individual, with the treatment being based on a non-Western diagnosis that may differ among individuals with a particular biomedical condition. Thus, using a single treatment for all trial participants might well provide inappropriate treatment to a large fraction of participants, and would certainly not reflect actual acupuncture practice. Finally, acupuncture is already available to the public therefore one priority for patients is to know how it compares with other currently available treatments. This is especially critical because the research process is lengthy and an estimate of the relative value of acupuncture compared with other treatments would be useful for third party reimbursement and more rapid integration of acupuncture in mainstream care.

While this approach contains some practical advantages, it also contains some risks. For one thing, many experts in biomedicine, including behavioural medicine, accept the current model of research into a pharmacological agent: it should first be tested for mechanism of action, dosage and safety, then tested in a few patients in tightly controlled situations, and only then tested in a broader population under more realistic conditions (Glasgow et al 2006). While it could be argued that these individuals hold orthodox views without merit, they often serve on panels that review medical research grant applications and research funding recommendations or decisions.

There is another aspect of the debate that is more difficult to evaluate. Some proponents of research into whole systems of medicine, including traditionally based systems of acupuncture, say that acupuncture works by combining synergistic effects — which are usually referred to as 'specific' (e.g. needling) and 'non-specific' (e.g. practitioner enthusiasm, process of making a diagnosis) effects of a treatment. These proponents hold that it is those synergistic effects combined, rather than specific effects of individual components, that have clinically important effects. The distinction between specific and non-specific effects is rather artificial, and probably not helpful for a complex intervention like acupuncture: the process of making a diagnosis, for example, might quite possibly have 'specific' therapeutic effects. Following this argument, one might predict that moxibustion, cupping and acupuncture needling, by themselves might not be useful treatments for persons with lumbar pain, but together, they would be effective. So, there is a different understanding of 'specific effects' in the context of a whole system, which, according to proponents of this viewpoint, cannot be teased apart. A logical consequence of this reasoning is that it would be difficult to demonstrate the biological mechanisms behind whole systems of medicine. Without knowing the mechanisms, it is difficult to know what treatment is optimal for which particular types of patient or diagnosis. This uncertainty could put a disproportionately large burden on these so-called 'pragmatic' or 'practical' trials, which are generally not designed to look for 'optimal treatment' parameters. It opens the Pandora's box of questions regarding precisely how tight or loose the patient selection criteria should be, what components of the whole system should be permitted in the treatment, what the minimum qualifications of the participating practitioners should be, how many treatments should be permitted, and other nuances of treatment design. Finally, if the whole system (for example acupuncture) did not perform well compared to other standard treatments in properly conducted studies of a particular condition, its continued use would not be justified.

A FIELD GUIDE TO CATALOGUING CLINICAL TRIALS

Even though all clinical trials include patients, treatments, and assessments of whether the patients are getting better, there are many features of clinical trials, such as exactly what type of treatment each of the groups will receive, that vary considerably between studies. Some of these differences are due to the nature of the condition under study, while others reflect some differences in the overall purpose of the trials.

One feature of trial design, randomly assigning participants to each treatment while concealing the treatment assignment before it is actually made, is considered extremely important in ensuring that the assignment to treatment is unbiased. There is no reason why this design feature cannot be implemented in all clinical trials of acupuncture. Randomised and concealed allocation prevents selection bias, and helps to ensure that differences between the treatment groups at baseline are not responsible for any differences in the outcomes after treatments (Friedman et al 1998).

Another possible bias that may distort the results of a trial results from systematic inaccuracies in measuring the outcomes of treatment. If participants and their healthcare providers do not know what treatment the study participants are receiving (i.e. they are 'masked' or 'blinded'), their expectations about the treatment should not influence the study outcomes. This is one of the reasons for the emphasis on placebo pills and 'sham' interventions, even when two 'real' treatments are being compared with each other. Of course, not all treatments lend themselves to being camouflaged, and acupuncture is a good example: this is a recurring problem in acupuncture research.

As with all other forms of research, we are interested in whether the findings of clinical trials are 'valid', that is, whether we can believe them or not. There are actually two types of validity and it is important to understand each of them. Internal validity refers to whether or not we can believe that the results from a particular study are accurate for the population that was studied. We believe that there is good internal validity when a study is designed and carried out so that serious biases that could easily distort the findings from that study, such as selection and measurement bias, are avoided. In this case, the changes can be attributed to the intervention.

However, just because a study has good internal validity does not mean its results are expected to hold true for other patients or when a different form of acupuncture is used. The term 'external validity' refers to whether those results can be generalised to other patient populations, and to a different type of acupuncture. An example will make this clearer. A study by Meng et al (2003) of older patients with back pain found that bi-weekly treatments of acupuncture for 5 weeks added to usual medical care were associated with improvements in back-related function compared to usual care only. Whether the results of this study could be generalised to individuals under 60 or those who might have been injured at work or from auto accidents is unknown and thus, the external generalisability of the study to different populations is not clear. Researchers generally give first priority to internal validity, since if the trial's result is not internally valid there is little point in considering whether it applies to other situations.

One problem of external generalisability that has arisen in trials of acupuncture (and other CAM therapies) is that the people who are willing to participate in trials are different from people who would routinely seek these therapies. Thus, the results of the trial might not be widely applicable. One way to circumvent this challenge is to conduct a partially randomised study comparing two treatment options in which persons who have a preference for a treatment receive that treatment and those who do not, are randomly assigned to one of the options (Brewin & Bradley 1989). Such studies could allow a comparison of whether patient preferences actually made a difference in the outcomes of treatment. Witt et al (2006a) have recently published a study of acupuncture for neck pain that includes this design and results of this trial are described in Box 7.6.

To assist the reader in understanding the array of clinical trial designs, a few definitions are in order. In Box 7.1, we provide some definitions of trial designs where acupuncture might be evaluated. Some of these designs are suitable for studies where acupuncture is compared with other active therapies and will be discussed further in this chapter, while others are more suitable for looking at the 'specific effects' of components of acupuncture such as needling, and these will be discussed in Chapter 8. Several of these trial definitions can be seen as a yin-yang polarity. For example, efficacy and effectiveness trials differ on the degree to which persons recruited for a trial are actually encouraged to receive the treatment. Explanatory and pragmatic trials differ regarding whether there is an intention to answer a biological or a practical question.

Finally, active control equivalent trials and superiority trials differ regarding whether the 'experimental' treatment is predicted to be similar to or better than the control treatment. Table 7.1 assists the reader in

> **Box 7.1** Definition of some types of clinical trials (Herman et al 2005, Jadad & Rennie 1998)

- Efficacy trial: A trial conducted to see whether there is a therapeutic effect in an ideal, highly controlled setting with optimal administration of treatment. These trials are designed to include participants willing to adhere to the treatment regimen so they can determine whether the treatment works among those who receive it. In some cases, people are asked to do activities prior to randomisation that suggest whether they may adhere to the treatment regimen (e.g. make a number of visits to the study clinic, keep a diary). These studies have high internal validity. It is worth noting that the use of 'sham' or 'placebo' controls does not itself constitute an efficacy study.
- Effectiveness trial: A trial conducted to see whether there is a therapeutic effect when the intervention is delivered as it would be in practice in the real world. These trials are usually simpler in design than efficacy trials as they allow participants to accept or reject the intervention and may include flexible treatment protocols and broader inclusion criteria. These studies have high external validity. Again it is worth noting that 'effectiveness trials' may or may not involve 'sham' or 'placebo' controls – the definition is not concerned with that point.
- Explanatory trial (fastidious trial): A trial undertaken to establish the mechanism by which a therapy such as acupuncture may work. It controls for non-specific elements in order to evaluate the specific effect (or 'active ingredient') of a treatment. Explanatory trials of acupuncture typically evaluate the effects of needling 'in the correct location' compared to some form of 'sham' acupuncture. This type of trial will be discussed in more detail in Chapter 8. Typically, these trials have stringent inclusion criteria and 'objective outcomes' if possible. These design characteristics lead to high internal validity. The term 'explanatory trial' should not be confused with 'efficacy trial'.
- Pragmatic trial (practical trials, management trials): A trial designed to describe the overall benefits of a routine treatment, without separating the treatment out into specific and non-specific components. These trials tend to employ broader inclusion criteria and controls receiving another treatment (i.e. active controls).
- Comparative trial: A clinical trial comparing two or more 'real' treatments for a particular condition. Such trials could be undertaken with a more efficacy or a more effectiveness approach, depending on the other aspects of the trial.
- Superiority trial: A clinical trial designed to test whether one treatment is superior to another treatment (or to a placebo or sham treatment).
- Active control equivalent study (non-inferiority trial): A clinical trial designed to test whether a new treatment is roughly equivalent to another treatment. Such trials are not universally accepted because in order to be

valid, they require showing that the comparison treatment is efficacious in previous clinical trials that are similar to the current study in terms of the study population, settings and other key factors. This type of trial also requires an unusual approach to analysing the data and generally requires larger sample sizes than a superiority trial.

- Cost-effectiveness: an analysis undertaken alongside a clinical trial to determine the costs of producing a change in a particular health outcome. When health outcomes are expressed in terms of costs for increased quality of life (typically 'quality adjusted life years'), the analyses are actually 'cost-utility analyses'.

understanding how efficacy and effectiveness trials differ by highlighting some key features in these trials. In practice, however, many studies of acupuncture and other therapies are hybrids that contain some features of each design.

Table 7.1 Classic features of efficacy and effectiveness trials of acupuncture

	Efficacy trial	Effectiveness trial
Research question	Does the treatment work under ideal conditions?	Is there a therapeutic benefit when the treatment is given under everyday conditions?
Setting	Specialised research setting	Usual clinical practice
Patients/exclusion criteria	Homogeneous group of patients with numerous exclusions	Heterogeneous group of patients with few exclusions
Acupuncture intervention	Single-point prescription	Based on what acupuncturists would normally provide
Other interventions	None or clearly defined	Variable, depending on acupuncturist's judgement in the context of patient needs
Typical control group	'Sham' controlled	Usually not 'sham' controlled
Assessments	Elaborate, often includes 'objective' outcomes	Sparse, often includes 'subjective' outcomes
Follow-up period	Short	Longer
Validity	High internal validity	High external validity
Generalisability	Low	High

Adapted from Jadad 1998 and March et al 2005.

METHODS OF ASSESSING COMPARATIVE EFFECTIVENESS AND COST-EFFECTIVENESS

Regardless of at which point in the research process they are undertaken, clinical trials comparing acupuncture to other available treatments or acupuncture as an adjunct to other available treatments are an important part of evaluating the role of acupuncture in contemporary healthcare. They are often ideal studies for collecting information on cost-effectiveness, since the costs of the treatments can be accurately measured. The principal research questions asked in studies of acupuncture compared to standard care are whether acupuncture is better than standard care, whether it is equivalent to standard care or whether acupuncture is an effective adjunct to standard care. In some studies, standard care consists of the best available care, while in others, it consists of 'usual care', that is whatever care the patient would have received in the absence of participation in the trial.

In actual practice, there are a number of basic designs that can be used to answer these broad questions.

Comparative trials with sham controls

Sham controls can be included in the group receiving standard care if the researcher is concerned that patients' expectations of acupuncture could lead to bias in measuring the outcome. This design resembles more of an efficacy study. In fact, it is even possible to randomly assign patients to receive acupuncture and placebo medication or a medication treatment and sham acupuncture. For example, Hesse et al (1994) have compared acupuncture with a β-blocker as a treatment for prophylaxis of migraine headache in a smallish trial asking whether acupuncture was equivalent to β-blocker in its therapeutic effects. In this trial, people randomised to acupuncture were given a placebo medication and people assigned to metoprolol were touched with the blunt end of a needle. This trial was described as an active control equivalent trial wherein the study was carried out under identical conditions to those that had earlier shown that metoprolol was better than placebo (e.g. dosage, duration of treatment, use of outcomes, and patient characteristics). However, the study was too small and not analysed appropriately to be certain that these conclusions were robust.

An example of a trial asking whether acupuncture is a useful adjunct to physiotherapy for adults with knee pain is currently being conducted in the UK by Hay et al (2004). In this three-arm trial, older adults with knee pain are being randomised to receive acupuncture plus physiotherapy, simulated acupuncture plus physiotherapy or physiotherapy alone. In this design, people receiving acupuncture will get six bi-weekly treatments of acupuncture over 3 weeks and acupuncturists will be required to select local and distal points from a pre-specified list. In a US study asking a similar question (Farrar 2006), people with osteoarthritis of the knee are being randomised to receive acupuncture plus physical therapy or simulated acupuncture plus physical therapy.

Pragmatic effectiveness trials

Interestingly, there have been relatively few pragmatic clinical trials of acupuncture. Pragmatic trials are considered a strong design for acupuncture studies because they allow the acupuncturist to deliver the type of care that most resembles what they do in practice. They also include a broad array of participants who might be interested in trying acupuncture and they also avoid the vexing issue of designing a suitable sham control. They also look at longer-term outcomes and are likely the most appropriate designs for undertaking economic analyses. These trials will appeal to patients and some doctors and insurers because they answer questions relevant to everyday practice. They may be helpful to acupuncturists by testing what is actually practised. However, they are less likely to assist acupuncturists in identifying the most effective acupuncture care. Some major issues in designing pragmatic trials include deciding what to include in the treatment and comparison protocols as well as what constraints should be put on the patient population (MacPherson 2004).

Three large pragmatic trials of acupuncture for pain (headache, persistent or chronic back pain) in primary care patients have been published and are described more fully in Boxes 7.2–7.4. Two of the trials were conducted in the UK's National Health Service while one of them was conducted in a large integrated healthcare organisation in the US. The UK trials were funded after the National Health Service first determined that acupuncture for the treatment of pain in primary care populations was a research priority and then requested researchers to submit proposals for pragmatic trials to address this issue. The US trial was funded shortly after Washington state enacted a law requiring health insurers to pay for at least some treatments given by all licensed health providers, including acupuncturists. Two of these trials included constraints on the practice of acupuncture. The headache trial focused on acupuncture needling only, while the US chronic back pain trial prohibited Chinese herbs and acupressure.

While pragmatic trials of acupuncture might be expected to be more common in primary care, Box 7.5 describes the results of a small pragmatic trial of chronic daily headache undertaken in a tertiary care setting.

Mixed explanatory and pragmatic trials

Some newer trials include elements of both explanatory and pragmatic trials. In 2000, the German health authorities commissioned a series of

Box 7.2 Pragmatic trial of acupuncture for headache conducted in primary care in the UK (Vickers et al 2004)

Vickers et al (2004) designed this pragmatic trial to see whether adding access to acupuncture improved care for primary care patients with chronic headache. The study recruited 401 patients with chronic headaches from 30 general practices in 12 areas of England and Wales and randomised them to receive referral for up to 12 acupuncture treatments over 3 months or continued usual care. Physiotherapists who had completed at least 250 hours of training in traditional Chinese medicine, and had practised for a median of 12 years, treated patients in the acupuncture group. Among those randomised to a referral for acupuncture, 90% received acupuncture, with a median of nine treatments. The point prescriptions were individualised for the patient. Patients reported headache score, quality of life and medication use at baseline, 3 months and 12 months, while healthcare utilisation was reported every 3 months. Patients in the acupuncture group reported significantly lower headache scores and fewer headaches (equivalent of 22 fewer headaches per year) and improvements in several aspects of quality of life (physical role function, energy, changes in health). Compared to controls, those randomised to acupuncture used 15% less medication, made 25% fewer visits to general practitioners and took 15% fewer sick days from work. The authors concluded that acupuncture leads to persisting, clinically relevant benefits for primary care patients with chronic headache.

Box 7.3 Pragmatic trial of acupuncture for low back pain conducted in primary care in the UK (Thomas et al 2006)

Thomas et al (2006) designed a trial to determine whether referral to a short course of traditional acupuncture improved patient outcomes at 12 and 24 months compared to primary care alone. The study recruited and randomised 241 patients from 43 general practitioners in York, England, to one of the two study arms. Twice as many patients were randomised to referral to acupuncture, which consisted of up to 10 acupuncture treatments employing individualised treatments over a 3-month period, as to continued usual care. Six traditionally trained acupuncturists who were registered with the British Acupuncture Council and had at least 3 years' experience provided the acupuncture care. Nearly all (94%) patients randomised to referral to acupuncture actually received treatment. The primary outcome measure was pain, with secondary measures of medication use, back-related dysfunction, safety and satisfaction. At 2 years, patients in the acupuncture group reported a clinically important reduction in pain with a benefit that had been statistically and clinically weaker at 12 months. There were no benefits in back-related dysfunction at any time, while medication use was 19% lower in the acupuncture group at 24 months. No serious or life-threatening events were reported. The authors concluded that referral for a short course of acupuncture appears safe and acceptable to patients and has long-term benefits on pain.

Box 7.4 Pragmatic trial of traditional Chinese acupuncture for low back pain among primary care patients in Washington State, USA (Cherkin et al 2001)

Cherkin et al (2001) randomised 262 primary care patients with chronic low back pain in western Washington State to receive a course of traditional Chinese medical acupuncture, a course of therapeutic massage or self-care educational materials in addition to continued access to conventional care. The study was designed to measure treatment effects on back pain and dysfunction at 4, 10 and 52 weeks. In the acupuncture and massage groups, up to 10 treatments over 10 weeks were permitted. The acupuncture protocol, which was administered by seven experienced acupuncturists with traditional training, permitted individualised treatment but proscribed the use of Chinese herbal medicine and acupressure. Most patients randomised to acupuncture (94%) or massage (95%) received at least one treatment with an average of eight treatments per person in both groups. At the 10-week follow-up, the massage group had reduced pain and superior function compared to the self-care group with the acupuncture group in between. By the 1-year follow-up, the massage group had less pain and better function than the acupuncture group. The massage group used the fewest medications and had the lowest costs of non-study treatment-related back care. The authors concluded that traditional Chinese medical acupuncture was relatively ineffective, although they noted that the study acupuncturists felt constrained by the protocol for 70% of the patients for at least one study visit.

Box 7.5 Pragmatic trial of acupuncture for chronic daily headache conducted in a tertiary care clinic, North Carolina, USA

Coeytaux et al (2005) conducted this small pragmatic trial that was designed to see whether acupuncture was an effective adjunct to specialty headache medical management for people with chronic daily headache in a tertiary care clinic at a university hospital in North Carolina. The study randomised 74 people with chronic daily headache to receive 10 sessions of individualised acupuncture over 6 weeks or medical management only. The acupuncture was delivered by an acupuncturist and physician trained in China in both acupuncture and Western medicine. Patients in the acupuncture group reported greater improvement on a standardised headache questionnaire, on several domains of a standard quality-of-life instrument and on a question about suffering due to headaches.

large clinical trials evaluating needle acupuncture for chronic low back pain, osteoarthritis of the knee, migraine and tension headache to evaluate the benefits, if any, of acupuncture (Streitberger et al 2004). Three series of multi-centre trials were designed to meet the needs of the funders, which included at least 6 months of follow-up and a sham control group (Brinkhaus et al 2006, Diener et al 2006, Linde et al 2006, Melchart et al 2005, Scharf et al 2006, Witt et al 2005, 2006a, 2006b). The trials we are concerned with here are the GERAC (German Acupuncture) and the ART trials (Acupuncture Randomised Trials), which have many similarities.

Both sets of trials included three arms: they compared verum acupuncture (patients receiving the true treatment) with sham acupuncture (off-point, off-meridian, superficial needling) and with either, in the GERAC trials, standard conventional care which was predefined according to guidelines, or, in the ART trials, a wait-list group which was permitted to use medications. In both cases, treatment was given from a selection of predefined points agreed by consensus after consulting acupuncture experts and (in the GERAC trials) acupuncture texts. This was an attempt to ensure 'optimal' treatment by combining recommendations with some individualisation.

In the GERAC trials, in another example of a somewhat pragmatic design, patients who responded only partially to the initial course of treatment were given the option of five more treatments. To improve the generalisability of the studies, a large number of physician acupuncturists participated in both groups of trials.

Even though the trials were largely undertaken to see whether acupuncture should continue to be reimbursed by insurers, a practical question of great interest, it is interesting that sham controls were required in all trials. This suggests that the insurers were applying the policy that a treatment must be shown to have a specific effect beyond the placebo effect before it is acceptable. This policy is imported from the thinking behind acceptance of new pharmaceutical products, but may not be appropriate for acupuncture. The results of the studies have given the insurers some difficulty in interpretation: most of them (Linde et al 2006, Melchart et al 2005) found that acupuncture was greatly superior to usual care, but not significantly better than sham acupuncture.

In the migraine trial, Diener et al (2006) reported no statistically significant difference between the three groups (acupuncture, sham acupuncture or standard therapy) in the initial three-way comparison. While the authors make the argument that verum acupuncture and standard therapy give similar results, the study was not originally designed or analysed as an active control equivalent study. The conclusion 'no difference was found between the treatments' is not the same as saying 'the treatments are equivalent'.

Preference trials

A preference trial is one in which patients' preference for a particular treatment is taken into account in some way, with only those having no strong preferences being randomised to the two alternative treatments.

Those who have a preference for the treatment receive it and are followed as part of a parallel non-randomised cohort study. Clearly, inferences cannot be made with the same strength from the changes in groups of people who were not randomised to the treatment they received. However, by comparing outcomes from those people who were randomised to acupuncture with those from people who were part of the cohort study, one can determine whether the results of the randomised trial might be relevant for those who have a definite preference for acupuncture.

Preference trials are appropriate for many questions related to acupuncture research, because they accurately reflect daily practice (where patients generally make their own decision to opt into or out of treatments), because expectation might influence the effectiveness of the treatment, and because it may be ethically inappropriate to allocate patients randomly to acupuncture or an alternative treatment when they have overriding preference for one or the other. However, only limited conclusions may be drawn from the results because often it is not possible to avoid the measurement bias from the patient's expectations.

There is a series of German randomised trials of acupuncture in routine care (Acupuncture in Routine Care, ARC), which consist of a non-randomised cohort arm in parallel with a randomised trial. These preference trials asked people with a variety of health conditions, including cervical and lumbar pain, headache and osteoarthritis, if they were willing to be randomised. If so, they were randomised to receive either immediate acupuncture or delayed acupuncture after 3 months. If they did not agree to randomisation, they were enrolled in the cohort study and treated immediately. Box 7.6 describes the results of the ARC study of acupuncture for neck pain. Interestingly, the results suggest that the effects of acupuncture outside a clinical trial are little if any different from those of acupuncture in a randomised controlled trial.

Box 7.6   Acupuncture for patients with chronic neck pain: a patient preference trial (Witt et al 2006a)

Witt et al (2006a) conducted a 'preference' study of acupuncture for chronic neck pain in routine care. They recruited 14 161 patients from 4005 physician acupuncturists. Of those, 1880 patients were randomised to acupuncture, 1886 to the delayed acupuncture control, and 10 395 patients did not consent to randomisation and received acupuncture immediately in the non-randomised cohort study undertaken alongside the trial. Acupuncture treatment included up to 15 acupuncture sessions over 3 months. Among trial participants, acupuncture was superior to no acupuncture at the end of 3 months. In addition, the proportion of treatment responders was similar in both the immediate acupuncture arm of the trial and the non-randomised cohort study.

Cost-effectiveness studies

As healthcare expenses climb, studies that collect information on both costs and benefits (or harms) of treatments are valuable in helping make the best use of resources in the most equitable manner. Acupuncture is inexpensive in equipment, though expensive in practitioner time. Possible areas to be considered for cost savings with acupuncture include a reduced need for drugs, a reduced need for referral for other secondary care, and reduced costs of adverse effects of other treatment, such as gastrointestinal haemorrhage caused by non-steroidal anti-inflammatory drugs.

Acupuncture is likely to be used as an additional treatment in patients who have not responded to other care, for example for musculoskeletal conditions. In this case, the relevant question is whether the benefit gained from acupuncture is worth the additional cost. In other cases, acupuncture might be offered as an alternative treatment, in which case the relevant research question is how the outcomes and costs of the two treatments compare. The benefit may be expressed in terms of monetary value, which amounts to a 'cost-benefit' analysis. More usually, the economic evaluation is usually performed as a 'cost-effectiveness' or 'cost-utility' analysis, i.e. the cost incurred in improving the quality of life. This is assessed by a standard method, the Quality Adjusted Life Year (QALY) which is crude but can be applied to all conditions and all interventions. The QALY is the number of additional years of life gained (regarded as one in conditions treated by acupuncture, which does not prolong life) multiplied by the health status measured on a standard scale from zero (death) to one (full active health). Conventional medical treatments typically cost significantly less than £30 000 per QALY, and those costing more are only considered in exceptional cases.

There are actually few economic analyses of acupuncture. A systematic review of economic analyses of complementary medicine by White & Ernst (2000) identified four studies of acupuncture that included measures of costs, only two of which were clinical trials (the preferred venue for conducting valid economic analyses because actual costs can be measured). However, none of these studies was actually designed to measure costs prospectively and thus, there are always concerns that the costs may not have been measured with equal accuracy in both groups (White 1996). More recently, Herman et al (2005) examined cost-effectiveness studies of complementary (and alternative) medicine conducted since 1999 and identified three acupuncture clinical trials that included economic analyses (Liguori et al 2000, Paterson et al 2003, Wonderling et al 2004).

Boxes 7.7 and 7.8 describe the results from two cost-effectiveness analyses undertaken as part of the large pragmatic trials described in Boxes 7.2 and 7.3. A cost-effectiveness analysis from the chronic neck pain trial of the ARC studies has recently been published (Willich et al 2006) and found results similar to those described in Boxes 7.7 and 7.8.

Deciding whether a treatment is worth the cost depends on the perspective(s) from which the analysis is undertaken. For example, society

Box 7.7 Cost-effectiveness of acupuncture for chronic headache (Wonderling et al 2004)

In the cost-effectiveness analysis that accompanied the trial described in Box 7.2, the authors found that average total costs were higher for the acupuncture group because of the costs of acupuncture itself. However, the formal economic analysis was undertaken in terms of cost per QALY. This incremental measure of cost-effectiveness was found to be £9180 per QALY, but may be an underestimate, because it did not consider cost savings associated with lower use of prescription drugs and higher work productivity. The authors conclude that if healthcare decision-makers are willing to pay up to £30 000 to gain one QALY, then acupuncture for chronic headache is very likely to be cost-effective.

Box 7.8 Cost-effectiveness of acupuncture for persistent low back pain (Ratcliffe et al 2006)

This cost-effectiveness analysis was conducted as part of the clinical trial described in Box 7.3. The costs of care were higher in the acupuncture group, with the average incremental gain per QALY being £4241. The authors note that acupuncture is likely to be cost-effective if healthcare decision-makers set the threshold for cost-effectiveness at £20 000 per QALY gained.

will be willing to pay more for a treatment that has a higher chance of enabling the patient to return to profitable work. However, return to work will not be relevant for the insurer or health service who will have to balance the costs of competing demands. By contrast, the individual patient will probably put a high premium on having symptoms relieved and function restored. The duration of the benefit has a powerful influence on the value of the treatment.

REMAINING CHALLENGES AND POTENTIAL STRATEGIES

Readers will have noticed the variation in choice of the comparison group in the studies that have been summarised in this chapter. This is often a difficult decision to make, and depends entirely on framing a precise and focused research question, which in turn depends on the condition, and may have to be a balance between what one would theoretically like to know and what is achievable and ethical. For example, medication is not very effective at preventing migraine headaches and therefore not often offered: acupuncture could be compared with no treatment. But medication can be very effective in treating an acute episode of migraine and it would be unethical to compare acupuncture with anything but usual treatment. For another example, back pain may not be particularly well managed with the treatments available in primary care, and society may be interested to know whether it would be worth spending additional resources on new treatments; in this case, acupuncture might be compared both to massage and to manipulation in the same study.

Patient selection

There are a number of remaining design challenges in clinical trials comparing acupuncture to other forms of care. One important question is how much to constrain the eligibility criteria for a study. In general, if the trial is testing the efficacy of an intervention under ideal conditions, then more stringent selection criteria are appropriate. However, if the trial is more about the value of acupuncture in routine care compared to other forms of care, broader inclusion criteria are preferred.

Acupuncture treatment

Important challenges arise in specifying the treatment under study in both explanatory and pragmatic trials. Within the context of explanatory trials, a number of creative solutions have been proposed to researchers beyond using a fixed treatment protocol for all individuals (Sherman & Cherkin 2003a, 2003b) and some of these are discussed in greater detail in Chapter 9. Within the context of pragmatic trials, a number of questions logically arise before the protocol can be fully described.

Will there, for example, be any limits on the styles of practice to be included in a particular study? Or on the elements of treatment that may be included (for example, excluding herbal medicine or self-care recommendations)? Or the qualifications and experience of the practitioners? Wrestling to make protocol constraints reasonable becomes especially important when investigating acupuncture in countries or communities where there is substantial variation in practice. To date, all pragmatic studies have included some constraints on the nature of the treatments provided. Constraints on the number of treatments in these trials probably reflect what insurers are willing to reimburse. Constraints on the elements of a particular style of acupuncture may reflect what providers commonly use (e.g. needle acupuncture among UK physiotherapists). The proscription against Chinese herbal medicine in pragmatic trials in the US has reflected the impossibility of getting regulatory approval to conduct research on Chinese herbal medicine in the individualised way it is typically practised. Most Western trials of a particular 'style' of acupuncture have focused on traditional Chinese medicine or on contemporary styles of acupuncture, such as trigger point needling.

As mentioned in the section above on mixed trials, one way to decide on a protocol for treatment is for a committee to ask experts for their opinions and then agree a consensus. There are some more elaborate methods for consensus of experts, which may be more reliable: they involve asking experts their opinions, feeding back the opinions of the other experts (anonymously), then again asking their opinions. The feedback takes the form of a live discussion in the 'nominal group' method (MacPherson & Schroer 2007), and simply summaries of opinions in the Delphi method which can be conducted by mail or email. However, with all these methods, there is no way to ensure that the consensus that is eventually achieved is anything other than a consensus of ignorance. The only reliable way is by direct comparison of the methods in clinical trials.

Once a pragmatic trial of acupuncture has been completed, it is important to describe the treatments provided so that readers can evaluate how representative they appear of acupuncture treatments for the condition under study (Sherman et al (2001) and MacPherson et al (2004) are examples of such reports). Comparisons of trial treatments to treatments for the same condition from a randomly selected sample of practitioners might allow a more formal assessment of how representative these treatments are of usual practice.

Many new clinical trials designed to evaluate the use of acupuncture as an adjunct to usual care actually include three study arms: acupuncture, sham acupuncture and usual care (for example the German GERAC and ART trials). Such studies allow one to answer two useful questions in the same study: does acupuncture treatment provide clinically useful benefits beyond usual care, and what are the relative contributions of acupuncture 'needling' and other aspects of acupuncture care? Each question addresses 'stakeholders' with different interests in the outcomes of acupuncture research. While the first question may appeal more to patients, acupuncture practitioners and some biomedical healthcare providers, the second is considered more important by many biomedical researchers and many physicians. The first question may be of more use to insurers in deciding to fund acupuncture on the grounds that it is superior to usual care. However, this decision may be undermined by subsequent studies showing acupuncture and sham acupuncture to be similar in benefit. The 'real' acupuncture arms of many of these studies have included a list of approved acupuncture points from which practitioners could select appropriate points (Haake et al 2003, Linde et al 2006, Molsberger et al 2006) but, in principle, there is no reason why even less constrained treatments could be included.

Qualitative research in quantitative trials

One newer trend in CAM clinical research is the addition of qualitative research as part of clinical trials (Conboy et al 2006). For example, one study explored the practitioner's approach to be based on building a therapeutic relationship; individualising care; and facilitating the active engagement of patients in their own recovery (MacPherson et al 2006). The use of qualitative methods to obtain information on the experience of treatment in the context of a trial may help us better interpret the results, especially in comparison to acupuncture care outside of a trial, and to see if there are other important outcomes of care that were not measured in the trial. This understanding can also be used to improve the design of subsequent studies.

TRANSLATING RESEARCH INTO CLINICAL PRACTICE

The results of pragmatic trials comparing acupuncture with usual care can more easily be generalised to the results that one would anticipate obtaining in practice at large. For example, the study of acupuncture for neck pain in a national sample of patients in Germany by Witt et al (2006a) demonstrated clinically similar results in people randomised to acupuncture in a clinical trial and those who chose acupuncture without being randomised. Such studies may provide the scientific rationale for policy decisions about access to acupuncture or reimbursement by health insurers. However, given the wide variety of treatments that could be administered in such studies, it is hard to imagine how these studies can lead to changes in the way acupuncture is practised unless future studies randomise people to different styles of acupuncture or to treatment arms permitting only certain elements of acupuncture care, so that different types of treatments can be compared to each other. Even in such studies, many details of the treatment protocol, which are considered essential to the success of a treatment, would likely be customised for each patient. Therefore the results of such studies would contain many uncertainties in their application to clinical practice, as it would usually be difficult to know which aspects of treatment contributed to its success.

Research resources

Fletcher R H, Fletcher S W, Wagner E H 1996 Clinical epidemiology: the essentials. Williams and Wilkins, London

Friedman L M, Finberg C D, DeMets D L 1998 Fundamentals of clinical trials. Springer, London

Hulley S R, Cummings S R (eds) 1988 Designing clinical research: an epidemiologic approach. Williams and Wilkins, London

MacPherson H 2004 Pragmatic clinical trials. Complementary Therapies in Medicine 12:136–140

References

Bombardier C, Maetzel A 1999 Pharmacoeconomic evaluation of new treatments: efficacy versus effectiveness studies? Annals of the Rheumatic Diseases 58(suppl 1):I82–I85

Brewin C R, Bradley C 1989 Patient preferences and randomised clinical trials. British Medical Journal 299:313–315

Brinkhaus B, Witt C M, Jena S et al 2006 Acupuncture in patients with chronic low back pain: a randomized controlled trial. Archives of Internal Medicine 166:450–457

Cherkin D C, Eisenberg D, Sherman K J et al 2001 Randomized trial comparing traditional Chinese medical acupuncture, therapeutic massage, and self-care education for chronic low back pain. Archives of Internal Medicine 161(8):1081–1088

Coeytaux R R, Kaufman J S, Kaptchuk T J et al 2005 A randomized, controlled trial of acupuncture for chronic daily headache. Headache 45:1113–1123

Conboy L A, Wasserman R H, Jacobson E E et al 2006 Investigating placebo effects in irritable bowel syndrome: a novel research design. Contemporary Clinical Trials 27:123–134

Diener H C, Kronfeld K, Boewing G et al 2006 Efficacy of acupuncture for the prophylaxis of migraine: a multicentre randomised controlled clinical trial. Lancet Neurology 5:310–316

Farrar J T 2006 Efficacy of acupuncture with physical therapy for knee osteo-arthritis. Ongoing clinical trail identified in ClinicalTrials.gov

Fønnebø V, Grimsgaard D, Walach H et al 2007 Research complementary and alternative therapies — the gatekeepers are not at home. BMC Medical Research Methodology 7:7

Friedman L, Furberg C D, Demets D L 1998 Fundamentals of clinical trails. Springer, New York

Glasgow R E, Davidson K W, Dobkin P L et al 2006 Practical behavioral trials to advance evidence-based behavioral medicine. Annals of Behavioral Medicine 31:5–13

Haake M, Muller H H, Schade-Brittinger C et al 2003 The German multicenter, randomized, partially blinded, prospective trial of acupuncture for chronic low-back pain: a preliminary report on the rationale and design of the trial. Journal of Alternative and Complementary Medicine 9:763–770

Hay E, Barlas P, Foster N 2004 Is acupuncture a useful adjunct to physiotherapy for older adults with knee pain?: the 'acupuncture, physiotherapy and exercise' (APEX) study. BMC Musculoskeletal Disorders 5:31

Herman P M, Craig B M, Caspi O 2005 Is complementary and alternative medicine (CAM) cost-effective? A systematic review. BMC Complementary and Alternative Medicine 5:11

Hesse J, Mogelvang B, Simonsen H 1994 Acupuncture versus metoprolol in migraine prophylaxis: a randomized trial of trigger point inactivation. Journal of Internal Medicine 235(5):451–456

Jadad A 1998 Randomized controlled trials. A users guide. BMJ Group, London

Levin J S, Glass T A, Kushi L H et al 1997 Quantitative methods in research on complementary and alternative medicine. A methodological manifesto. NIH Office of Alternative Medicine. Medical Care 35(11):1079–1094

Liguori A, Petti F, Bangrazi A et al 2000 Comparison of pharmacological treatment versus acupuncture treatment for migraine without aura — analysis of socio-medical parameters. Journal of Traditional Chinese Medicine 20:231–240

Linde K, Streng A, Hoppe A et al 2006 Treatment in a randomized multicenter trial of acupuncture for migraine (ART migraine). Forschende Komplementarmedizin 13:101–108

MacPherson H 2004 Pragmatic clinical trials. Complementary Therapies in Medicine 12:136–140

MacPherson H, Schroer S 2007 Acupuncture as a complex intervention for depression: a consensus method to develop a standardised treatment protocol for a randomised controlled trial. Complementary Therapies in Medicine 15(2):92–100

MacPherson H, Thorpe L, Thomas K et al 2004 Acupuncture for low back pain: traditional diagnosis and treatment of 148 patients in a clinical trial. Complementary Therapies in Medicine 12:38–44

MacPherson H, Thorpe L, Thomas K 2006 Beyond needling – therapeutic processes in acupuncture care; a qualitative study nested within a low back pain trial. Journal of Alternative and Complementary Medicine 12(9):873–880

March J S, Silva S G, Compton S et al 2005 The case for practical clinical trials in psychiatry. American Journal of Psychiatry 162:836–846

Melchart D, Streng A, Hoppe A et al 2005 Acupuncture in patients with tension-type headache: randomised controlled trial. British Medical Journal 331:376–382

Meng C F, Wang D, Ngeow J et al 2003 Acupuncture for chronic low back pain in older patients: a randomized, controlled trial. Rheumatology (Oxford) 42:1508–1517

Molsberger A F, Boewing G, Diener H C et al 2006 Designing an acupuncture study: the nationwide, randomized, controlled, German acupuncture trials on migraine and tension-type headache. Journal of Alternative and Complementary Medicine 12:237–245

Paterson C, Ewings P, Brazier J E et al 2003 Treating dyspepsia with acupuncture and homeopathy: reflections on a pilot study by researchers, practitioners and participants. Complementary Therapies in Medicine 11:78–84

Ratcliffe J, Thomas K J, MacPherson H 2006 A randomised controlled trial of acupuncture care for persistent low back pain: cost effectiveness analysis. British Medical Journal 333:626

Scharf H P, Mansmann U, Streitberger K et al 2006 Acupuncture and knee osteoarthritis: a three-armed randomized trial. Annals of Internal Medicine 145:12–20

Sherman K J, Cherkin D C 2003a Challenges of acupuncture research: study design considerations. Clinical Acupuncture and Oriental Medicine. An International Journal 3:200–206

Sherman K J, Cherkin D C 2003b Developing methods for acupuncture research: rationale for and design of a pilot study evaluating the efficacy of acupuncture for chronic low back pain. Alternative Therapies in Health and Medicine 9:54–60

Sherman K J, Cherkin D C, Hogeboom C J 2001 The diagnosis and treatment of patients with chronic low-back pain by traditional Chinese medical acupuncturists. Journal of Alternative and Complementary Medicine 7(6):641–650

Streitberger K, Witte S, Mansmann U et al 2004 Efficacy and safety of acupuncture for chronic pain caused by gonarthrosis: a study protocol of an ongoing multi-centre randomised controlled clinical trial. BMC Complementary and Alternative Medicine 4:6

Thomas K J, MacPherson H, Thorpe L et al 2006 Randomised controlled trial of a short course of traditional acupuncture compared with usual care for persistent non-specific low back pain. British Medical Journal 333:623

Vickers A, Cassileth B, Ernst E et al 1997 How should we research unconventional therapies? A panel report from the Conference on Complementary and Alternative Medicine Research Methodology, National Institutes of Health. International Journal of Technology Assessment in Health Care 13(1):111–121

Vickers A J, Rees R W, Zollman C E et al 2004 Acupuncture for chronic headache in primary care: large, pragmatic, randomised trial. British Medical Journal 328:744–747

White A 1996 Economic evaluation of acupuncture. Acupuncture in Medicine 14:109–113

White AR, Ernst E 2000 Economic analysis of complementary medicine: a systematic review. Complementary Therapies in Medicine 8(2):111–118

Willich S N, Reinhold T, Selim D et al 2006 Cost-effectiveness of acupuncture treatment in patients with chronic neck pain. Pain 125:107–113

Witt C, Brinkhaus B, Jena S et al 2005 Acupuncture in patients with osteoarthritis of the knee: a randomised trial. Lancet 366:136–143

Witt C M, Jena S, Brinkhaus B et al 2006a Acupuncture for patients with chronic neck pain. Pain 125:98–106

Witt C M, Jena S, Selim D et al 2006b Pragmatic randomized trial evaluating the clinical and economic effectiveness of acupuncture for chronic low back pain. American Journal of Epidemiology 164:487–496

Wonderling D, Vickers A J, Grieve R et al 2004 Cost effectiveness analysis of a randomised trial of acupuncture for chronic headache in primary care. British Medical Journal 328:747

Investigating the components of acupuncture treatment

8

Peter White, Klaus Linde and Rosa N. Schnyer

OVERVIEW

This chapter focuses on the investigation of the components of acupuncture treatment and examines some of the problems associated with this particular area of research. It examines the tension between the conventional medical model of assessing efficacy by the use of the randomised placebo-controlled trial and a fresh and more global approach that seeks to build and expand on the conventional reductionist paradigm. This innovative view seeks to embrace, rather than screen out, the elements of treatment which many conventional researchers regard as 'background noise'. In this emerging view, the interplay between patient, practitioner, the needle and even the diagnostic process are all regarded as integral parts of the whole treatment. Thus to break this unit down into separate entities is to negate a treatment which has developed over millennia. This more 'global' approach might also be useful as a tool to assess therapies other than acupuncture.

INTRODUCTION

Acupuncture continues to increase in popularity with more and more people turning to this ancient therapy as time goes on. This increasing popularity and acceptance of acupuncture, however, is occurring in spite of relatively little sound or strong evidence to support the efficacy of acupuncture for many conditions. People are therefore continuing to return for treatment with little proof, in scientific terms, of whether acupuncture works or not.

The question of 'does it work' is not always straightforward to answer and there are several ways to look at this. Two elements which are particularly important are effect versus efficacy (see section on effect and efficacy below). Which is more important largely depends on the viewpoint of the interested party but there might very well be a difference between these two. Conventional scientists are very often much more interested in efficacy, i.e. 'Does acupuncture perform better than a placebo?' because this tends to suggest that there is some specific active ingredient or element to the treatment that can be separated and pinpointed. Patients, on the other hand, tend to be more concerned with effect, i.e. 'Will the treatment make me better?' and are less concerned with the details as to why or how this improvement occurs. Acupuncture trials often show very large effects whereby patients seem to gain a great benefit from treatment but, equally often, efficacy tends to be marginal when acupuncture is tested against a 'placebo' treatment. This phenomenon would suggest at least a dual action to explain how acupuncture might work, i.e. a 'specific' effect (illustrated by efficacy) and a 'non-specific' effect, these two together demonstrating the overall clinical effect.

It is important for several reasons to be able to answer the question 'Does acupuncture work?' as well as other related questions that add to our knowledge base. First, from an ethical perspective, when a health professional is asked by a patient whether acupuncture 'works' or if a health professional decides to recommend acupuncture treatment, this must be done in an informed way. Simply relying on anecdotal evidence is far from satisfactory and is likely to provide biased information. The correct use of resources must also be a consideration here and the use of public money, whether for healthcare or research (e.g. National Health Service, NHS; National Institutes of Health, NIH), must be justified. Similarly, it would be considered unethical to encourage patients to spend their own money in the private sector on a treatment that has evidence of no effect. This ethos has, in part, driven the desire to isolate the 'active ingredient' in any given treatment from its non-specific element. 'Non-specific' (placebo) effects are considered to be a relevant component of all healthcare interventions. However, as stated in the House of Lords' sixth Science and Technology Report, 'any discipline whose practitioners make specific claims for being able to treat specific conditions should have evidence of being able to do this above and beyond the placebo effect' (www/parliament.the-stationery-office/co.uk/pa). The report considers this especially true for therapies that seek coverage by health insurance and funding bodies such as the NHS in the UK and the NIH in the US. Practitioners of all disciplines are being encouraged to justify what they do, hence evidence-based practice is important, particularly in the current climate of litigation. Last, from a research perspective, if efficacy is proven it would be reasonable to try to understand how this treatment works, for the sake of improving treatment, enhancing benefits and developing other treatments along similar lines. If efficacy cannot be proven, research on mechanism would justifiably be viewed as a waste of resources.

In summary, it has conventionally been seen as important to be able to break down the effect of acupuncture treatment into its component parts, the 'specific' and 'non-specific' elements in order to better understand how it works and to provide more informed advice to patients. This chapter examines different ways to gather and interpret evidence on this question looking first from a purist and conventional 'scientific' point of view and then from a broader perspective.

THE CONVENTIONAL SCIENTIFIC APPROACH

The conventional researcher would test acupuncture by conducting a placebo-controlled trial, based on logic that assumes there is one active ingredient in a treatment. In a drug trial for example, this would be the active chemical in a tablet. In an acupuncture trial, by analogy, the active ingredient is usually considered to be the action of the needle on the acupuncture point. All other parts of the treatment process are thought to be, in effect, background noise which needs to be screened out or controlled for. In this way the active element of treatment can be isolated. Therefore if patients are allocated to one of two groups, both of which are treated in exactly the same way with the exception that one of the groups has the active ingredient and the other does not, then these two groups can be compared. If there is a difference between these groups in terms of effect, then logically speaking, this can only be attributed to the presence or absence of the active element (assuming the trial is correctly set up, minimising bias). If there is no difference, then it is assumed that the treatment being tested has no effect, i.e. there is no 'specific effect'. Efficacy is therefore not demonstrated and hence the conclusion is that acupuncture is simply a placebo treatment. One of the challenges to this logic, as will be discussed later, is its circular reasoning: without being certain of what constitutes the 'active ingredient' of acupuncture, it is difficult to design an appropriate 'inactive' control.

There have been a great many trials conducted that have attempted to assess the efficacy of acupuncture and many of these have demonstrated either minimal or no efficacy when compared to placebo intervention (Assefi et al 2005, Gallacchi et al 1981, Gaw et al 1975, Linde et al 2005, Mendelson et al 1983). The conventional scientist would therefore suggest that in these cases, acupuncture has no place in the treatment of the particular condition being tested.

Whether this evaluation is correct or not will also depend on many other factors, a major one being that of bias, i.e. was the trial set up so as to be objective and balanced? Other factors include whether the methodology was appropriate to answer the question being posed and whether the treatment was adequate, given the current state of knowledge.

Potential sources of bias in RCTs and problems with validity

BLINDING

The measurement of outcomes in clinical trials is often prone to bias, particularly if outcomes are subjective such as pain, function or quality of life. Therefore, it is desirable that as many parties involved in a trial are unaware (blinded) as to which group a participant was allocated. Because practitioners are an integral part of the treatment process in an acupuncture trial and delivers a manual intervention, it is virtually impossible to blind them. Acupuncture is a fluid treatment modality, requiring practitioners to react to changes in symptoms and adapt treatment accordingly. This might lead the practitioners, especially if they have a vested interest in the outcome, to systematically treat one group of patients differently from another. They might be very enthusiastic with the acupuncture group and not so with the control, thus imparting their own viewpoint to the patient. This in turn might influence outcome. Equally, if patients know to which group they have been allocated, they might also bias results particularly if they have a strong opinion about the treatment under question. One method to address this potential bias would be to ensure that the researcher and practitioner are not one and the same. Outcomes should also be measured by a blinded assessor and if this is not possible then patient-completed measures should be used and completed without input from the researcher. Similarly, analyses should be performed by a statistician blinded to the allocation. Many people believe that double-blind automatically means that providers and patients are blinded. However, often trials in which patients and outcome assessors are blinded but not providers are also described as double-blind. Readers should not be confused by this but must always check to ascertain who actually was blinded in a clinical trial. At the end of the treatment period, a simple check can be performed to ensure that blinding was adequate, i.e. to ask the participants to record whether they felt that their intervention had been real or control. In a parallel arm trial, there should be no statistical difference between the two groups in how they answer this question, although it should be acknowledged that even if the interventions are in fact identical, some subjects would cite them as being 'different' just by random chance alone.

TREATMENT

The nature of the treatment regime could also introduce bias and particularly so if this is sub-standard. Clearly a poor treatment would be less likely to be able to demonstrate efficacy. There are a number of trials involving acupuncture interventions where there can be no doubt that the 'true' acupuncture intervention was inadequate. For example, three trials for neck pain used only one treatment session for a chronic condition which is far from normal practice (Kreczi & Klingler 1986, Lundeberg et al 1991, Thomas et al 1991). One method to minimise this problem would be to ensure that the treatment regimen has been through a process of consultation with relevant experts. The question of which 'type' of treatment should be employed is open for debate. So far, there is little evidence that individualised treatment strategies are superior to more standardised approaches, however an individualised treatment would tend to reflect everyday care. Equally there is no evidence to suggest that there is any superiority in terms of effect between a Westernised and a traditional Chinese medicine format.

RANDOMISATION AND CONCEALED ALLOCATION

Failure to randomly allocate subjects to treatment group could also be a major source of bias, which can lead to gross overestimation of the effectiveness of treatment (Schulz et al 1995). When assessing efficacy it is important that both groups are, as far as possible, identical in every aspect. This is best achieved by randomly allocating patients to each group. If this is not done the researcher could allocate patients to each group on the basis of patient preference or on criteria such as whether it was felt a subject would obtain better results from one form of treatment relative to another. Furthermore, certain 'known' prognostic factors can be spread equally between groups by employing a system of stratification for key variables (e.g. baseline pain levels), thus ensuring balance. Randomisation therefore ensures that both known and, hopefully, unknown prognostic factors are equally distributed (Ernst & White 1997). A frequently used technique for concealing allocation from practitioners and investigators, in trials of acupuncture, involved sealed envelopes which contain the allocation information and are opened only after inclusion. While adequate in principle this technique is not fully safe therefore an increasingly used technique involves phoning an independent central randomisation centre.

INTENTION-TO-TREAT ANALYSIS

In placebo-controlled trials researchers try to minimise the risk of a false-positive result (considering the intervention as superior to placebo while, in reality, it is not). In the past researchers sometimes excluded patients in the intervention group who had a bad outcome and patients in the control group who had a good outcome from the analysis. Obviously, this severely biases the results. This can also be the case if patients drop out from the study for reasons which differ between groups (for example if there are many side effects from the treatment). Therefore, placebo-controlled trials are analysed according to the intention-to-treat principle, that is, all patients randomised (or in some trials, only all patients who at least started treatment) are included in the analysis in the group to which they were allocated, and if post-treatment or follow-up data are lacking they are replaced, for example, with baseline data or the last recorded data available.

INCLUSION/EXCLUSION CRITERIA

The make-up of the recruited patients must be appropriate for the question being asked. This is also important in terms of generalisation, i.e. being able to extrapolate the results of a trial to the general population. An efficacy study must therefore recruit patients in an appropriate way so as to target participants most likely to meet the study criteria. The inclusion and exclusion criteria must be well thought out and justifiable. Failure to consider these factors may result in an inappropriate group and would therefore be another source of bias.

SAMPLE SIZE

Finally, too small a sample size has been a major problem in many acupuncture trials and therefore the number of patients recruited must be large enough to adequately answer the question. In the past, there was little funding and most trials were performed at a single centre; trials were often strongly depended on the enthusiasm, capacities and resources of single investigators or small groups. In consequence the majority of acupuncture trials probably included less than 50 patients. This can provide very useful information if the study is designed as a pilot in order to inform a subsequent larger trial, however a 'definitive' trial must be adequately powered. In order to find significant differences between acupuncture and sham interventions in small studies, effects must be very large (or variability very low). And most findings from rigorous large trials suggest that differences (if any) are small for many conditions.

DEFINITIONS AND TERMINOLOGY

Placebo

The placebo is an important element when evaluating efficacy. It is generally defined as an inactive substance (drug or procedure) designed to satisfy or 'please' the patient. This means that it has no *intrinsic* therapeutic value. In the context of a clinical trial to evaluate efficacy it is important to assess whether there is some intrinsic or 'active' element to the treatment in question (often assumed to be acupuncture needling) and whether this is responsible for the improvement. The alternative (conventional) explanation for an observed clinical effect is that it is not due to an 'active ingredient' associated with needling but is assumed to be something else such as the patient's will to improve, the context of the treatment, the process of diagnosis, the use of explanations, the lifestyle advice, etc. Thus, comparing acupuncture needling to an intervention which appears to be the same in all respects, but has no 'active' ingredient, effectively controls for all these other elements and is vital to answer the question of efficacy.

Therein lies a problem. In a drug trial, the active ingredient to be tested is usually a chemical of some sort and it is a fairly simple matter to produce a tablet which looks the same as the real drug but does not contain the chemical in question. In the case of complex physical treatments such as surgery, chiropractic manipulations or acupuncture, this is very much harder and aspects of the interventions not considered crucial to the procedure are often used to serve as placebos. For example, in a trial of arthroscopic knee surgery patients in the placebo group only received a skin incision (Mosely et al 2002).

Designing suitable controls for acupuncture is problematic for two reasons. First, it is not known what the 'active' ingredient of acupuncture is. It could be the insertion of a needle into an acupuncture point, the manipulation of the needle to generate *De Qi* sensation, the pressure exerted over the acupuncture point when locating it or a whole range of components, those listed as well as others, acting separately or in concert. Second, because acupuncture is a manual treatment involving an invasive element, it is extremely difficult to design a convincing placebo which fully mimics the real intervention yet does not stimulate an acupuncture point in some way. Various novel attempts have been made to achieve this which has resulted in a great many acupuncture controls (Box 8.1).

Effect and efficacy

Effect can be defined as the overall improvement from a baseline value as a result of receiving a course of treatment. For example if patients experience an overall 50% reduction in their pain from the start of the treatment to the end of treatment, then this would be the effect and is independent of the control arm. Efficacy on the other hand is an evaluation of whether acupuncture is better than a placebo (equivalent in all respects but inert). Efficacy tells us whether it is the intrinsic therapeutic action of needling itself that causes the improvement or whether the change in clinical picture is due to some other element.

Specific and non-specific effects

The 'non-specific' effects (sometimes called placebo effects) can be very powerful indeed and are usually a net result of many different factors. The

Box 8.1   Sham interventions in randomised clinical trials of acupuncture (Dincer & Linde 2003)

In 2003 Dincer and Linde (2003) reviewed the sham interventions used in 47 randomised trials of acupuncture for chronic pain and a variety of other conditions. Trials were collected from systematic reviews and from PubMed searches. Details of patients, interventions, sham interventions and outcomes were extracted in a standardised manner. In two trials the sham intervention consisted of superficial needling of the true acupuncture points, four trials used true acupuncture points which were not indicated for the condition being treated, in 27 trials needles were inserted outside true acupuncture points, five trials used non-penetrating 'placebo needles' and nine trials used pseudo-interventions such as switched-off laser acupuncture devices. True and sham interventions often differed in a variety of other variables, such as manipulation of needles, depth of insertion, achievement of *De Qi*, etc. There was no clear association between the sham intervention used and the results of a trial, for example, differences between true and sham acupuncture were similar in trials with and without skin penetration in the sham group. In summary, it is obvious that randomised clinical trials of acupuncture have used a great variety of sham interventions as controls. The authors concluded that summarising all the different sham interventions as 'placebo' controls seems misleading and scientifically unacceptable.

context in which the treatment is given may very well have a profound effect on outcome. Acupuncture is a manual treatment involving ritual, physical contact and invasive perturbations that are independent of needle placement. Such non-specific effects are generally believed to generate large 'placebo' effects. Other factors that might play a role could be the interaction between the patient and practitioner, the appearance and demeanour of the practitioner and perhaps even the appearance of the clinic in which the treatment is given to name a few. The expectation of the patients, i.e. what they believe will happen, might also have an influence. All of these factors may well feed into the overall effect experienced by patients, but all are usually considered 'non-specific'. In contrast, the 'specific' effect is usually considered to be that caused by the 'active element' of acupuncture treatment or the intrinsic therapeutic action of the needle and its influence on an acupuncture point (see efficacy above). Any overall 'effect' of acupuncture experienced by patients will comprise both a 'specific' and 'non-specific' component. An assessment of efficacy (through the use of placebo controls) therefore seeks to split those components and evaluate the influence of each. The difference in the outcome of the group of patients receiving the true treatment (verum) and those receiving the placebo treatment is considered the 'specific' effect (see Fig. 8.1).

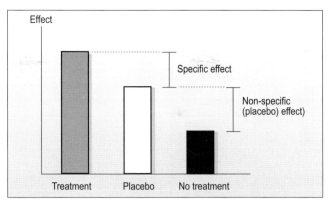

Fig 8.1 The conventional concept of 'specific' and 'non-specific' (placebo) effects.

It should be pointed out that the 'specific' effect under examination will depend on the hypothesis being tested, which can vary from experiment to experiment, i.e. it will not always be based on testing the effect of the acupuncture needle on the acupuncture point. For example, a study might be designed to test the hypothesis that treatment in a quiet and tranquil setting will achieve better results than treatment on a busy ward. The setting is the independent variable and is thus the 'specific' effect in this context. Many practitioners of acupuncture define the specificity of the treatment in a much broader sense which includes elements that are conventionally considered to be 'non-specific'. Therein lies a major difference in assumptions between some researchers of traditional acupuncture and other researchers with a biomedical background (see Chapter 9).

Natural history of the condition and regression to the mean

In any group of patients, there will be changes which occur naturally over time, regardless of the intervention given. This will be due to the natural history of the disease (symptoms will often wax and wane) or regression to the mean which is the tendency of extreme values (such as pain) to return to more 'normal' levels. Often all such changes over time observed in the placebo group are called 'non-specific' or placebo effects. For example, the often cited 35.2% in the most famous publication on the topic, 'The powerful placebo' by Henry Beecher (1955), is simply the average change over time in the placebo control group of a number of arbitrarily collected trials. It is obvious that such an approach is problematic. If patients in the placebo group of a trial who suffer from common cold become free of symptoms after 4 weeks, most people would probably attribute this improvement to the spontaneous course of the illness rather than being an effect of the placebo intervention. To separate placebo or 'non-specific' effects of an intervention from the natural history of disease, regression to the mean, or the effects of co-interventions, an untreated control group is needed (Hrobjartsson & Gotzsche 2001).

COMMONLY USED CONTROL PROCEDURES IN ACUPUNCTURE RESEARCH

Studies into acupuncture have been conducted over many years but it is only as we have come to understand more about acupuncture that we have been able to alter and refine trial design in order to gain more meaningful results. The model of the randomised controlled trial (RCT) has typically been the mainstay in terms of methodology but the fact that there has been no proven placebo for acupuncture has been a problem and has often confounded research findings.

Use of 'non-acupuncture' points (sham acupuncture)

Many early researchers, not unreasonably, assumed that acupuncture would only work when a needle was inserted into an acupuncture point. It therefore seemed logical that insertion of a needle into a non-acupuncture point would be a placebo and so several trials were conducted in this way (Assefi et al 2005, Christensen et al 1984, Forbes et al 2005, Lee et al 1975, Melchart et al 2005). When acupuncture failed to perform better than this control it was assumed that acupuncture had no efficacy. The problem in part was the lack of a coherent theory to explain how acupuncture worked from a Western scientific paradigm. The present-day understanding of non-specific effects of needling suggests that placing a needle anywhere in the body induces physiological effects through a variety of mechanisms including local alteration in circulation and immune function as well as neurophysiological and neurochemical responses. Box 8.2 describes one of these mechanisms as an example (diffuse noxious inhibitory control) (Le Bars et al 1991).

This means that there was a strong likelihood that the chosen 'placebo' was not a placebo at all and this might obviously have affected the results and conclusions of the trial, creating a strong chance of a false-negative outcome (a type II error).

Minimal acupuncture

To minimise the physiological effects of 'sham' acupuncture interventions, many researchers tried not only to insert the needles at non-acupuncture points, but also more superficially, without stimulation or manipulation to avoid eliciting De Qi sensations. These types of sham acupuncture are often called 'minimal acupuncture'. While it seems plausible that minimal acupuncture should be less active than a more intense

Box 8.2   Diffuse noxious inhibitory control (DNIC) (Le Bars et al 1991)

DNIC has been used to explain the non-segmental effects of acupuncture (Le Bars et al 1991). Basically, Le Bars suggests that dorsal horn neurons in the spinal cord are inhibited by a nociceptive afferent signal applied to any other part of the body. Therefore any applied painful or noxious stimulus (such as an acupuncture needle) will attenuate existing pain even in extra-segmental areas. It is suggested that this works by both peripheral and central systems. The peripheral system works via A delta and C fibres and indeed the propagation of 'De Qi' is a sign of activation of the A delta fibres (Andersson 1993). If this sensation is blocked by the local injection of procaine, acupuncture is ineffective (Ceniceros & Brown 1998). The central mechanism is via descending inhibition from brainstem structures such as the Nucleus Raphe Magnus. In support of the involvement of 'higher' structures in this aspect of pain control is the fact that stimulation of the para-aqueductal grey (PAG) in the midbrain will inhibit responses of the spinal cord neurons to noxious stimuli (Andersson 1993). It is also suggested that endogenous opioids may participate in the DNIC mechanism (Bing et al 1990).

and full-depth sham acupuncture intervention it still is clearly not physiologically inert and might still have an effect through diffuse noxious inhibitory controls (DNIC).

Non-penetrating techniques

Other researchers have tried additional ways to mimic acupuncture in the control arm whilst simultaneously trying to minimise the 'specific' effect. Techniques such as blindfolding the patient and then pricking the skin with a cocktail stick, or the end of a guide tube have been tried (Molsberger & Hille 1994, White et al 2000). Again this would seem reasonable but the problem with this approach is that it is obvious to the patient that 'something underhand' is going on, as clearly it would not be normal clinical practice to blindfold patients. Also, the patient would not be able to see the needle in use. This might generate a different set of 'non-specific' effects. Also it is not known if the act of pricking the surface of the skin might have a 'specific' therapeutic effect or not.

Another non-invasive technique was employed which involved the application of mock electrical stimulation to acupuncture points (White et al 2004). This was usually achieved by using a decommissioned acupuncture stimulation unit or a transcutaneous electrical nerve stimulation (TENS) unit and fixing sticky electrodes to the surface of the skin, over the acupuncture point. Patients were led to believe that the electrodes stimulated the acupuncture point. A similar approach is the use of a switched-off laser acupuncture device. Whilst the intervention is inert, the problem with this is that again the 'non-specific' effects of this technique might be very different from real acupuncture. The outcome and integrity of any clinical trial may well be dependent upon the credibility of the control (Borkovec & Nau 1972, Zaslawski et al 1997).

A third non-invasive technique, developed more recently involves the use of dummy needles which look as though they have pierced the skin yet do not do so (Park et al 2002, Streitberger & Kleinhenz 1998) (see Box 8.3). It has the advantage of giving the same visual cues as real acupuncture and so the 'non-specific' effects associated with the patient's expectancy should be similar. The disadvantage of this technique is that it does cause a 'pricking' sensation and it has been suggested by some practitioners/researchers that this might stimulate the acupuncture point and therefore is not a placebo. Also because it employs a novel mechanism to hold the needle in place, this might arouse suspicion in some patients. Furthermore, this mechanism is not suitable for use on certain parts of the body (e.g. certain points on the fingers).

Box 8.3   Streitberger needle (Streitberger & Kleinhenz 1998)

This needle (Streitberger & Kleinhenz 1998) works exactly like a 'theatrical stage dagger'. The tip of the needle is blunt and the handle is hollow. As the needle is pushed against the skin, it causes a pricking sensation but as increased pressure is applied, the shaft of the needle disappears into the handle, mimicking a 'stage dagger'. This gives the impression that the needle is actually entering the skin. The needle is held in position by a mechanism including a small adhesive plastic ring and adhesive tape. The ring (approximately 6 mm in diameter) is placed over the acupuncture point and held in position on the body by the tape. The needle passes through the tape, through the middle of the 'O' ring and then touches the skin. The needle is therefore effectively held in position at two places, i.e. at the tape and at the skin. To aid consistency and credibility the tape and 'O' ring are also used with real needles that are identical in appearance.

It is clear that the issue of what is a placebo, in relation to acupuncture, is a much more complex question than originally thought. As we learn more about this technique, it might become apparent that it is not possible to design a placebo control in the conventional sense of the word. More work is needed to understand how acupuncture and placebos work before any firm conclusions can be drawn on this subject.

Assessing the credibility of the control

Where the control differs substantially from the treatment actually being examined, it is of prime importance that this credibility must be routinely assessed (Margolin et al 1998, Petrie & Hazleman 1985, Staebler et al 1994, Vincent 1990, Vincent & Lewith 1995). If this is not assessed and a study shows that there is a difference between acupuncture and a placebo, in favour of the active treatment, it could be argued that perhaps acupuncture is simply a more convincing placebo and therefore has a greater effect. It is therefore necessary to employ measures to assess equipoise of intervention, i.e. to check that the treatments are viewed by the patient as being similar, or equally credible to each other. This can be ascertained by comparing the expectancy of effectiveness of the real versus placebo treatment such as with the Borkovec and Nau 'credibility rating' (Borkovec & Nau 1972) or the newer 'credibility and expectancy' questionnaire (Devilly & Borkovec 2000).

THE BROADER VIEW — ARE ASSUMED NON-SPECIFIC EFFECTS OF ACUPUNCTURE ACTUALLY ACUPUNCTURE SPECIFIC?

For many years now acupuncture researchers have invested considerable thought and resources into finding the optimal placebo which is both indistinguishable from 'true' acupuncture and physiologically inert. While the development of better sham interventions should remain an important objective we should not be over-optimistic that this will resolve the problem of trials, in that sham acupuncture that is not inert is more likely to yield marginal or contradictory results. There is a growing opinion that complex treatments such as acupuncture cannot be easily broken down into its constituent parts because of the complicated interplay between many different elements (Paterson & Dieppe 2005, Ritenbaugh et al 2003, Verhoef et al 2005). Indeed some practitioners would go as far as to suggest that the patient, practitioner and the needle all form one unit and therefore are incapable of being viewed independently. Furthermore it is possible that these different elements interact so that the overall effect is greater than the simple sum of its constituent parts. If true, this would tend to further limit the scope for an evaluation based on reducing acupuncture to its component parts to those contexts where acupuncture is practised as a more simple intervention, perhaps for an acute condition such as for post-operative nausea.

All placebo effects are the same — or not?

Statements such as the one from the House of Lords' sixth Science and Technology Report cited in the introduction to this chapter implicitly assume that either all placebo responses are the same or that their size fluctuates only randomly. However, there is some evidence that some (physiologically inert) placebos are better than others (Kaptchuk et al 2000). In placebo research there are a number of trials using the so-called balanced placebo design (Kleijnen et al 1994). In such four-armed studies two treatments (for example, a pain killer and acupuncture) are compared with respective placebos (a drug placebo and a sham acupuncture intervention). An example of the findings of the trial might be as in Fig. 8.2: treatment A is clearly superior to its placebo (placebo A) while treatment B is the same as its placebo (placebo B). If these findings would come from two separate trials one would conclude that treatment A is clearly better than placebo while treatment B is not. The difference in overall effectiveness would typically be explained by differences in patient population. However, if coming from a four-armed trial the interpretation is more difficult. Overall, treatment B seems to be more effective than treatment A. The results further suggest that the size of 'non-specific' effects differs between the two placebos. But how should one define the difference between two 'non-specific' effects? It might laughably be called a 'specific non-specific' effect of placebo B but this is clearly confusing and unwieldy. This issue leads on to a fundamental problem of the placebo concept, or at least, of its common interpretation.

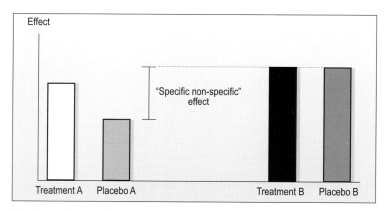

Fig 8.2   Findings of a hypothetical four-armed randomised trial.

Meaning response/context effect

A number of experts in the area of placebo research propose that the term 'placebo effect' should be replaced by concepts such as 'meaning response' or 'context effect' (Di Blasi & Kleijnen 2003). The meaning response is defined as the physiological or psychological effects of meaning in the origins or treatment of illness (Moerman & Jonas 2002). Any intervention is associated with expectations, intentions, understandings, or values, depending on individual patients and providers. Neurophysiological research has clearly shown that, for example, the expectation of a patient does not only modify the reporting of a patient but modifies the biological processes underlying pain perception in the brain (Pariente et al 2005). Epidemiological research has confirmed that factors such as expectation of a positive outcome, optimism or support have long-term impact on hard clinical end points independently of other predictors (Price et al 2006). It is obvious that the complex ritual of an acupuncture intervention with its repeated provider contacts, the possible micro trauma of needling and its (for a Westerner) 'exotic nature', is associated with quite different meanings and expectations than, for example, the prescription of a drug. In this concept a) it seems plausible to expect that acupuncture could be associated with a more powerful meaning response than a drug in many (but probably not all) patients; and b) some of these effects might be considered not undifferentiated noise but 'specific' and 'real' meaning responses provided they are integral to, and characteristic of, the acupuncture intervention. The term 'context effect' points to a similar understanding, as it implies that the context of a healthcare intervention can be highly variable but possibly influences the outcome of an intervention in a relevant manner.

Possible effects of co-interventions

An acupuncture treatment for a chronic disease is not only associated with frequent provider contacts but typically also with lying in a quiet room, hopefully relaxed, after the needles have been inserted. In a stressed headache patient this relaxation might contribute to the overall effect of an acupuncture intervention. Such an effect can hardly be interpreted as a meaning effect. Almost all sham interventions for acupuncture try to keep rest time, frequency of sessions, etc. comparable to the true treatment.

Direct physiological effects of the sham intervention

In addition to the meaning response and to potential effects of co-interventions the direct physiological effects of sham intervention discussed above might contribute to the overall effect observed in acupuncture trials.

Effects associated with an intervention

When considered together, meaning responses, effects of co-interventions and direct physiological effects might make sham interventions for acupuncture very powerful. The available evidence suggests that at least in chronic pain and a number of other conditions these effects might contribute more to the overall benefit than so-called 'specific' needling effects due to the correct location of points or achieving De Qi. Fig. 8.3 emphasises that different kinds of effects probably interact and therefore simple trials designed to isolate the needling components would be prone to fail.

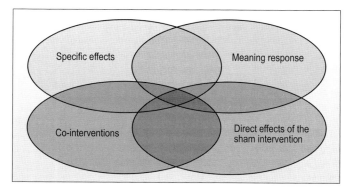

Fig 8.3 Different components contributing to the total effect of an acupuncture intervention.

Characteristic and incidental effects

The way to conceptualise what conventionally has been called 'placebo' effects as described above is not the only approach to address the problem. For example, Paterson and Dieppe (2005) differentiate characteristic and incidental effects. Characteristic factors are theoretically derived, unique to a specific treatment, and believed to be causally responsible for the outcome. However, they argue that some of what are normally considered incidental effects could be characteristic for a specific treatment. This is highlighted by other research whereby three elements of the acupuncture treatment process were highlighted as being integral to the whole process and important to outcome, i.e. the therapeutic relationship, individualised care and facilitating the active participation of patients in their own recovery (MacPherson et al 2006). While many of these processes of care would normally be considered 'non-specific', this research highlighted areas of the therapeutic relationship that were actually specific to acupuncture. The authors discuss for example the way acupuncturists use explanations from Chinese medical theory to build a stronger understanding in the patients about why they are ill and, in this context, what they might be able to do to enhance their self-care. Thus the therapeutic relationship can be considered to have aspects to it that are specific to and characteristic of acupuncture. A fuller description can be found in Box 9.7 in Chapter 9.

FUTURE RESEARCH

We would emphasise that we consider it crucial, for the future of acupuncture, to continue to investigate this modality using the randomised controlled trial for a range of questions including efficacy, correct point location, skin penetration, needling depth, and achieving *De Qi*, to test for a 'specific' difference. However, if such trials constantly fail to show differences, it will be important to examine the concept of the 'specific' effect in relation to acupuncture, i.e. is it actually possible to isolate a specific effect? At present it must be emphasised that we are unsure if a true 'placebo' for acupuncture exists or will ever be attainable, although work does continue in this field. It could be said therefore that efficacy trials are simply comparisons of two therapies one of which may lack certain elements considered important. To quantify the size of the effects associated with the sham or control interventions, additional 'no treatment' control groups are desirable as often as possible, although an additional arm will of course increase the cost of trials. Trials investigating whether manipulations of the context of an acupuncture intervention are needed, as are pragmatic trials comparing different types of acupuncture, e.g. individualised versus standardised acupuncture and finally, trials which compare acupuncture to current conventional treatment are important in order to place the effect of acupuncture in perspective. When considering acupuncture as a complex intervention, perhaps the time has come to revisit the 'importance' of the question of pure efficacy and to ask other questions that are more patient centred and patient relevant and also questions that are economically driven (for cost-effectiveness, see Chapter 7). Only by viewing a range of evidence from different types of trials will it be possible to gauge how 'useful' this treatment is in the context of other conventional therapies.

SUMMARY

In summary, the difficulties encountered in assessing efficacy may have arisen for several reasons:

- It might simply be that acupuncture has no (or very minimal) efficacy for many conditions and its effects are mainly non-specific. This would be the logical conclusion from many of the reductionist trials but does not account for the very large clinical effects often seen with acupuncture.
- There is an inherent difficulty in measuring any complex intervention such as acupuncture. The many aspects of the encounter are an integral part of the whole and therefore must be taken into account. Indeed the 'whole' might be greater than the sum of its component parts.
- A randomised controlled trial to test efficacy implies controlling for non-specific effects and eliminating the 'active ingredient' from the control group. Therefore, as it is not known what specificity is in acupuncture, researchers are unable to pinpoint this active ingredient and design appropriate trials.
- We are asking the wrong questions as it pertains to acupuncture: the value of acupuncture might be in how it modifies the trajectory of illness and the patient's ability to heal. At this point in time, our measures may not be sensitive enough or studies may not have sufficient long-term follow-up to assess the real differences between control and verum acupuncture interventions.

Research resources

Everitt B S, Pickles A 1999 Statistical aspects of the design of clinical trials. Imperial College Press, London, p 336

Lewith G, Jonas W B, Walach H 2002 Clinical research in complementary therapies. Churchill Livingstone, Edinburgh, p 376

Mason S, Tovey P, Long A 2003 Evaluating complementary therapies: methodological challenges of randomised controlled trials. British Medical Journal 325:832–834

Pocock S J 1983 Clinical trials, a practical approach. Wiley, Chichester, p 266

White P 2004 Methodological concerns when designing trials for the efficacy of acupuncture for the treatment of pain. In: Cooper E, Yamaguchi N (eds) Complementary and alternative approaches to biomedicine. Kluwer Academic Publishers, New York, p 217–227

References

Andersson S 1993 The functional background in acupuncture effects. Scandinavian Journal of Rehabilitation Medicine 29(suppl):31–60

Assefi N, Sherman K, Jacobsen C et al 2005 A randomised clinical trial of acupuncture compared with sham acupuncture in fibromyalgia. Annals of Internal Medicine 143(1):10–19

Beecher H 1955 The powerful placebo. Journal of the American Medical Association 159:1602–1606

Bing Z, Villanueva L, Le Bars D 1990 Acupuncture and diffuse noxious inhibitory controls: naloxone-reversible depression of activities of trigeminal convergent neurons. Neuroscience 37(3):809–818

Borkovec T, Nau S 1972 Credibility of analogue therapy rationales. Journal of Behavior Therapy and Experimental Psychiatry 3:257–260

Ceniceros S, Brown G R 1998 Acupuncture: A review of its history, theories, and indications. Southern Medical Journal 91(12):1121–1125

Christensen C, Laursen L, Taudorf E et al 1984 Acupuncture and bronchial asthma. Allergy 39:379–385

Devilly G, Borkovec T 2000 Psychometric properties of the credibility/expectancy questionnaire. Journal of Behavioral Therapy 31:73–86

Di Blasi Z, Kleijnen J 2003 Powerful therapies or methodological bias? Evaluation & the Health Professions 26:166–179

Dincer F, Linde K 2003 Sham interventions in randomised clinical trials of acupuncture — a review. Complementary Therapies in Medicine 11(4):235–242

Ernst E, White A R 1997 A review of problems in clinical acupuncture research. American Journal of Chinese Medicine 25(1):3–11

Forbes A, Jackson S, Walter C et al 2005 Acupuncture for irritable bowel syndrome: A blinded placebo controlled trial. World Journal of Gastroenterology 11(26):4040–4044

Gallacchi G, Muller W, Plattner C et al 1981 Akupunktur und Laserstrahlbehandlung beim Zervikal und Lumbalsyndrom. Schweizerische Medizinische Wochenschrift 111(37):1360–1366

Gaw A C, Chang L W, Shaw L C 1975 Efficacy of acupuncture on osteoarthritic pain. A controlled, double-blind study. New England Journal of Medicine 293(8):375–378

Hrobjartsson A, Gotzsche P 2001 Is the placebo powerless? An analysis of clinical trials comparing placebo with no treatment. New England Journal of Medicine 344:1594–1602

Kaptchuk T J, Goldman P, Stone D et al 2000 Do medical devices have enhanced placebo effects? Journal of Clinical Epidemiology 53:786–792

Kleijnen J, de Craen A, van Everdingen J et al 1994 Placebo effect in double-blind clinical trials: a review of interactions with medications. Lancet 344:1347–1349

Kreczi T, Klingler D 1986 A comparison of laser acupuncture versus placebo in radicular and pseudoradicular pain syndromes as recorded by subjective responses of patients. Acupuncture and Electro Therapeutics Research 11(3–4):207–216

Le Bars D, Villanueva L, Willer J et al 1991 Diffuse noxious inhibitory controls (DNIC) in animals and man. Acupuncture in Medicine 9(2):47–56

Lee P K, Anderson T W, Modell J H et al 1975 Treatment of chronic pain with acupuncture. Journal of the American Medical Association 232(11):1133–1135

Linde K, Streng A, Jurgens S et al 2005 Acupuncture for patients with migraine. Journal of the American Medical Association 293(17):2118–2125

Lundeberg T, Eriksson S V, Lundeberg S et al 1991 Effect of acupuncture and naloxone in patients with osteoarthritis pain. A sham acupuncture controlled study. The Pain Clinic 4(3):155–161

MacPherson H, Thorpe L, Thomas K 2006 Beyond needling – therapeutic process in acupuncture care: A qualitative nested study within a low back pain trial. Journal of Alternative and Complementary Medicine 12(9):873–880

Margolin A, Avants S K, Kleber H D 1998 Investigating alternative medicine therapies in randomized controlled trials. Journal of the American Medical Association 280(18):1626–1628

Melchart D, Streng A, Hoppe A et al 2005 Acupuncture in patients with tension type headache: randomised controlled trial. British Medical Journal 331:376–379

Mendelson G, Selwood T S, Kranz H et al 1983 Acupuncture treatment of chronic back pain. A double-blind placebo-controlled trial. American Journal of Medicine 74(1):49–55

Moerman D, Jonas W 2002 Deconstructing the placebo effect and finding the meaning response. Annals of Internal Medicine 136:471–476

Molsberger A, Hille E 1994 The analgesic effect of acupuncture in chronic tennis elbow pain. British Journal of Rheumatology 33(12):1162–1165

Mosely J, O'Mally K, Peterson N et al 2002 A controlled trial of arthroscopic surgery for osteoarthritis of the knee. New England Journal of Medicine 11(347):81–88

Pariente J, White P, Frackowiak R et al 2005 Expectancy and belief modulate the neuronal substrates of pain treated by acupuncture. NeuroImage 25:1161–1167

Park J, White A, Stevinson C et al 2002 Validating a new non-penetrating sham acupuncture device: two randomised controlled trials. Acupuncture in Medicine 20(4):168–174

Paterson C, Dieppe P 2005 Characteristic and incidental (placebo) effects in complex interventions such as acupuncture. British Medical Journal 330:1202–1205

Petrie J, Hazleman B 1985 Credibility of placebo transcutaneous nerve stimulation and acupuncture. Clinical and Experimental Rheumatology 3(2):151–153

Price S, Mercer S, MacPherson H 2006 Practitioner empathy, patient enablement and health outcomes: a prospective study of acupuncture patients. Patient Education and Counseling 63:239–245

Ritenbaugh C, Verhoef M, Fleishman S et al 2003 Whole systems research: a discipline for studying complementary and alternative medicine. Alternative Therapies in Health and Medicine 9(4):32–36

Schulz K, Chalmers I, Hayes R et al 1995 Empirical evidence of bias. Journal of the American Medical Association 273:408–412

Staebler F E, Wheeler J, Young J et al 1994 Why research into traditional Chinese acupuncture has proved difficult. Strategies of the Council for Acupuncture, UK, to overcome the problem. Complementary Therapies in Medicine 2(2):86–92

Streitberger K, Kleinhenz J 1998 Introducing a placebo needle into acupuncture research. Lancet 352(9125):364–365

Thomas M, Eriksson S V, Lundeberg T 1991 A comparative study of diazepam and acupuncture in patients with osteoarthritis pain: a placebo controlled study. American Journal of Chinese Medicine 19(2):95–100

Verhoef M, Lewith G, Ritenbaugh C et al 2005 Complementary and alternative medicine whole systems research: beyond identification of inadequacies of the RCT. Complementary Therapies in Medicine 13(3):206–212

Vincent C 1990 Credibility assessment in trials of acupuncture. Complementary Medical Research 4(1):8–11

Vincent C, Lewith G 1995 Placebo controls for acupuncture studies. Journal of the Royal Society of Medicine 88(4):199–202

White A, Resch K L, Chan J et al 2000 Acupuncture for episodic tension-type headache: a multicentre randomised controlled trial. Cephalalgia 20:632–637

White P, Lewith G, Prescott P 2004 Acupuncture versus placebo for the treatment of chronic mechanical neck pain. Annals of Internal Medicine 141:911–919

Zaslawski C, Rogers C, Garvey M et al 1997 Strategies to maintain the credibility of sham acupuncture used as a control treatment in clinical trials [see comments]. Journal of Alternative and Complementary Medicine 3(3):257–266

9

Acupuncture practice as the foundation for clinical evaluation

Rosa N. Schnyer, Stephen Birch and Hugh MacPherson

There is a rising demand for acupuncture services in communities across the globe; acupuncture is increasingly being used not only in private offices, but also in hospitals and community clinics, in refugee camps and rural health clinics, in North America and Europe, in Africa and Latin America. The use of acupuncture spans a broad range of conditions, including acute and chronic pain, stroke rehabilitation, endometriosis, post-traumatic stress, management of side effects of chemotherapy, depression, and irritable bowel syndrome. Research in acupuncture has seen an almost equally rapid growth, and clinically it has focused also on a variety of conditions. In spite of an increased number of well-conducted, large randomised clinical trials the evidence for the efficacy of acupuncture continues to be inconclusive and contradictory. Why? The aim of this chapter is to summarise the key characteristics of acupuncture practice and define the challenges that these characteristics present to research. In addition, we provide an overview of some of the work that has been conducted to date to address some important methodological issues and we outline some of the challenges that still lie ahead.

ACUPUNCTURE AS A COMPLEX INTERVENTION

Acupuncture is a complex, multimodal, interactive, treatment intervention. The patient, the practitioner and the treatment form an integral unit, a system in which an interactive process of diagnosis and treatment dynamically develops as part of a feedback loop. Treatment is generally tailored to the individual patient and continuously becomes adjusted to the clinical features, experience and response of the patient. A good analogy for describing the acupuncture clinical encounter is that of a living organism composed of mutually interdependent parts (patient, environment, acupuncture point, needle stimulation, verbal and non-verbal cues). The properties and functions of this organic system, and thus the effects of treatment, are determined by the relations between the individual components of the intervention. The integrity and efficacy of an acupuncture treatment are contingent upon the various, interdependent parts (see Box 9.1 for an example of a clinical encounter).

Acupuncture is a richly heterogeneous discipline. The vast body of knowledge and scope of practice is the result of a dynamic process, in which traditional theories have evolved over time and are constantly being transformed and redefined by clinical experience within historical and cultural contexts. Treatment with acupuncture for a specific condition

---

Box 9.1   The acupuncture clinical encounter

John has had problems with his right shoulder for the last 7 months. It hurts with reaching behind and with lifting the arm in front of him and has been causing increasing limitation of activity. The traditionally trained acupuncturist inquired about many things such as how he sweats, especially that he sweats a little at night, his sleep, whether the pain is worse with heat or cold, activity or rest, about his occasional back pain and his need to get up twice a night to urinate. John was pleased by the extensive questioning and was a bit surprised when she looked at his tongue, felt the pulses at his wrists and concluded that he had a combination of 'patterns' present that was causing or irritating the shoulder pain. The main pattern was one of weakness of 'Kidney *yin*', coupled with 'stagnation of Liver *Qi*'. This was complicated by 'Cold Stagnation' (called 'Bi') in the Small Intestine channel. She briefly explained how the pain was related to a variety of niggling complaints that John hardly gave a second thought to, but which were clearly relevant clinically. She then needled points on his hands, near his ankles, on top of his feet and finally on the shoulder itself. After removing the needles John found that he was more relaxed, that he felt more refreshed and energised and that his arm moved more easily with less pain.

John had problems with his shoulder 6 years earlier and had seen a physiotherapist acupuncturist at that time. This acupuncturist had performed treatment quite differently since he followed a more contemporary style of treatment. After asking a few more questions about the shoulder problem, how it started, whether there had been any traumas to the shoulder, the acupuncturist examined the shoulder and found an exquisitely painful point centred on the scapula that caused the pain of the shoulder to temporarily increase. After needling this point he then added another needle at the elbow and on the hand between the finger and thumb 'for good measure' he said. When the needles were removed 10 minutes later he could move his arm more easily with less pain in the shoulder.

therefore, can vary greatly depending on the specific treatment method and generally involves more than one single modality. Acupuncturists have described the process of care they provide as composed intrinsically of more than only the actual needling. Engaging patients actively in their own healing process and building a solid therapeutic relationship can motivate lifestyle changes and reinforce the potential for long-term positive outcomes (MacPherson et al 2006). Besides relief from presenting complaints, acupuncture patients have valued improvements in other more general physiological areas and in their psychosocial adaptability (Cassidy 1998). Traditionally, acupuncturists are trained to cultivate a quality of attentive presence, which in conjunction with the somatosensory experience of the actual needling may provide patients with the acknowledgement necessary to integrate fragmented aspects of their illness experience.

Acupuncture treatment can involve other forms of stimulation besides the use of needles, for example manual, mechanical, thermal, electrical stimulation can be used to elicit changes in outcome. Dietary and lifestyle recommendations are often an integral part of treatment, and it is not uncommon to combine Chinese herbal medicine with acupuncture. Knowing what constitutes normal practice is helpful in building a map of the complexity and diversity of acupuncture (see Box 9.2 for a snapshot description of practice in two US states).

Box 9.2 Variation in training and practices of licensed acupuncturists in the USA (Sherman et al 2005)

Sherman and colleagues (2005) randomly selected licensed acupuncturists in Massachusetts and Washington States and interviewed them as well as asking them to record information on 20 consecutive patient visits. They found that most acupuncturists in both states had 3 or 4 years of academic acupuncture training and had received additional 'postgraduate' training as well. Acupuncturists treated a wide range of conditions, including musculoskeletal problems (usually back, neck, and shoulder) (33% in Massachusetts and 47% in Washington), general body symptoms (12% and 9%, respectively) such as fatigue, neurological problems (10% and 12%, respectively) (e.g. headaches), and psychological complaints (10% and 8%, respectively) (especially anxiety and depression). Traditional Chinese medicine (TCM) was the predominant style of acupuncture used in both states (79% and 86%, respectively). Most visits included a traditional diagnostic assessment (more than 99%), regular body acupuncture (95% and 93%, respectively), and additional treatment modalities (79% and 77%, respectively). These included heat and lifestyle advice (66% and 65%, respectively), most commonly dietary advice and exercise recommendations. Chinese herbs were used in about one-third of visits. Although most patients self-referred to acupuncture, about one-half received concomitant care from a physician.

PLURALISM OF TRADITIONAL ACUPUNCTURE

The practice of acupuncture is defined by a pluralism of clinical conceptual frameworks, divergent approaches to the selection of acupuncture treatment points, multiple needling techniques, and a diversity of opinions regarding adequate number and frequency of treatments. The various acupuncture treatment styles have evolved by way of emphasising specific clinical theories, applying traditional and modern concepts, and developing particular sets of clinical skills over others. In very general terms, acupuncture treatment styles can be grouped into two categories. The first includes traditionally based systems of acupuncture (which include any styles that have developed directly from Chinese medicine, or which have adapted traditional concepts and techniques). Examples of traditionally based systems of acupuncture include traditional Chinese medicine (TCM) and traditional Japanese acupuncture. The second includes contemporary systems of acupuncture that integrate various biomedical and psychological ideas or techniques with selected components of Chinese traditional medicine. Examples of contemporary styles include trigger point acupuncture and segmental acupuncture. These categories are of course a continuum, and it is sometimes rather arbitrary to ascertain what styles fit into which category. Different styles in either category may utilise general body points, scalp points or microsystems (e.g. ear or hand acupuncture); may include diverse types of needle stimulation (e.g. electro-stimulation, microcurrent, laser, ion pumping cords, etc.), or may incorporate specific adjunctive techniques (e.g. moxibustion, injection of points, application of colours and sounds).

The concept of *Qi*

The popularity of acupuncture in the West and the emergence of Chinese medicine research highlight the tension between a systemic and a mechanistic view of the natural world. This tension has been a recurring theme in the history of science (Capra 1996) and has been shaped by cultural, social and political trends. In acupuncture research, at the heart of this tension resides *Qi*, the most fundamental, misunderstood and controversial concept in traditional Chinese medicine. The uses and meanings of this concept which permeates traditional Chinese culture and life (Huan & Rose 2001), have evolved and changed over time. Equivocally and simplistically, it has been loosely translated as 'energy', an analogy that gives acupuncture plausibility but limits scientific inquiry and biases research. Kaptchuk refers to *Qi* as the capacity of life to maintain and transform itself (Kaptchuk 2000); Wiseman describes *Qi* as anything perceptible but intangible (Wiseman & Boss 1990); Sivin states that *Qi* is both what animates change in the material world and the material in which change takes place (Sivin 1987). The entire complex of natural stimulus and human response is *Qi*.

The idea of *Qi* as a single concept does not really match our current understanding of natural phenomena. Inadvertently, those interested in acupuncture as an alternative to biomedicine have perpetuated a pre-scientific view of acupuncture by reviving vitalistic ideas that assume a non-physical entity, force or field that has to be added to natural laws. Together these perspectives have maintained the notion that Chinese medicine principles are incompatible with modern science and have created a split between the scientific community and practitioners of acupuncture. We lack a common language, one that neither reduces Chinese medicine terms to familiar words that fit biomedical expectations, nor defines acupuncture in metaphysical terms. A new working definition of *Qi*, considers it not a force but a model, a framework for organising correlations, a theory for predicting observations. Thinking of '*qi* as a generative matrix in which all things interact with all other things through the exchange of information' (providing) 'the information needed to maintain the stability of a complex system' (Birch & Felt 1999), can begin to resolve the perceived conflict between traditional ideas and biomedical concepts.

The channel system: a signalling network?

Qi is thought to be distributed and circulated by a network of channels that connects the surface of the body with the internal organs, serving as a two-way communication system that conveys messages to the surface about internal malfunctioning and alerts the internal organs about surface phenomena that might be threatening to move deeper into the system (Seem 1987). This is the matrix of information exchange as mentioned above. Although the actual physical existence of these channels is still under investigation and is the subject of much debate (Ahn et al 2005, Lee et al 2005), clinically their relevance resides in providing a map of the inner landscape of the patient, which consists of a complete set of functions that reflect *Qi*-based relationships among physiological and psychological events. Acupuncture points, located along the channels are considered hubs of this entire functional network. Traditionally they are not considered to be anatomically based, but rather places where *Qi* comes in and wanders out (Liangsheng 1997). They generally correspond to depressions or crevices between bones and sinews, places of access on the surface of the body where the *Qi* and blood of the channels and network vessels are thought to collect (Wiseman & Feng 1998). Recently, researchers have found that acupuncture points correspond to connective tissue planes (Langevin & Yandow 2002) and postulate that needle manipulation transmits a mechanical signal to connective tissue cells via mechanotransduction, producing several changes that propagate along connective tissue planes (Langevin & Yandow 2002), see Chapter 10 for more detail. This may explain local, remote and long-term effects of acupuncture (Langevin et al 2002). According to the connective tissue model, the interaction between connective tissue and acupuncture stimulation could occur even at the smallest connective tissue areas (Langevin & Yandow 2002). More research is needed to determine whether the correspondence to connective tissue planes is an artefact of the particular needling techniques used in the experiments rather than actual properties of the acupuncture points themselves.

If in fact acupuncture sets in motion important auto-regulatory mechanisms, in order to establish efficacy (above and beyond placebo effects) more sensitive measures of change or an assessment of change over a longer time period may be required. Why? Because acupuncture not only seems to affect a wide range of symptoms, but also it seems to increase people's adaptability to stress and sense of well-being. Acupuncture's greatest impact on clinical outcomes may hinge upon how it modifies the trajectory of illness, rather than on how it changes, short-term narrowly defined biomedical outcomes (see Chapter 5).

Specificity of the location of acupuncture points

Although many people think of acupuncture points as having very precise locations and indications (i.e. one point for one symptom or disease), traditionally they are selected and combined, literally to adjust the 'irrigation' system of *Qi* flow and thus balance *Yin* and *Yang* (Beinfield & Korngold 1991). The points can be understood to offer optimal access to the *Qi* network, and their exact anatomical locations are just approximate landmarks where this access can be reached. Among practitioners in Japan the points are thought to reflect disturbances that need correcting. These points are often called 'live' points, sites of activation of the tissues in response to the underlying disturbances. Finding the actual 'live' point for a particular patient involves finding them by palpation; live points can present as subtle signs at the skin level (dryness, sponginess, stickiness), palpable 'holes', resistance or hardness when applying pressure, or sensitivity, discomfort or pain upon deep palpation. Different types of stimulation can produce different effects. Zaslawski conducted a study to explore how specific the locations of points are and the application of needle manipulation (see Box 9.3).

Theoretical underpinnings

The basis of clinical decision-making in traditional Chinese medicine resides in the recognition of observable patterns in nature and in the way humans interact with their environment. These observations take place through our naked senses and can be described by their sensory qualities. By observing that some events occur simultaneously or synchronously with other events and that these events share specific qualities among them, it was possible for the Chinese to systematise these

Box 9.3 Specificity of point locations and needle manipulation (Zaslawski et al 2003)

Zaslawski and colleagues (2003) conducted a small pilot to evaluate site specificity and application of needle manipulation. Thirteen volunteers were randomised to one of five different interventions: deep needling 1) with or 2) without manual needle rotation of acupoint Large Intestine 4 (LI-4) or 3) with or 4) without manual needle rotation at a non-acupoint located on the medial side of the second metacarpal; or 5) inactive laser to LI-4 used as a control. All interventions were administered for 21 minutes. The main outcome measure was the pressure pain threshold measured with an algometer, before and after intervention at 10 sites (acupoints and non-acupoints) across the body. Pressure pain threshold increased at all 10 sites following needling of LI-4 with manipulation compared with one site after needling LI-4 without manipulation. Needling the non-acupoint with manipulation resulted in statistically significant increases at six sites, compared with none in the absence of manipulation. No significant changes in mean pressure pain threshold followed inactive laser. Although needling LI-4 with manipulation produced greater increases than those for the other interventions, needling the non-acupoint with manipulation was as effective as needling LI-4 with manipulation at one measurement site.

This study concluded that both manipulation and site of needling contributed significantly to the elevation of pressure pain threshold following acupuncture. Psychological and physiological non-specific effects appeared to play a minimal role in changes to pressure pain threshold.

observations as patterns and to discover other links. The process of gathering clinical data in Chinese medicine involves confirming observations, correlations and questions and organising them into frameworks that constitute refined theories of correspondence.

Acupuncture treatment is determined by a range of unique diagnostic and clinical reasoning processes that emphasises the contextual and qualitative nature of a patient's illness, and which aims at integrating and synthesising a large number of variables (Kaptchuk 2000, Schnyer et al 2005). Diagnosis consists of weaving all information into a dynamic clinical picture that includes the etiological, physiological and pathological mechanisms of the illness (Kaptchuk 2000, Schnyer et al 2005). Diagnostic categories in Chinese medicine are not fixed disease entities, but rather clinical metaphors, coordinates that help us navigate the individual's experience of distress; guidelines that allow us to collect and organise patient data, and then select and apply treatment. In medicine, we know *Qi* by what it does, by how it behaves, and by how it unfolds. Movement, warmth, shape, transformation, containment, in sum all metabolism and signalling is an attribute of *Qi*. When *Qi* is insufficient, there is poor organ function, weakness; when *Qi* accumulates, obstruction follows.

Health is defined as the balance between *Yin* and *Yang*, two complementary representations of the dynamic equilibrium of *Qi*. *Yin*, which is nourishing, grants the qualities of rest, tranquility, and quiescence (Kaptchuk 2000). When *Yin* is insufficient, fluids and blood are depleted (Wiseman & Feng 1998); patients lack the qualities of receptivity and contemplation and become easily agitated, unsettled or nervously uneasy (Kaptchuk 2000), brittle, dry and overheated. *Yang*, which by contrast is activating, causes transformation and change, providing the capacity to engage life, to react, and to respond. When *Yang* is insufficient, there is a reduction in the warming and activating power of the body (Wiseman & Feng 1998). The balance between *Yin* and *Yang* depends on the adaptability of an organism. Sickness is the result of a hypo function or diminished capacity of any physiological process and decreased resistance or a hyper function or obstruction of any physiological process and increased reactivity (Beinfield & Korngold 1991). The *Yin Yang* theory of correspondence is used to organise, catalogue and label an enormous amount of sensory information as is the five-phase theory based on seasonal correspondences, and other Chinese medicine theories.

Diagnostic and treatment processes

Acupuncturists who base their practice on traditional Chinese medicine do not produce a single categorical diagnosis, but rather contextual descriptions of clinical patterns. Patterns, which can be thought of as dynamic representations of the clinical experience of the patient's imbalance, are experienced through the senses and then identified qualitatively. Symptoms are assessed on the basis of how they manifest and how specifically they interfere with a person's life and behaviour. For example, a mild, recurrent headache that manifests primarily at the vertex of the head, which is exacerbated at the end of the day and from exhaustion, and which is accompanied by irritability and fear, a weak, thin pulse and a pale, thin tongue is approached clinically in a different way than an intense, recurrent, acute headache that manifests on the right temple, which is exacerbated by food, which is accompanied by violent outbursts of anger and which presents with a full, bounding, fast pulse and a thick, yellow coating on the tongue.

Traditionally, an acupuncturist is trained to assess the data gathered during examination by using a matrix that organises clinical signs into one of several, interrelated but different theoretical frameworks such as the Eight Principles and Five Phases. Since *Qi* can only be known by what *Qi* does, a traditional acupuncturist is meant to develop the skills to assess *Qi* changes by observing not only how a symptom develops, where it resides, how it moves and what makes it change for better or for worse, but also by attending to subtle cues in demeanour, behaviour, colour, speech and voice. The clinical relevance of any symptom depends on the overall presentation and experience of the patient. Diagnosis involves the assessment of the process and the experience of distress and how that distress manifests in the patient's temperature, abdomen, pulse, tongue, etc. Furthermore, different symptoms acquire relevance depending on the constitution of the patient, the living environment, and lifestyle habits.

Information required for assessment traditionally is gathered through the Four Examinations: questioning, observation, palpation and listening/smelling. As mentioned previously, different treatment styles emphasise different diagnostic skills and techniques. In actual practice some practitioners faithfully apply traditional assessment methods alone, while others combine the traditional four examinations with the use of measuring instruments, such as Ryodoraku (Nakatani & Yamashita 1977) and Electroacupuncture according to Voll (EAV) (Voll 1975).

The information gathered through examination is reorganised within a particular theoretical framework, differentiated and synthesised to identify predominant signs and symptoms according to particular patterns, and to select treatment based on these patterns. Again, the 'diagnoses' produced by pattern differentiation are working metaphors, and are only appropriate as long as they produce the desired clinical results; they are constantly refined by the ongoing treatment outcome itself. When dealing with internal medicine issues or complex medical problems (as opposed to musculoskeletal complaints) in traditional Chinese acupuncture, the focus is to correct imbalances at a functional level, incorporating the presenting symptoms and the constitutional predisposition of the patient in the selection of treatment. In classical Japanese meridian acupuncture the emphasis is on regulating the *Qi* and addressing the root imbalance, rather than on stimulating anatomical or physiological functions, therefore the needling stimulation is minimal and correcting the symptoms is of secondary importance. In some forms of traditional acupuncture (Jarret 2001) the aim is to correct constitutional problems by identifying and clearing stagnation and by transferring *Qi* among various physiological and psychological functional areas; the point indications may include psychosocial relationships.

The central role of the Chinese medicine diagnostic framework in traditional acupuncture has not been well integrated yet into clinical research.

Contemporary styles of acupuncture

New approaches to acupuncture treatment have developed that use points based on neuromotor function, alignment with major nerves, trigger point areas or anatomical location. In these styles, the biomedical diagnosis is sufficient to design a treatment (Filshie & White 1998, Ulett 1992) and the point selection depends on the framework chosen by each practitioner. Other approaches reinterpret biomedical concepts and combine them with a particular model based on traditional theories and/or empirical experience (Matsumoto & Euler 2002), for example Kiko Matsumoto's style of acupuncture. Some practitioners select points and techniques that have worked for specific conditions (Mori 1979, Paldan & Lee 1993) while others propose original ideas and methods of diagnosis and treatment that neither reject nor accept traditional concepts, for example the French system of auriculotherapy developed by Nogier (1983). Yet others accept traditional principles but prefer to make the process of diagnosis and point selection more objective and use various instruments to quantify diagnostic measures as mentioned above (Kenyon 1983, Nakatani & Yamashita 1977). Some systems are practised as simple interventions and use correspondences to some form of homunculus as the basis of treatment, for example the foetus as an ear acupoint correspondence map, or the hand and nose microsystems. All these contemporary styles vary broadly in the way they adapt and modify a traditional system, or use the biomedical model; therefore the challenge of integration into a research model varies accordingly.

DEVELOPING AN ACUPUNCTURE RESEARCH METHODOLOGY

Acupuncture can be described as a continually evolving set of practices with well-articulated conceptual frameworks. A thorough understanding of these theoretical frameworks, whether traditionally or biomedically based, can provide a solid foundation on which to evaluate clinical outcomes. This perspective requires us to be clear about certain fundamental questions. What approach to acupuncture should we be prioritising for clinical evaluation? Considering the broad diversity of treatment options, how can we be assured that the style of treatment to be tested in a clinical trial of acupuncture is consistent with the specific research questions, aims, design and methods of the study (Schnyer & Allen 2002)? Are different styles and techniques patient specific or condition specific? To what extent do we aim to control for idiosyncratic treatment style differences among practitioners? Can we be assured of adherence to the treatment protocol? How does a researcher go about selecting a treatment protocol? To what extent should the acupuncture intervention be modified or constrained when seeking to improve the rigour of the research? Can we generalise the results of acupuncture clinical trials to other practice styles? All these are important questions in acupuncture research that necessitate an approach informed by clinical practice and experience.

These questions present some significant methodological challenges to clinical research. The solutions will depend on the research question and setting chosen by the researchers and the style of acupuncture that is being evaluated. There is a spectrum here. On the one hand acupuncture can be practised as a complex intervention on a more traditional basis, which would be more appropriate for chronic long-term conditions as described above (Allen et al 2006, Birch & Jamison 1998, Wayne et al 2005). On the other hand acupuncture can be practised as a simple intervention, perhaps as an adjunct to a conventional modality, which would be more appropriate for such short-term conditions as post-operative nausea (Vickers 1996) or acute dental pain (Lao et al 1999). This spectrum, from complex to simple, is a useful guide in understanding the implications for research, particularly for the design of clinical trials and for the drawing up of a trial treatment protocol. Moreover the spectrum of complex vs. simple is helpful when considering replicability of the acupuncture in different settings or with different patient groups. Additionally it is helpful with regard to generalisability of one's findings, that is, the extent that the findings can be transferred to different contexts and settings.

Developing an acupuncture trial treatment protocol

In the field of acupuncture research, there has been a trend towards using treatment protocols for trials that have a simplified form of acupuncture, often with a focus on pre-selected components that are assumed to be the 'active' ingredients. For example, a particular group of acupuncture points may be delivered to each patient in the same way at each treatment session. Other possibilities include the provision for each patient of a fixed set of points along with a series of optional points that can be chosen by the practitioner on the basis of clinical judgement, i.e. partially individualised. The tighter the specification, the easier the interpretation of the results of trials, in that one can identify more precisely the parameters of treatment that one can attribute the outcome to. One disadvantage of these types of studies for traditional acupuncture is the low ecological validity, i.e. a poor reflection of actual clinical practice, therefore it is more difficult to generalise findings to normal practice. Also it is a challenge to know, prior to a trial designed to establish whether there is an effect, what components are optimally active. If there is a negative outcome to a trial with a tightly specified intervention, then interpretation may lead to a 'negative conundrum' (MacPherson & Schroer 2007): was the acupuncture over-simplified to the extent of reducing its impact, or was it that the acupuncture just didn't work? A treatment protocol at the other end of the spectrum might involve a very loose specification of the acupuncture. While this may be more readily generalised to routine care, the problem might be that the acupuncturists incorporate various styles into treatment or additional therapeutic modalities, such as herbs, nutritional supplements, massage and manipulation, only some of which are underpinned by Chinese medical theory. The more diverse that practice is, the less clear what it is that one can attribute change to. In this case, a negative outcome could indicate a dilution effect due to some components being less effective than others, such that the outcome underestimated the potential impact, or it may indicate that the acupuncture just didn't work.

Therefore the challenge regarding the nature of the trial treatment protocol is a trade off, and needs careful consideration at the design stage of clinical evaluation (see Fig. 9.1).

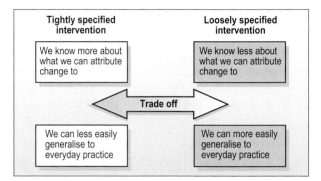

Fig 9.1   Trade off between a tightly and a loosely defined acupuncture trial treatment protocol. (Adapted from MacPherson & Schroer 2007.)

The extent that standardisation of acupuncture is appropriate in a treatment protocol for an acupuncture trial is clearly an important consideration. The simpler the conceptualisation of acupuncture, the easier this standardisation becomes. For example the use of P-6 for postoperative nausea (Vickers 1996) or LI-4 for local pain after dental surgery (Lao et al 1999) are clearly simple interventions. The parameters of treatment with just one acupuncture point for a single condition used identically for all patients can be simply specified. The other end of the spectrum is the individualised treatment for a chronic condition where the history, aggravating factors and constellation of symptoms are likely to vary from individual to individual. It is problematic to try and establish a protocol to treat all patients with the same chronic condition in a way that would gain wide acceptability among acupuncturists.

The need to standardise an acupuncture treatment protocol in explanatory trials is associated with the desire to raise internal validity, ideally minimising all but one (independent) variable, and thereby establishing a stronger relationship between cause (treatment) and effect (outcome). Not only does standardisation help one know the specifications of treatment and what one can attribute effects to, it also facilitates replication of the study. However the practice of individualisation in traditional acupuncture appears difficult to reconcile with standardisation. Treatment is normally tailored to the individual patient and dynamically develops over time. The danger of standardisation is that it might result in the integrity of the acupuncture to be unintentionally compromised. Solutions to this potential limitation of standardisation have varied, depending on national contexts, local norms of practice, and the demands of funding agencies. In the USA, Schnyer and colleagues have developed a manualisation approach which aims at attaining both

> **Box 9.4** Developing a treatment manual for a clinical trial: manualisation (Schnyer & Allen 2002)
>
> Developing a treatment manual for a clinical trial is known as manualisation. Schnyer & Allen (2002) have set out the processes and procedures for manualisation as a means of promoting standardisation and flexibility in acupuncture trials. They discuss how a manual will specify the acupuncture theoretical and conceptual framework that supports the study hypotheses, the treatment design and the guidelines for its implementation. It will clearly specify which system, style and techniques are being tested in a particular study as well as provide explicit decision algorithms for diagnosis and treatment. Treatment manualisation is a methodology that has been widely used in psychotherapy research (Wilson 1996) and allows the systematic administration of individualised protocols. It aims to provide replicability and standardisation, while maintaining fidelity to complex, interactive treatment interventions. By using a treatment manual one can more easily implement a protocol for training and evaluating practitioner competence and adherence to treatment. It leads to a transparent and repeatable intervention tailored to the characteristics of individual patients. Manualisation has been successfully employed in several clinical trials of acupuncture. However, it has not been shown that manuals increase the treatment efficacy or diminish outcome variance; to conclusively answer this question would require expensive and elaborate trials that compare manualised versus non-manualised flexible treatment interventions (Klein 1997). Manualisation has the potential to impede clinical flexibility and increases training costs (Dobson & Shaw 1988); it is a very helpful tool to help describe and refine acupuncture treatment interventions employed in clinical trials. Rather than promote the adoption of a universal style of acupuncture treatment, it can be used in a way that supports richness of a diverse tradition.

flexibility of treatment and standardisation; this approach is set out in Box 9.4.

Acupuncture researchers have opted for a spectrum of responses to standardisation. These can be broadly categorised into five types, with increasing scope for individualisation. First there is the cookbook or formulaic approaches, where the protocols specify the same set of points (or perhaps even a single point) that are used for every patient at every consultation. This was typical of many trials of acupuncture until recently (Lao et al 1995). Second there are the protocols that specify a prescribed set of acupuncture points to be used for every patient at every visit, along with a set of optional points that are selected for optional use by the practitioners (Linde et al 2005). The third type of protocols provide specific guidelines for diagnosis and treatment design within a pre-specified framework, yet allow flexibility to tailor the treatment to the individual needs of the patient, as described in manualisation above (Allen et al 2006, Manber et al 2004). The fourth type of protocols are the ones that allow freedom for the practitioner to treat as they normally would, but set limits on which auxiliary modalities are provided as well as lifestyle advice and other supportive care (Cherkin et al 2001). The fifth type of protocols is the ones that are designed to reflect as accurately as possible the acupuncture that is delivered in normal practice, with no constraints on the full range of treatment options available to acupuncturists (Thomas et al 2006, Vickers et al 2004). The decision on the level of standardisation will depend on the research question and the methods to answer the question. Explanatory trials are more commonly associated with more highly standardised protocols, while pragmatic trials are more commonly associated with flexible protocols.

Implicit to questions of standardisation is the question of identifying what constitutes 'best practice'. For explanatory trials, and following the convention in drug evaluation, the ideal is to deliver optimal acupuncture. The reason for pre-trial drug testing is to establish precisely the ideal conditions for the drug treatment, including the optimal dose. However pre-trial testing of acupuncture will not help in identifying optimal acupuncture, as sample sizes will be far too small to establish differences between components of treatment. For acupuncture, when practised as a complex intervention, there are many different components that make up a treatment, and a rigorous evaluation to select only those that are active is not feasible. This is a Catch-22 situation, we cannot know whether there are 'active' components until we have done a trial, yet we need to *a priori* select the presumed active components in order to test them in a trial. The same problem is associated with determining the parameters for the control arm, where the aim might be to utilise only points that are therapeutically inactive. Consequently researchers have used a variety of methods to establish treatment protocols. These methods include reviews of both the clinical and trial literature, though the utility of the former is limited by the immense diversity of options and the latter by the paucity of rigorous research. Expert opinions have also been used, although the extent that experts can identify 'best practice' is not clear. Consensus methods of eliciting professional opinion also have a place, and have the advantage of overcoming the problem of one expert's opinion being overly influential (MacPherson & Shroer 2007, Schnyer et al 2006, Stux & Birch 2001). As an example Stux & Birch (2001) have provided one solution to the challenge of identifying good practice by setting out a process for identifying relevant and irrelevant acupuncture points for a clinical trial (see Box 9.5).

Box 9.5 Selection and validation of acupuncture points: the BRITS method (Stux & Birch 2001)

The Birch Relevant and Irrelevant Treatment Selection method or BRITS method (Stux & Birch 2001) has provided an easily applied standardisable approach to selecting and validating relevant and irrelevant acupuncture points. The BRITS method consists of conducting an extensive review of the literature, including research papers and treatment texts directly related to the method or tradition of practice being tested, to confirm that all acupuncture points to be treated in a study are recommended for the treatment of a specific condition in a reasonable proportion of sources. The same system can be used to determine irrelevant points that are to be used in the controlled arm of the study. The literature review is best enhanced by practitioners' surveys and a panel of experts to assess whether practitioners concur. A weakness of the BRITS method is that it failed to point out the need to critically assess the sources and the shortcomings of using the limited literature available in English, most of which are tertiary sources. Also the process of point selection in traditional acupuncture is not usually made in the absence of a conceptual framework. Finally there is no literature — or clinical experience — that directly identifies unequivocally 'irrelevant' points. There is also increasing evidence from trials that the use of what might be defined by experts as irrelevant sham points has potentially therapeutic properties (see Chapter 8) (Stux & Birch 2001).

Underpinning the quest for 'best practice' is a dependence on English language textbooks and curricula of acupuncture courses in the West. How confident can we be that the theories that acupuncturists have been taught in the West are the best basis for clinical evaluation? Scheid (2006) argues that TCM diagnoses that are currently widely accepted in the West may not be entirely traditional or even Chinese in their origin. Textbooks of Chinese medicine may set out that a particular condition is normally associated with treatment strategies that should be geared towards a specific syndrome or syndromes. Scheid takes the treatment of menopause as his exemplar which in the West is commonly taught to be caused by Kidney deficiency. He cites a study (Zell et al 2000) in which nine TCM practitioners diagnosed 25 patients on the same day, predominantly diagnosing Kidney *Yin* deficiency. However from analysis of the development of textbooks in China, it emerges that a Kidney-oriented diagnosis for menopause was put forward for the first time in the 1960s. This was in response to a growing Westernisation of TCM, and an opportunistic translation of knowledge of hormone deficiency into Kidney deficiency to provide TCM with added legitimacy in China. Scheid argues that this translation is problematic, as it is primarily a biomedicalised approach to menopause that ignores social and cultural differences in the way menopause is experienced. Taylor (2004) has a more wide-ranging critique of 'TCM' as it is known in the West, identifying the process of Westernisation of Chinese medicine that has taken place during the twentieth century. The importance of these anthropological studies is that they highlight the challenge of establishing 'best practice' in clinical trials.

For more pragmatic trials, the ideal is to deliver to patients what might be called 'representative' acupuncture. One approach to this is to simply select acupuncturists on the basis of their training and years of experience, perhaps from a particular professional association. While this overcomes many of the challenges of trying to determine 'best practice' it is not entirely unproblematic. In particular just because the acupuncture is representative, it might not be as good as it could be. It will only be as good as the education provided by the schools and colleges, much of which is based on acupuncture sources that are not original (Scheid 2006). Moreover with the huge diversity of styles, and with many practitioners practising more than one style (Dale 1997), there are additional problems associated with potential variations in effectiveness, with attributability and with replication. Given the huge investment required for clinical trials, the case can at least be made to be selective about which acupuncturists participate and to provide pre-trial training to enhance outcomes.

INTEGRATING CLINICAL KNOWLEDGE INTO RESEARCH

Acupuncture research based on the biomedical drug model may be workable when acupuncture is conceptualised as a simple intervention; however the drug model is not methodologically congruent when acupuncture is conceptualised as a complex intervention. The increased demand for access to acupuncture services by the general public is alone insufficient to assess its potential contribution to healthcare. It is necessary to develop an appropriate model of research grounded on a sound framework, consistent with Chinese medicine and which effectively expands on the biomedical research model. The exploration of the mechanisms by which acupuncture works needs to include innovative hypothetical models. Traditional theories and clinical practice point to acupuncture as a way of setting in motion a complex auto-regulatory matrix and indicate that acupuncture may have an effect in various physiological systems simultaneously. The evaluation of acupuncture effects in clinical trials needs to include Qi-based and patient-centred outcomes. By identifying relevant indicators of functionality, well-being and healing in acupuncture we can begin to determine at what level and in what way acupuncture contributes to positive patient responses.

Rather than completely embrace traditional acupuncture concepts and theories as absolute, or totally reject them as anachronistic cultural artefacts, we could use research as an opportunity to challenge our assumptions on both sides of the spectrum. Systematically assessing one of the oldest literate medicines in the world is likely to expand and enrich our medical knowledge. In order to integrate traditional Chinese medicine principles with scientific concepts, however, we need to find a common language and develop a model that can generate testable hypotheses. For this process of integration to be a true collaborative effort that maintains the integrity of Chinese medicine as a medical system, acupuncturists need to participate in as well as inform research. Acupuncturists need to engage in determining where the various styles fit into the oral and literate traditions and to assess which theories and techniques are clinically useful, for what patients and in what conditions.

Systematically mapping out the diagnostic and clinical reasoning process of divergent styles of treatment, will help evaluate the validity and reliability of the Chinese medicine assessment process (Schnyer et al 2005, Zaslawski et al 2003). In addition, for explanatory trial research it is necessary for clinicians to help inform what constitutes the specific, attributable effects of acupuncture, above and beyond non-specific therapeutic factors that are common to all clinical encounters (i.e. attention, empathy, the belief in the efficacy of the treatment, relief from daily stress, being in a relaxing environment and lying down for half an hour).

Reliability and validity of the acupuncture diagnostic process

Integrating the Chinese medicine diagnostic process in clinical trials would help determine if there are any valuable correlations between biomedical and Chinese medicine-defined disease categories that may help us better understand patients' response to treatment. In order to accomplish this integration, it is necessary to operationalise the assessment process for research purposes, which requires the development of reliable and valid diagnostic instrumentation in the form of assessment questionnaires. Reliability can be established when there is concordance between practitioners in diagnosis and/or treatment parameters. Validity is established when the results are shown to accurately reflect what is being measured. If reliability can be properly established then there is an opportunity to use a double screening method to select patients for a trial on the basis of both their conventional medical diagnosis and their acupuncture diagnosis (Lao et al 2001); or to use the acupuncture diagnosis to evaluate variance in treatment response on the basis of patient differences. This targeting would be especially useful where we have some confidence that patients with a biomedical condition are more responsive to acupuncture because they also have a specific Chinese medical diagnosis. We present a study of women with recurrent cystitis to illustrate the potential for such additional screening (see Box 9.6). However, this study has a major weakness: it does not mention whether the inter-rater agreement of the diagnostic categories and methods was conducted and whether reliability among raters was found. If the diagnostic categories have not been shown to be reliable the validity of the results of this study are under question.

Several small studies have evaluated the reliability of the Chinese medicine assessment process (Birch 1998, Hogeboom et al 2001, Kalauokalani et al 2001, Ogawa 1978, Zaslawski 2003, Zhang et al 2003, 2004) or some of its components (Debata 1968, King et al 2002a, 2002b, Kurosu 1969, Matsumoto 1968, Walsh et al 2001, Zhang et al 2005). In a small reliability study of TCM diagnosis and treatment in chronic lower back pain a high rate of agreement existed among five of seven acupuncturists; however, there was a great variation in the number and location of recommended acupuncture points (Hogeboom et al 2001). In another

Box 9.6 Differential outcomes depending on the TCM diagnosis (Alraek & Baerheim 2003)

Alraek & Baerheim (2003) evaluated the effectiveness of acupuncture for recurrent cystitis and compared outcomes for three TCM diagnostic categories. Ninety-eight patients were randomly allocated to acupuncture or no treatment. The primary outcome was the number of cystitis attacks over a 6-month monitoring period. Of the acupuncture group, 22 patients were diagnosed with Spleen deficiency, 18 with Kidney deficiency, and 18 with Liver *Qi* stagnation. Of the Kidney group, 78% had remained cystitis free over the 6 months compared to 45% in the Spleen group, 44% in the Liver group, and 17% in the non-treated group. The Kidney group was statistically significantly improved compared to all other groups ($p < 0.05$). All three acupuncture groups fared better than the non-treated group ($p < 0.01$). Sub-analysing for cystitis with detected bacteria yielded comparable results, with significantly reduced residual urine over time only in the Kidney group (Alraek & Baerheim 2003).

similar small study six TCM acupuncturists evaluated the same six patients with chronic low back pain on the same day; most acupuncturists included in their selection of patterns the combination (*Qi*/Blood Stagnation with Kidney deficiency) and the acupuncture point (UB 23) for every patient. However, consistency across acupuncturists regarding diagnostic details and other acupoints was poor. Differences in diagnoses and treatment recommendations were associated more with the variability in judgements of practitioners, rather than with actual differences in the patients. At the University of Maryland, Zhang and colleagues conducted a prospective survey of three licensed acupuncturists with at least 5 years' experience, who separately assessed 40 patients with rheumatoid arthritis. The rate of agreement among practitioners with regard to the TCM diagnosis was only 28.2% (25.6–33.3%; with Kappas ranging from 0.23 to 0.30) (Zhang et al 2005). Since there will be some agreement by chance, Kappa is a measure of agreement between practitioners that is beyond chance. MacPherson and colleagues (2004) as part of a pragmatic trial of acupuncture for low back pain mapped levels of agreement between one of the six trial acupuncturists and the other five for three predefined syndromes, *Qi* Stagnation, *Bi* Syndrome and Kidney deficiency, and found Kappa levels between zero ('same as chance') and 0.67 ('good') (MacPherson et al 2004).

One of the challenges of determining 'reliability' in Chinese medicine is the inherent variability in how acupuncturists practise. Different practitioners may have different methods of re-establishing self-regulation at the whole person level. It can be expected that there may not be just one correct diagnosis for an individual patient. For some patients there may be more than one legitimate approach to diagnosis, and more than one legitimate and effective treatment plan. Poor inter-rater reliability may be either due to errors in the clinical judgements made by individual practitioners, or a failure of the analytic process to consider multiple legitimate conclusions as instances of inter-rater agreement (Schnyer et al 2005). There is an inherent difficulty in establishing inter-rater reliability when one has the possibilities of the many diagnostic categories that practitioners normally use, as one would require unfeasibly large sample sizes. A first step towards establishing reliability might be to develop an intake form specific to a particular style of diagnosis and treatment that contains all the information needed to make a *Qi*-based diagnosis (with face and content validity) that reflects what practitioners actually do in clinical practice (ecological validity). An example of such an intake form to systematically record a Chinese medicine assessment has been described in Box 6.7 in Chapter 6 (Schnyer et al 2005). The validity and reliability of this instrument is currently being tested. It remains to be seen whether a systematically developed intake form combined with training of the practitioners may yield better reliability of the Chinese medicine assessment process.

Redefining what is specific to acupuncture — the practitioner perspective

When traditional acupuncturists discuss the need to control for non-specific factors of the acupuncture clinical encounter in explanatory trial research settings, they are frequently baffled by the notion that some integral aspects of the acupuncture treatment itself are considered to be non-specific and that needling itself is expected to be the only specific 'active' component. When acupuncture is understood as a complex intervention, with multiple components that are driven by theoretical considerations integral to acupuncture, it can be expected that the characteristic components of treatment that involve more than needling are therapeutically active.

In their research, Paterson & Dieppe (2005) have observed that elements of treatment that might be characterised as non-specific (incidental) in drug trials might be specific (characteristic) to acupuncture trials. They argue therefore that it might not be meaningful to split complex interventions into specific and non-specific components. For example the thoughtful silence that accompanies the taking of the pulse, the palpation of the abdomen and channels, and the attentive listening and shared exploration of the meaning of symptoms, are all considered by most practitioners to be essential to (and characteristic of) the acupuncture treatment. They are the way in which a clinician might probe the response of the *Qi* of the patient to an external stimulus, the means of assessing the correct quality of the potential intervention (i.e. point, needle stimulation), the method to evaluate the best treatment and techniques that may bring the system back into balance. In Box 9.7 we present a qualitative study that explores acupuncturists' perspectives on treatment processes, and also consider whether components of care are specific or not to acupuncture.

> **Box 9.7** Aspects of acupuncture beyond needling that are specific to acupuncture (MacPherson et al 2006)
>
> This study by MacPherson et al (2006) was nested within a pragmatic clinical trial of acupuncture for low back pain. Six participating acupuncturists treated up to 25 patients each, with the protocol allowing acupuncture to be provided as it normally would. Following the treatment phase of the trial, the acupuncturists were interviewed using a topic guide to obtain an account of their experiences of providing acupuncture care to patients. Data were collected and analysed for both *a priori* and emergent themes. This study focused on practitioners' accounts of the goals and processes of care and describes the strategies employed in addition to needling and other hands-on treatments.
>
> This qualitative study raised questions about what exactly is 'specific' and what is 'non-specific' to acupuncture. The therapeutic relationship was found to have both specific and non-specific dimensions: some of the rapport building and communication was non-specific, such as engendering empathy, while some was specific to acupuncture such as the utilisation of appropriate explanations from the traditional Chinese medicine model, for example explanations about the cause of ill health or the reasons for exacerbations. The diagnostic processes, which included palpation to identify points, not only enhanced the therapeutic relationship generally, but at the same time had potentially specific (theory-related) and therapeutically active aspects. Key components that the practitioners used to help patients maintain longer-term benefits had to do with the way they facilitated patients' active involvement. Only through a shared understanding and ongoing dialogue, based in part on the traditional Chinese model of health and illness, could patients maximise their opportunities for changes in attitudes and behaviours, leading to a more supportive self-care over the longer term. An outcome of this study was that to consider needling to be the only active component in such circumstances is likely to lead to an underestimate of the clinical effect.

Priming of the *Qi* in acupuncture treatment as a specific component

The patient–practitioner interaction in acupuncture is intrinsic to the process and likely to impact on treatment effects. The practitioner's intention is to affect the patient's *Qi* and this includes the patient's attitude towards treatment. Literally, by interacting with patients in a specific way, either by approaching them gently or with resolve for example, practitioners are evaluating their response to a particular stimulus, to a certain quality of *Qi*; they are implicitly assessing the potential for a *Qi*-based factor that might facilitate treatment. The quality of presence of the practitioners during the treatment and their ability to use their intention, their attentive presence, their *Qi* as a tool for further influencing a change in the patient's *Qi*, is as important as the points selected or the stimulation provided. The overall (verbal and non-verbal) patient–practitioner interaction can constitute a 'priming' of the *Qi*, a pre-needling event that facilitates the processing of the subsequent event (needling) and it is intrinsic and specific to acupuncture's clinical efficacy. We are not referring here to the priming of the *Qi* as a form of verbal communication, but rather a form of physiological concordance. Although experimental evidence is not yet present we believe that there is a relationship between simultaneous changes in physiological measures such as heart rate, skin conductance, blood pressure, respiratory rate, etc. between the patient and the practitioner, which enables access to the signalling system activated by acupuncture. Even in the complete absence of any verbal cues, therapeutic advice, empathic attention, reframing, positive suggestions, encouragement and appreciation, a practitioner of acupuncture is specifically trained to access and transform the *Qi* of the patient before proceeding with the actual needling. From the *Qi*-based perspective of the acupuncture clinician, the specific components of treatment include this 'priming of *Qi*'. If the hypothesis of a physiological concordance as a mediator of the acupuncture treatment effects can be proven experimentally, the definition of placebo will need to be redefined: the 'priming of *Qi*' (which includes the palpation, observation, listening/smelling and questioning inherent in acupuncture treatment) will need to be considered as a specific component of treatment, rather than as a non-specific (i.e. placebo) factor.

TRANSLATING CLINICAL SKILLS INTO THE RESEARCH SETTING

Acupuncturists should participate from the beginning in the design of the study in order to help assure that the study questions are consistent with clinical practice and with the proposed treatment style under investigation. The selection of the acupuncture treatment style should be hypothesis driven, that is it should postulate a testable research question that is informed by clinical practice and experience. For more explanatory trials, where the design requires reduced variability of treatment, a particular style or combination of styles should be selected for testing in the study. Literature reviews and surveys of experienced practitioners in the particular condition and style of treatment, can help determine the representative treatment options (Schnyer & Allen 2002, Schnyer et al 2006). Formal consensus methods have been used, such as the nominal group technique, to elicit opinions of acupuncturists (MacPherson & Schroer 2007, Webster-Harrison et al 2002).

In our experience, the assumption that being a good clinician will automatically translate into being a good practitioner in an explanatory trial research setting has not been found to be useful. The more experienced the clinicians, the more unlikely they are to follow a treatment protocol, no matter how flexible. On the other hand, new practitioners sometimes lack the clinical skills to correctly implement an experimental treatment algorithm. Practitioners face great difficulty and conflict of interest when asked to perform sham procedures which can appear to clash with the ethics of undivided loyalty to patient care (Miller & Kaptchuk 2004). Treatment interventions that aim at blinding the practitioners (Allen et al 1998, Manber et al 2004) as a way of reducing practitioner expectancy effects have been used, though they are not a reliable form of blinding and compromise ecological validity. It is therefore usually necessary to train acupuncturists to prepare them for participating in research, regardless of their years of clinical experience.

Training of the treating acupuncturists in clinical trials should include a thorough review of the conceptual framework that informs the treatment selection, the diagnosis and treatment algorithm, and the guidelines for treatment implementation (Schnyer et al 2001), as well as the systematic use of assessment, treatment record and outcome measures. If the trial is explanatory with a placebo control arm, the acupuncturist should receive training on the placebo control intervention and on how to maintain equal input across active and control groups. Further instruction can include the biomedical condition under study, evidence on acupuncture so far for the treatment of that condition and details on the inclusion and exclusion criteria. All this information can be compiled into a treatment manual (Schnyer & Allen 2002) and a minimum one day workshop should be conducted to induct practitioners into the processes and procedures of the trial. Periodic supervision of treatment records, regular meetings to assess reliability of the methods employed, observation of treatments, and assessment of fidelity, can all help minimise any drift away from the treatment protocol that is common in many clinical research settings.

SUMMARY

Acupuncture clinical research needs to be informed by the actual clinical practice of acupuncture. Given that acupuncture is a complex, multimodal, interactive, treatment intervention, which stems from a rich and diverse tradition, acupuncture presents several methodological challenges to research. The unique diagnostic and clinical reasoning process that characterises traditional styles of acupuncture has not been systematically mapped out; we lack a common language that reflects an integration of an expanded biomedical model, consistent with the medicine's theoretical principles.

Because the practice of acupuncture is highly heterogeneous, research protocols employed in clinical trials must articulate which specific aspects of the theoretical foundations of Chinese medicine serve as the basis for the selection of any particular treatment protocol, whether consistent with traditional theories or based on innovative contemporary adaptations. Our ability to separate complex versus simple styles of treatment, may enable us to determine appropriate research methodology to answer specific research questions. Greater funding of pragmatic study designs would help us design better explanatory trials.

If, as practitioners believe, acupuncture involves more than just actual needling, it will be necessary to develop a testable hypothesis that reflects a clear articulation of what actually takes place during an acupuncture treatment. Only then will we be better able to assess acupuncture as a complex treatment intervention and assist in determining what is indeed specific to an acupuncture treatment. Research into the mechanism of acupuncture can help inform clinical research; clinical research can help guide basic research into the mechanisms of acupuncture. Clinical practice should provide the foundation for both basic and clinical research. In order to inform research, practitioners of acupuncture need to become involved and help articulate relevant research questions, assist in the development of best practice guidelines, participate in the design of treatment protocols and guide the operationalisation of the Chinese medicine diagnostic process.

Research resources

Birch S, Felt R 1999 Understanding acupuncture. Churchill Livingstone, London

Hsu E 1999 The transmission of Chinese medicine. University of Cambridge, Cambridge

Scheid V 2002 Chinese medicine in contemporary China: plurality and synthesis. Duke University Press, North Carolina

Taylor K 2004 Chinese medicine in early communist China (1945–1963): medicine in revolution. Routledge, London

Unschuld P 1985 Medicine in China: a history of ideas. University of California Press, Berkeley

References

Ahn A, Wu J, Badger G et al 2005 Electrical impedance along connective tissue planes associated with acupuncture meridians. BMC Complementary and Alternative Medicine 5(1):10

Allen J, Schnyer R, Hitt S 1998 The efficacy of acupuncture in the treatment of major depression in women. Psychological Science 9:397–401

Allen J, Schnyer R, Chambers A 2006 Acupuncture for depression: A randomized controlled trial. Journal of Clinical Psychiatry 67:1665–1673

Alraek T, Baerheim A 2003 The effect of prophylactic acupuncture treatment in women with recurrent cystitis: Kidney patients fare better. Journal of Alternative and Complementary Medicine 9(5):651–658

Beinfield H, Korngold E 1991 Between heaven and earth, a guide to Chinese medicine. Ballantine Books, New York

Birch S 1998 Preliminary investigations of the inter-rater agreement reliability of traditionally based acupuncture diagnostic assessments. In: An exploration with proposed solutions of the problems and issues in conducting clinical research in acupuncture. Exeter Publishers, Exeter

Birch S, Felt R 1999 Understanding acupuncture. Churchill Livingstone, London

Birch S, Jamison R 1998 Controlled trial of Japanese acupuncture for chronic myofascial neck pain: assessment of specific and nonspecific effects of treatment. Clinical Journal of Pain 14(3):248–255

Capra F 1996 The web of life. Random House, New York

Cassidy C 1998 Chinese medicine users in the United States. Part II: Preferred aspects of care. The Journal of Complementary and Alternative Medicine 4(2):189–202

Cherkin D, Eisenberg D, Sherman K et al 2001 Randomized trial comparing traditional Chinese medical acupuncture, therapeutic massage, and self-care education for chronic low back pain. Archives of Internal Medicine 161(8):1081–1088

Dale J 1997 Acupuncture practice in the UK. Part 1: report of a survey. Complementary Therapies in Medicine 5:215–220

Debata A 1968 Experimental study on pulse diagnosis of rokubujoi. Japan Acupuncture and Moxibustion Journal 17(3):9–12

Dobson K, Shaw B 1988 The use of treatment manuals in cognitive therapy: experience and issues. Journal of Consulting and Clinical Psychology 56(5):673–680

Filshie J, White A 1998 Medical acupuncture. Churchill Livingstone, Edinburgh

Hogeboom C, Sherman K, Cherkin D 2001 Variation in diagnosis and treatment of chronic low back pain in traditional Chinese medicine acupuncturists. Complementary Therapies in Medicine 9:154–166

Huan Z H, Rose K 2001 A brief history of qi. Paradigm, Brookline

Jarret L 2001 Nourishing destiny: The inner tradition of Chinese medicine. Spirit Path Press, Stockbridge

Kalauokalani D, Sherman K, Cherkin D 2001 Acupuncture for chronic low back pain: diagnosis and treatment patterns among acupuncturists evaluating the same patient. South Medical Journal 94(5):486–492

Kaptchuk T 2000 The web that has no weaver: understanding Chinese medicine, 2nd edn. Contemporary Books (McGraw-Hill), Chicago, IL

Kenyon J 1983 Modern techniques of acupuncture. Vol. 1. Thorsons, Wellingborough

King E, Cobbin D, Ryan D et al 2002a The reliable measurement of radial pulse: characteristics. Acupuncture in Medicine 20(4):150–159

King E, Cobbin D, Ryan D 2002b The reliable measurement of radial pulse: gender differences in pulse profiles. Acupuncture in Medicine 20(4):160–167

Klein D 1997 A psychotherapeutic context for clinical trials is promising, but manualization is not. Archives of General Psychiatry 54(10):929–930

Kurosu Y 1969 Experimental study on the pulse diagnosis of rokujuboi II. Japan Acupuncture and Moxibustion Journal 18(3):26–30

Langevin H, Yandow J 2002 Relationship of acupuncture points and meridians to connective tissue planes. Anatomical Record 269(6):257–265

Langevin H, Churchill D, Cipolla M 2002 Mechanical signaling through connective tissue: a mechanism for the therapeutic effect of acupuncture. FASEB Journal 15(2):2275–2282

Lao L, Bergman S, Langenberg P et al 1995 Efficacy of Chinese acupuncture on postoperative oral surgery pain. Oral Surgery, Oral Medicine, Oral Pathology, Oral Radiology, and Endodontics 79(4):423–428

Lao L et al 1999 Evaluation of acupuncture for pain control after oral surgery: a placebo-controlled trial. Archives of Otolaryngology – Head & Neck Surgery 125(5):567–572

Lao L, Ezzo J, Berman B et al 2001 Assessing clinical efficacy of acupuncture: considerations for designing future acupuncture trials. In: Stux G, Hammerschlag R (eds) Clinical acupuncture: scientific basis. Berlin, Springer Verlag, p 187–209

Lee M et al 2005 Differences in electrical conduction properties between meridians and non-meridians. American Journal of Chinese Medicine 33(5):723–728

Liangsheng W T 1997 Yellow emperor's cannon of internal medicine. China Science and Technology Press, Beijing

Linde K, Streng A, Jurgens S et al 2005 Acupuncture for patients with migraine: a randomized controlled trial. Journal of the American Medical Association 293(17):2118–2125

MacPherson H, Schroer S 2007 Standardising a complex intervention: a consensus method to define the characteristic components of treatment for use in a randomised controlled trial of acupuncture for depression. Complementary Therapies in Medicine 15(2):97–100

MacPherson H, Thorpe L, Thomas K et al 2004 Acupuncture for low back pain: traditional diagnosis and treatment of 148 patients in a clinical trial. Complementary Therapies in Medicine 12(1):38–44

MacPherson H, Thorpe L, Thomas K 2006 Beyond needling – therapeutic processes in acupuncture care; a qualitative study nested within a low back pain trial. Complementary Therapies in Medicine 12(9):873–880

Manber R, Schnyer R, Allen J et al 2004 Acupuncture: a promising treatment for depression during pregnancy. Journal of Affective Disorders 83:89–95

Matsumoto K, Euler D 2002 Kiiko Matsumoto clinical strategies. Vol. 1. Kiiko Matsumoto International, Natick, MA

Matsumoto T 1968 Experimental study on fukushin (abdominal palpation). Japan Acupuncture Moxibustion Journal 17(3):13–16

Miller F, Kaptchuk T 2004 Sham procedures and the ethic of clinical trials. Journal of the Royal Society of Medicine 97:756–758

Mori H 1979 Shinkyu no tameno Shindan to Chiryo. Ido no Nippon Sha, Yokosuka

Nakatani Y, Yamashita K 1977 Ryodoraku acupuncture. Osaka Ryodoraku Research Institute, Osaka

Nogier P 1983 From auriculotherapy to auriculomedicine. Maisonneuve, Saint-Ruffine

Ogawa T 1978 To establish new 'Chinese medicine': Searching for the contemporary significance of the 'meridian controversy' (in Japanese). Chinese Medicine 1(2):151–158

Paldan D T, Lee M R 1993 Tung's acupuncture by Dr Ching Chang Tung. Blue Poppy Press, Boulder

Paterson C, Dieppe P 2005 Characteristics and incidental (placebo) effects in complex interventions such as acupuncture. British Medical Journal 330:1202–1205

Scheid V 2006 Not very traditional, nor exactly Chinese, so what kind of medicine is it? TCM's discourse on menopause and its implications for practice, teaching and research. Journal of Chinese Medicine 82:5–20

Schnyer R, Allen J 2002 Bridging the gap in complementary and alternative medicine research: manualization as a means of promoting standardization and flexibility of treatment in clinical trials of acupuncture. Journal of Complementary and Alternative Medicine 8(5):623–634

Schnyer R, Allen J, Hitt S et al 2001 Acupuncture in the treatment of major depression: a manual for research and practice. Churchill Livingstone, London

Schnyer R, Conboy L, Jacobson E et al 2005 Development of a Chinese medicine assessment measure: an interdisciplinary approach using the Delphi method. Journal of Complementary and Alternative Medicine 11(6):1005–1013

Schnyer R, Wayne P, Kaptchuk T et al 2006 Standardization of individualized treatments in a randomized control trial of acupuncture for stroke rehabilitation. Journal of Alternative and Complementary Medicine 12:106–109

Seem M 1987 Bodymind energetics, towards a dynamic model of health. Thorsons Publishers, Rochester, Vermont

Sherman K et al 2005 The practice of acupuncture: who are the providers and what do they do? Annals of Family Medicine 3(2):151–158

Sivin N 1987 Traditional medicine in contemporary China. Center for Chinese Studies, University of Michigan, Ann Arbor

Stux G, Birch S, 2001 Proposed standards of acupuncture treatment for clinical studies. In: Stux G, Hammerschlag R (eds) Clinical acupuncture: scientific basis. Springer-Verlag, Berlin, p 171–185

Taylor K 2004 Divergent interests and cultivated misunderstandings: the influence of the West on modern Chinese medicine. Social History of Medicine 17(1):93–111

Thomas K, MacPherson H, Thorpe L et al 2006 Randomised controlled trial of a short course of traditional acupuncture compared with usual care for persistent non-specific low back pain. British Medical Journal 333(7569):623

Ulett G 1992 Beyond yin and yang. WH Green, St Louis, MI

Vickers A 1996 Can acupuncture have specific effects on health? A systematic review of acupuncture antiemesis trials. Journal of the Royal Society of Medicine 89:303–311

Vickers A, Rees R, Zollman C et al 2004 Acupuncture for chronic headache in primary care: large, pragmatic, randomised trial. British Medical Journal 328(7442):744

Voll R 1975 Twenty years of electroacupuncture diagnosis in Germany; A progress report. American Journal of Acupuncture 3:7–17

Walsh C, Corbin D, Bateman K et al 2001 Feeling the pulse: trial to assess agreement level among TCM students when identifying basic pulse characteristics. European Journal of Oriental Medicine 3(5):25–31

Wayne P, Krebs D, Macklin E et al 2005 Acupuncture for upper-extremity rehabilitation in chronic stroke: a randomized sham-controlled study. Archives of Physical Medicine and Rehabilitation 86:2248–2255

Webster-Harrison P, White A, Rae J 2002 Acupuncture for tennis elbow: an e-mail consensus study to define a standardised treatment in a GPs' surgery. Acupuncture in Medicine 20(4):181–185

Wilson G 1996 Manual-based treatments: The clinical application of research findings. Behavoral Research Therapy 34:295–314

Wiseman N, Boss K 1990 Glossary of Chinese medical terms. Paradigm Publications, Brookline, MA

Wiseman N, Feng Y 1998 A practical dictionary of Chinese medicine, 2nd edn. Paradigm Publications, Brookline, MA

Zaslawski C 2003 Clinical reasoning in traditional Chinese medicine: implications for clinical research. Clinical Acupuncture in Oriental Medicine 4(2–3):94–101

Zaslawski C J, Cobbin D, Lidums E et al 2003 The impact of site specificity and needle manipulation on changes to pain pressure threshold following manual acupuncture: A controlled study. Complementary Therapies in Medicine 11(1):11–21

Zell B, Hirata A, Marcus B 2000 Diagnosis of symptomatic postmenopausal women by traditional Chinese medicine practitioners. Menopause 7(2):129–134

Zhang G et al 2003 Assessing the consistency of traditional Chinese medical diagnosis: an integrative approach. Alternative Therapies 9(1):66–72

Zhang G, Bausell B, Lixing L et al 2004 The variability of TCM pattern diagnosis and herbal prescriptions on rheumatoid arthritis patients. Alternative Therapies 10(1):58–63

Zhang G et al 2005 Variability in the traditional Chinese medicine (TCM) diagnoses and herbal prescriptions provided by three TCM practitioners for 40 patients with rheumatoid arthritis. Journal of Alternative and Complementary Medicine 11(3):415–421

Physiological dynamics of acupuncture: correlations and mechanisms

10

Richard Hammerschlag, Hélène M. Langevin, Lixing Lao and George Lewith

OVERVIEW

The increasing Western acceptance of acupuncture as a safe and effective clinical practice has stimulated the testing of this traditional therapy in the twin forges of modern biomedicine: the randomised controlled trial (RCT) and the scientific laboratory. No matter that the East Asian system of medicine in which acupuncture is based has an explanatory model, diagnostic framework and treatment modalities that differ markedly from biomedicine. The dominant contemporary medical paradigm calls for acupuncture to be examined through Western lenses. The extent to which this approach generates 'images' of acupuncture that are clear and revealing, or are blurred and even distorted, forms the basis of ongoing debate (Ahn & Kaptchuk 2005, Hammerschlag 2003). The challenges, limited successes and lessons learned from evaluating acupuncture effectiveness and efficacy via RCTs are discussed elsewhere in this book (Chapters 7–8). The present chapter reviews a broad range of laboratory-based studies that have focused on the question, 'How does acupuncture work?'.

After exploring what is commonly meant by this question, from the perspectives of biomedicine and Oriental medicine, a range of potential benefits that derive from discovering answers are considered: from improvements in clinical practice as well as clinical trial designs to an enhanced understanding of physiological regulation in health and healing. A major section of the chapter is devoted to an overview of research that has probed the nature of acupuncture's functional anatomy, its acupuncture points and meridians. Research on morphological, bioelectrical, biochemical, biophysical and functional correlates of these

Oriental medicine-defined entities is examined to determine whether a physical basis for points and meridians is yet emerging and to assess the extent to which these descriptions may also provide clues to mechanism. We will see that much of the research purporting to examine 'mechanism' has assayed changes in biomarkers, e.g. neurohormones or other biochemicals, at sites considerably 'downstream' from where the needles are inserted. Such studies ask what biochemical or physiological changes can be measured when acupuncture is effective and thus provide 'correlational' data without revealing 'mechanism', i.e. how needling induces changes. With these distinctions in mind, the larger question becomes: to what extent can we begin to identify how the regulatory effects of acupuncture are initiated and mediated?

The chapter reflects a continuum of views of researchers in this field. At one end is a confidence that the mechanisms underlying acupuncture are explainable in terms of established biomedical constructs, in a manner that will facilitate the acceptance and integration of Oriental medicine into contemporary mainstream healthcare. At the other end is a conviction that exploration of acupuncture's traditional model, based on meridians and balancing the flow of *Qi*, will reveal important new aspects of physiological regulation that will expand our model of health and healing.

HOW DOES ACUPUNCTURE WORK? EXAMINING THE QUESTION

This chapter's central question, 'How does acupuncture work?' compels us to consider two differing paradigms: one molecular-based, the other 'energy'-based. In this light, it is helpful at the outset to examine what this question is asking. Since biomedicine and Oriental medicine offer differing sets of foundational principles as guides for answering the question (see Box 10.1), it is of interest to explore several commonly voiced responses that are based in these differing explanatory models.

When asked, 'How does acupuncture work?' many healthcare professionals as well as healthcare consumers are knowledgeable enough to respond quickly: 'By releasing endorphins'. Indeed, acupuncture-induced pain modulation has been linked to increased synthesis and release of encephalin, endorphin, and dynorphin as well as other endogenous substances in a wide variety of experimental studies, which have often led to detailed proposals of how acupuncture analgesia 'works' (Han 2003, Pomeranz 2001, White 2006) (see Box 10.2). Such findings, reinforced by brain imaging displays (Napadow et al 2006a), have enhanced the credibility of acupuncture, yet it is important to realise the limitations of such data for delineating mechanisms. Studies that detect change 'y' in response to intervention 'x' provide correlational or 'black box' data but reveal little direct information as to how the intervention induces the 'biomarker' changes. Hidden in the black box is the presumptive set of events that link needle insertion at an acupuncture point to the appearance of

---

Box 10.1 Framing the question, 'How does an intervention work?'

- From a biomedical perspective, pursuing how an intervention 'works' usually implies the aim of defining a sequence of molecular events. In the case of a drug, the concept of mechanism includes some combination of absorption, metabolic modification, recognition by specific receptors or target sites, initiation of biochemical and/or physiological events, and inactivation. Often forgotten is that the molecules involved, whether drugs or endogenous substances, can be described as aggregated fluctuations of atomic and subatomic energy as well as by the stick figure formulas found in textbooks of biochemistry and pharmacology.

- From a traditional Chinese medicine perspective, explanations of how acupuncture works are intrinsically related to how acupuncture heals. Relieving *Qi* stagnation or tonifying *Yin* is often reason enough. Only after rubbing shoulders with biomedicine have questions arisen concerning, for example, the anatomy and physiology of an acupuncture point or meridian. Just as biochemistry can be reframed in energetic terms, as considered above, it is intriguing to consider that information transmission triggered by acupuncture may well occur along molecular scaffolding and that the energetic fields that acupuncturists seek to regulate may be generated and monitored by cellular and sub-cellular mechanisms.

---

elevated levels of endogenous opioids in blood or cerebrospinal fluid. Little is known, for example, of the transduction events (involving transfer of mechanical, electrical and even more subtle forms of energy) by which the acupuncture needle initiates an informational signal. Nor are there any clear data regarding the nature of the acupuncture signal, how it is propagated or how it is received and responded to.

Ask the same question 'How does acupuncture work?', and members of the healthcare community familiar with the traditional acupuncture explanatory model may also choose to respond: 'By balancing the flow of *Qi*'. Relative to the response couched in 'endorphin release', evidence in support of the proposal that acupuncture balances *Qi* is more experiential than experimental. In several styles of acupuncture, practitioners compare pulse qualities before and after needling to provide an initial assessment of whether imbalances in *Qi* flow have been corrected. While pulse quality serves clinically as a surrogate marker of *Qi*, the measurement of *Qi* itself remains elusive. Without the ability to measure *Qi*, which in turn depends on an *a priori* knowledge of its nature, evidence that acupuncture corrects imbalances in *Qi* flow cannot be sought directly.

Box 10.2   Acupuncture analgesia: mediation by endogenous opioids and anti-opioids

Initial evidence of hormonal involvement:

- Time course of onset and decline of acupuncture analgesia in healthy volunteers is consistent with humoral rather than neural mediation (Research Group of Acupuncture Anesthesia PMC 1973).
- Perfusion of cerebrospinal fluid from rabbits with acupressure-induced analgesia to non-acupressured rabbits produces analgesia in recipients (Research Group of Acupuncture Anesthesia PMC 1974).

Similarities between acupuncture analgesia and morphine-induced analgesia:

- Pre-treatment with the morphine receptor blocker, naloxone, prevents acupuncture-induced analgesia (Mayer et al 1977, Pomeranz & Chiu 1976).
- Electroacupuncture analgesia and morphine analgesia show cross-tolerance (Han et al 1981).

Relation of electroacupuncture frequency (Hz) to type of endogenous opioid release:

- Low-frequency (2–10 Hz) electroacupuncture (EA) releases a different pattern of endogenous opioids than high-frequency (100–200 Hz) EA (Han 2003, Han et al 1981).

'Yin and Yang' of pain modulation: evidence for endogenous anti-opioids:

- Antiserum to cholecystokinin-8 (CCK-8) reverses EA tolerance (Han et al 1985).
- CCK-8 receptor deficient rats show enhanced EA (Lee et al 2003).
- CCK antisense RNA increases EA or morphine analgesia and converts low-responder rats to high responders (Tang et al 1997).

THE SEARCH FOR MECHANISM: THE NEEDLE OR THE MODALITY?

Thus far, the general consideration of how acupuncture works has focused on defining events triggered by, and correlated with, needle insertion. A broader view, beyond the scope of this chapter, could well be taken if mechanism is considered as the ground substance of the entire therapeutic encounter. Innovative studies establishing a role of endogenous opioids as mediators of the placebo response (Benedetti et al 2005) and explorations of unique brain responses to placebo acupuncture (Lewith et al 2005) are two examples of why physiological sequelae of needling will need to be interpreted within a more extensive context. What happens, for example, between sham insertion of a retractable needle and a brain image indicative of a placebo response is of major importance to understand as we seek to identify and enhance the contribution of placebo responses to outcomes in clinical practice. Since both acupuncture-induced analgesia and acupuncture-induced placebo responses may involve release of endogenous opioids, it is of interest to determine whether the verum (true treatment) and placebo/sham components of acupuncture analgesia are additive, synergistic or even antagonistic.

Practitioner intention, a component of acupuncture treatment that may contribute to clinical outcome, is another poorly controlled (and rarely considered) variable in clinical trials. In this context, researchers designing randomised, placebo-controlled trials of acupuncture need to be clear as to whether they are testing efficacy of the needle or efficacy of acupuncture. If the former, the research practitioners should be instructed to use a similar level of needling-associated intention when treating patients in either the verum or placebo groups. If the latter, practitioners should be coached to block their intention when administering placebo (sham) needling, so that the results will reflect a comparison of verum needling with intention versus sham needling without intention.

IMPORTANCE OF IDENTIFYING MECHANISMS OF ACUPUNCTURE

Progress toward an understanding of how acupuncture works will likely have benefits in several areas, notably improvements in clinical practice outcomes, a more rational design of control needling procedures for clinical trials and an expanded understanding of physiological regulation. Advances in each of these areas have the potential to enhance the credibility and consumer utilisation of acupuncture. Examples in each domain will be briefly considered.

Clinical practice

The emerging emphasis on 'translational research', the application of basic research findings to the treatment and prevention of human disease (Zerhouni 2005), is reflected in the outcome of basic research in acupuncture. An example involves developments in the use of electro-acupuncture. The addition of electro-stimulation to needles to facilitate acupuncture analgesia during surgery was a beneficial alternative for practitioners who were required to manually stimulate the needles over long periods of time. In this application of acupuncture, low-frequency and high-frequency electro-stimulation were found to mimic differing types of manual manipulation (Han 2003, Pomeranz 2001). Subsequent animal and human research revealed that low- vs. high-frequency stimulation releases different profiles of endogenous opioids and neurotransmitters, a finding that contributed to the redesign of commercially available electro-stimulation units used in contemporary clinical practice. Most units now include a setting that automatically toggles the frequency between low (2–10 Hz) and high (100–200 Hz) levels since this treatment produces a more effective degree of analgesia than either low or high frequency alone.

Clinical research

One of the most vexing problems in the design of clinical research is the uncertainty as to what constitutes an appropriate placebo or sham needling procedure (see Chapter 8). Since a placebo procedure, by definition, should mimic all external aspects of the real treatment but *not* mimic any of the internal (physiological) aspects, it follows that creation of an appropriate control procedure cannot occur until it is known 'what to avoid', i.e. until the mechanism of verum acupuncture is established (Hammerschlag & Zwickey 2006). The envisioned series of events is that an understanding of mechanism will inform appropriate design of sham needling procedures, which will lead to more definitive clinical trial results, which will produce a stronger evidence base for acupuncture and improve clinical practice.

Physiological regulation

As the emerging wisdom becomes gradually accepted that our endocrine, immune and nervous systems should no longer be considered as separate entities but as an intercommunicating whole (Wisneski & Anderson 2005), the biomedical community may take comfort in believing, at least, that all the major information-carrying systems of the body are known. It is in this context that we need to consider whether acupuncture acts via pathways already known or through a system that has remained below our biomedical radar. While a considerable body of evidence suggests that the acupuncture mediating system may be neural, with needles activating strategically positioned sensory nerve endings (see section on acupuncture points and meridians below), independent lines of research provide an alternative proposal: that the needle-initiating events occur within connective tissue (Langevin et al 2001a) whose planes are oriented in a manner that may follow traditional meridian pathways (Ahn et al 2005, Langevin & Yandow 2002).

Proposals of mechanisms subserving acupuncture phenomenology will need to consider the wide range of techniques that activate the acupuncture points and meridians. In addition to the Chinese-style needling, most commonly tested in clinical trials and basic science studies, there are styles of Japanese acupuncture that involve superficial (Birch & Jamison 1998) as well as non-invasive needling (Fukushima 1991). The latter, known as *Toyo Hari*, appears to affect acupoints 'energetically' in a manner similar to that occurring during external *Qigong* (one of acupuncture's sister modalities) administered at short and even long distances from the target (Chen 2004, Sancier 2001). Thus, while activation of the underlying system may occur by mechanical, electrical and even electromagnetic or other forms of stimuli, the identification and description of the system itself is likely to expand the present biomedical understanding of what one researcher has dubbed 'homeodynamic regulation' (Rubik 2002).

ACUPUNCTURE POINTS AND MERIDIANS: HOW ARE ACUPUNCTURE SIGNALS MEDIATED?

Despite several decades of multidisciplinary research, no generally accepted descriptions of acupuncture points (acupoints) and meridians have yet emerged in terms of Western anatomy and physiology. In the absence of a readily observable anatomical network, with clearly definable mapping to the classically defined meridians, the most frequently encountered proposal is that acupuncture is in effect an epiphenomenon of the nervous system (Cao 2002, Cho et al 2006, Ma 2004).

Considerations of neural pathways

The view of acupuncture points as sites where sensory nerve endings are most readily accessed and activated is based in part on anatomical findings, e.g. high densities of sensory nerve structures and an increased prevalence of nerve-vessel bundles penetrating the fascia have been observed at sites below dermal locations of classical acupoints (Heine 1988, Li et al 2004). Supporting evidence for this neural mediation view includes inhibition of acupuncture effectiveness at acupoints pre-injected with local anaesthetic (Chiang et al 1973); blockade of acupuncture 'action' distal to transection sites of spinal cord or nerve trunks in animals (Uchida et al 2000); and mimicking of acupuncture by direct electrical stimulation of peripheral nerves (Li et al 1998). Striking confirmation of neural involvement in acupuncture is also being provided by the emerging field of medical imaging (Napadow et al 2006a) (Box 10.3). Patterns of fMRI signals have been described for acupuncture-induced phenomena that are distinct from patterns evoked either by simple sensory stimulation, noxious stimuli or expectation (placebo) (Hui et al 2000, Pariente et al 2005).

While research findings pointing to a neural basis of acupuncture continue to accrue, a case can also be made that much of the supporting evidence for this view is correlational and indirect. For example, the observations of increased density of afferent nerve structures at

> ### Box 10.3 Brain imaging correlates of acupuncture
>
> - Patients' expectation of positive acupuncture effect (response to non-invasive sham acupuncture) causes greater brain activation than no expectation of effect (response to skin prick) (Pariente et al 2005).
> - Brain activity in response to acupuncture is distinct from activity in response to sharp pain (Hui et al 2000).
> - Acupuncture-induced clinical improvements in chronic pain (Harris et al 2006, Newberg et al 2005) and carpal tunnel syndrome (Napadow et al 2006b) correlate with changes in brain activity.
> - Whether traditional indications of acupuncture point function, e.g. improvement of sight or hearing, predict acupuncture-induced changes in specific brain regions, e.g. visual or auditory cortices, remains controversial: positive findings (Cho et al 1998, Li et al 2003); negative findings (Gareus et al 2002, Hu et al 2006).

acupoint sites require replication with validity and generalisability testing under blinded conditions. It can also be argued that local anaesthetic, transection and electrical stimulation may block or mimic acupuncture by acting on a yet-to-be-identified non-neural system via mechanisms independent of their actions on neural activity. Even the elegant fMRI images demand cautious interpretation. While the findings clearly suggest that the brain *monitors* acupuncture-related activity, it does not compel us to conclude that acupuncture-induced signals are solely neural events.

Considerations of non-neural pathways

If the evidence is not yet convincing for a neurally based model of acupuncture, are there other physiological systems that at least merit consideration as mediators of acupuncture effects? A reportedly novel system of histologically revealed ducts and corpuscles, for example, first described in the 1960s in relation to acupuncture, has been recently re-investigated (Shin et al 2005). While the morphology and ultrastructural features of this thread-like system have been visualised, claims of the system's relevance to acupoints and meridians have yet to be directly demonstrated. Another fluid-containing pathway proposed as an 'anatomical substrate' of meridians is the perivascular space, which has been tracked along portions of the Stomach and Gallbladder meridians in mice (Ma et al 2003). While portions of classically mapped meridians appear to follow major vascular structures, examinations of the 'anatomical substrate' are needed at sites where the respective courses of meridians and blood vessels diverge. Other recent studies, as cited above, have suggested a correspondence between acupuncture meridians and connective tissue planes, as visualised by ultrasound (Langevin & Yandow 2002). Findings that connective tissue comprises a network of extracellular matrix and cells which spans the whole body (Langevin et al 2004) and that connective tissue planes may be pathways of increased electrical conductance (Ahn et al 2005) suggest collagen-based connective tissue networks as an alternative to neural pathways as a basis of acupuncture phenomenology. Of added interest is that acupoints exhibit a stronger biomechanical 'needle grasp' compared with non-acupuncture points and that this response involves both the connective tissue matrix (Langevin et al 2001a, 2001b, 2002) and an active response of connective tissue fibroblasts (Langevin et al 2006). An interplay of signals between neural and connective tissue components, which could be triggered by mechanical or electrical perturbations during acupuncture, is further supported by the responsiveness of sensory neurons to biomechanical and chemical changes of the extracellular matrix that surrounds them (Ansel et al 1996). In this light, acupuncture-induced signalling may be envisioned as mediated via a neuro-fascial network of nervous system and connective tissue elements.

Biomedical correlates of acupuncture points and meridians

In considering the nature of an information-carrying system that acupuncture needles modulate, the wide variety of reported biomarkers of acupoints and meridians requires examination (see Box 10.4). From this literature, three examples of markers with differing physical properties: bioelectrical, biochemical and biothermal, will be described.

As alluded to above, considerable effort has been directed at determining whether acupoints and meridians can be identified on the basis of their bioelectrical properties. Despite decades of research, which has fostered a widespread belief that acupoints are dermal sites of decreased resistance/impedance (Becker et al 1976, Tiller 1989), and led to common clinical usage of battery-operated acupoint location devices, the evidence for electrodermal identification of acupoints has been questioned in several well-controlled studies (Martinsen et al 2001, McCarroll & Rowley 1979). This situation is due to a myriad of confounding variables, arising from physiology as well as instrumentation, from an almost total lack of attempted replicability of study design and results, and from the predominant use of healthy volunteers as subjects, in whom electrodermal differences between acupoints and non-point sites may not be marked (Tiller 1988). In contrast, a patient-based study design worth replicating, tests the Oriental medicine theory of somatotopic projection of the body onto the ear. In a blinded assessment of three groups of patients (current myocardial infarction (MI), prior MI, or angina) and a group of healthy controls, two ear points traditionally designated as representing the heart were found to be 'reactive' (conductivity $> 50\,\mu A$) in all three groups of patients at a markedly greater frequency than in the healthy controls.

Box 10.4   Biomedical correlates of acupuncture points and meridians

Bioelectrical correlates:

● Conductance maxima; resistance/impedance minima: positive evidence (Becker et al 1976, Colbert et al 2004, Tiller 1989); negative evidence (Martinsen et al 2001, McCarroll & Rowley 1979).

Biochemical correlates:

● Calcium ions (Guo et al 1991).
● Nitric oxide (Ma 2003).

Biophysical correlates:

● Bioluminescence (Edwards et al 1990, Litscher 2006, Lo 2002, Ovechkin et al 2001, Schlebusch et al 2005).

Functional correlates:

● Trigger points: positive (Melzack et al 1977); negative (Birch 2003).
● Pathways revealed by radioisotope markers: positive (Darras et al 1992, Kovacs et al 1992); negative (Simon et al 1986, Wu et al 1994).

Numerous other ear points tested showed no between-group differences (Saku et al 1993). The blinded design and 'reactive' point criteria had been developed previously for a study of patients with musculoskeletal pain (Oleson et al 1980). Ear points exceeding the conductivity threshold 'corresponded' to the painful musculoskeletal region on the body at a detection rate of 75%.

A second, more recently emerging candidate biomarker of acupoints and meridians is the multi-functional molecule, nitric oxide (NO). Since its initial identification as a modulator of blood vessels and its characterisation as a gas, NO has been the object of speculation as the biomedical equivalent of *Qi*, the unobstructed flow of which is essential in the Chinese view of health (Ralt 2005). The classical Chinese observation that '*blood* follows *Qi*' provides a literal description of the blood vessel dilation effect of NO, despite the confusion as to whether *Qi*' is actually flowing or is facilitating the flow of blood, just as NO itself does not flow but acts locally to regulate other cellular processes. Studies in rats (performed in a suitably blinded manner) have detected NO, its longer-lived metabolites and the neuronal form of its synthetic enzyme (NOS) at levels significantly higher in skin tissue associated with several different meridians (identified by their electro-dermal properties) compared to skin tissues from non-meridian regions (Ma 2003). More recent studies in hypertensive animals have demonstrated electro-acupuncture (ST36)-induced increases in peri-arteriolar NO and NOS that correlated with marked decreases in mean arterial pressure (Kim et al 2006).

A final, more speculative example of a putative biomarker of meridians is the reported emission of biophotons (thermal radiation) in the infrared range, either spontaneously (Ovechkin et al 2001) or in response to acupuncture (Lo 2002) or moxibustion (Schlebusch et al 2005). In each case, the infrared images revealed longitudinal entities corresponding to classically described meridians.

Speculations

Final considerations are merited for several theories of acupuncture-related mechanisms that as yet have little or no experimental support. Connective tissue-based proposals, for example, enter the realm of speculation on networks of collagen-linked fibres functioning as flexible liquid crystals that transmit bioinformation throughout the organism (Ho & Knight 1998, Oschman 2003). Such theories also build on findings that collagen fibres 'dock' at a myriad of cell surfaces (Vogel 2001) in a manner that would allow their proposed acupuncture-initiated 'information' to be transmitted through the cell membrane to modulate intracellular activity and function.

At a more bioenergetic level, the acupuncture system has been conceived as a manifestation of the biofield, a 'complex, extremely weak electromagnetic field of the organism' (Rubik 2002). This bioelectromagnetic (BEM) field allows the body to respond rapidly to relatively tiny perturbations, such as those produced by the acupuncture needle. Understanding how BEM fields are generated, maintained and modulated in the body is a central task for those who seek to establish an 'energy physiology' to ground the many emerging disciplines of energy medicine. One conjecture to explain therapeutic interactions with the biofield, either directly via the needle or non-invasively via *Toyo Hari* (see section on physiological regulation) and external *Qigong*, is impedance matching, a phenomenon akin to tuning an antenna to receive information at specific carrier frequencies (Hintz et al 2003).

Whether the 'acupuncture system' is eventually identified as a predominantly structural/biochemical or bioenergetic entity, a concept rooted in network theory seems helpful for guiding future research (Bell & Koithan 2006). If the extended meridian system is conceived as an interconnecting web, with acupuncture points as the sites of pathway crossings (or standing wave overlaps), then most acupoints would be network theory's *nodes*, while Oriental medicine's 'stronger' acupoints would represent network theory's *hubs*, i.e. sites of maximal path crossings or wave overlaps. In this view, the web or acupuncture system can be accessed and activated at sites anywhere on the body with acupuncture points representing the best sites of access, a concept that has important implications for acupuncture point specificity as well as the use of sham needling protocols in clinical trials.

SUMMARY

What this chapter reveals most clearly is how diverse the experimental approaches are that have been utilised to identify 'how acupuncture works'. It is not for lack of trying that the millennia-old, empirically developed system of acupuncture points and meridians has remained, from a Western perspective, more functional than physical. A comprehensive biomedical explanation remains elusive. The traditional system of acupuncture anatomy has yet to be either mapped onto a known biomedical system or adequately 'fit' into Western physiology as a 'homeodynamic' (Rubik 2002) complement to psychoneuroimmunological regulation. Future researchers grappling with the physiology of acupuncture need to bear in mind the importance of deconstructing this deceptively simple question, 'How does acupuncture work?'. First, the term 'acupuncture' must be unambiguously defined because of the multiplicity of practice styles. Physiology associated with one style of needling, e.g. electro-acupuncture, may not be generalisable to physiology of another style, e.g. superficial manual needling or non-penetrating *Toyo Hari* 'needling'. Similarly, the meaning of 'work' must be clarified, since measurements of biomarkers, e.g. changes in hormonal levels, will shed little light on how acupuncture 'signals' are transmitted from the skin surface to the site of hormone release. Finally, in crafting questions and research designs to explore the physiology of acupuncture, the importance of consulting with experienced acupuncture practitioners cannot be overstressed. Just as clinical research in acupuncture should be designed to closely reflect clinical practice, so too should studies of the physiology of acupuncture be informed by acupuncture's traditional explanatory model, its needling techniques and its needling-related phenomenology.

Research resources

Books

Kendell D E 2002 Dao of Chinese medicine: understanding an ancient healing art. Oxford University Press, Oxford

Stux G, Hammerschlag R 2001 Clinical acupuncture: scientific basis, 1st edn. Springer, Verlag

Articles

Andersson S, Lundeberg T 1995 Acupuncture — from empiricism to science: functional background to acupuncture effects in pain and disease. Medical Hypotheses 45(3):271–281

Cabyoglu M T, Ergene N, Tan U 2006 The mechanism of acupuncture and clinical applications. International Journal of Neuroscience 116(2):115–125

Dhond R P, Kettner N, Napadow V 2007 Neuroimaging acupuncture effects in the human brain. Journal of Alternative and Complementary Medicine (in press).

Kleinhenz J 1995 Acupuncture mechanisms, indications and effectiveness according to recent western literature. American Journal of Acupuncture 23(3):211–218

Korotkov K, Williams B, Wisneski L A 2004 Assessing biophysical energy transfer mechanisms in living systems: the basis of life processes. Journal of Alternative and Complementary Medicine 10(1):49–57

Langevin H M, Vaillancourt P D 1999 Acupuncture: does it work and, if so, how? Seminars in Clinical Neuropsychiatry 4(3):167–175

Lewith G T, White P J, Kaptchuk T J 2006 Developing a research strategy for acupuncture. Clinical Journal of Pain 22(7):632–638

Walling A 2006 Therapeutic modulation of the psychoneuroimmune system by medical acupuncture creates enhanced feelings of well-being. Journal of the American Academy of Nurse Practioners 18(4):135–143

Yung K T 2005 Birdcage model for the Chinese meridian system: part VI. Meridians as the primary regulatory system. American Journal of Chinese Medicine 33(5):759–766

References

Ahn A C, Kaptchuk T J 2005 Advancing acupuncture research. Alternative Therapies in Health and Medicine 11(3):40–45

Ahn A C, Wu J, Badger G J et al 2005 Electrical impedance along connective tissue planes associated with acupuncture meridians. BMC Complementary Alternative Medicine 5(1):10

Ansel J C, Kaynard A H, Armstrong C A et al 1996 Skin–nervous system interactions. Journal of Investigative Dermatology 106(1):198–204

Becker R O, Reichmanis M, Marino A A et al 1976 Electrophysiological correlates of acupuncture points and meridians. Psychoenergetic Systems 1:105–112

Bell I R, Koithan M 2006 Models for the study of whole systems. Integrative Cancer Therapies 5(4):293–307

Benedetti F, Mayberg H S, Wager T D et al 2005 Neurobiological mechanisms of the placebo effect. Journal of Neuroscience 25(45):10390–10402

Birch S 2003 Trigger point – acupuncture point correlations revisited. Journal of Alternative and Complementary Medicine 9(1):91–103

Birch S, Jamison R N 1998 Controlled trial of Japanese acupuncture for chronic myofascial neck pain: assessment of specific and nonspecific effects of treatment. Clinical Journal of Pain 14(3):248–255

Cao X 2002 Scientific bases of acupuncture analgesia. Acupuncture and Electro-therapeutics Research 27(1):1–14

Chen K W 2004 An analytic review of studies on measuring effects of external Qi in China. Alternative Therapies in Health and Medicine 10(4):38–50

Chiang C Y, Chang C T, Chu H L 1973 Peripheral afferent pathway for acupuncture analgesia. Scientia Sinica 16:210–217

Cho Z H, Chung S C, Jones J P et al 1998 New findings of the correlation between acupoints and corresponding brain cortices using functional MRI. Proceedings of the National Academy of Science of the USA 95(5):2670–2673

Cho Z H, Hwang S C, Wong E K et al 2006 Neural substrates, experimental evidences and functional hypothesis of acupuncture mechanisms. Acta Neurologica Scandinavica 113(6):370–377

Colbert A P, Hammerschlag R, Aickin M et al 2004 Reliability of the prognos electrodermal device for measurements of electrical skin resistance at acupuncture points. Journal of Alternative and Complementary Medicine 10(4):610–616

Darras J C, de Vernejoul P, Albarede P 1992 Nuclear medicine and acupuncture: a study of the migration of radioactive tracers at acupoints. American Journal of Acupuncture 20(3):245–256

Edwards R, Ibison M C, Jessel-Kenyon J et al 1990 Measurements of human bioluminescence. Acupuncture and Electro-therapeutics Research 15(2):85–94

Fukushima K 1991 Meridian therapy. Toyohari Medical Association, Tokyo

Gareus I K, Lacour M, Schulte A C et al 2002 Is there a BOLD response of the visual cortex on stimulation of the vision-related acupoint GB 37? Journal of Magnetic Resonance Imaging 15(3):227–232

Guo Y, Xu T, Chen J 1991 The study on calcium ion concentration specificity in meridian and acupoint in rabbit. Zhen Ci Yan Jiu 16(1):66–68

Hammerschlag R 2003 Acupuncture: on what should its evidence base be based? Alternative Therapies in Health and Medicine 9(5):34–35

Hammerschlag R, Zwickey H 2006 Evidence-based complementary and alternative medicine: back to basics. Journal of Alternative and Complementary Medicine 12(4):349–350

Han J S 2003 Acupuncture: neuropeptide release produced by electrical stimulation of different frequencies. Trends in Neuroscience 26(1):17–22

Han J S, Li S J, Tang J 1981 Tolerance to electroacupuncture and its cross tolerance to morphine. Neuropharmacology 20(6):593–596

Han J S, Ding X Z, Fan S G 1985 Is cholecystokinin octapeptide (CCK-8) a candidate for endogenous anti-opioid substrates? Neuropeptides 5(4–6):399–402

Harris R E, Gracely R H, McLean S A et al 2006 Comparison of clinical and evoked pain measures in fibromyalgia. Journal of Pain 7(7):521–527

Heine H 1988 Anatomical structure of acupoints. Journal of Traditional Chinese Medicine 8(3):207–212

Hintz K, Yount G, Kadar I et al 2003 Bioenergy definitions and research guidelines. Alternative Therapies in Health and Medicine 9(3):suppl A13–A30

Ho M W, Knight D P 1998 The acupuncture system and the liquid crystalline collagen fibers of the connective tissues. American Journal of Chinese Medicine 26(3–4):251–263

Hu K M, Wang C P, Xie H J 2006 Observation on activating effectiveness of acupuncture at acupoints and non-acupoints on different brain regions. Zhongguo Zhen Jiu 26(3):205–207

Hui K K, Liu J, Makris N et al 2000 Acupuncture modulates the limbic system and subcortical gray structures of the human brain: evidence from fMRI studies in normal subjects. Human Brain Mapping 9(1):13–25

Kim D D, Pica A M, Duran R G et al 2006 Acupuncture reduces experimental renovascular hypertension through mechanisms involving nitric oxide synthases. Microcirculation 13(7):577–585

Kovacs F M, Gotzens V, Garcia A et al 1992 Experimental study on radioactive pathways of hypodermically injected technetium-99 m. Journal of Nuclear Medicine 33(3):403–407

Langevin H M, Yandow J A 2002 Relationship of acupuncture points and meridians to connective tissue planes. Anatomical Record 269(6):257–265

Langevin H M, Churchill D L, Cipolla M J 2001a Mechanical signaling through connective tissue: a mechanism for the therapeutic effect of acupuncture. FASEB Journal 15(12):2275–2282

Langevin H M, Churchill D L, Fox J R et al 2001b Biomechanical response to acupuncture needling in humans. Journal of Applied Physiology 91(6):2471–2478

Langevin H M, Churchill D L, Wu J et al 2002 Evidence of connective tissue involvement in acupuncture. FASEB Journal 16(8):872–874

Langevin H M, Cornbrooks C J, Taatjes D J 2004 Fibroblasts form a body-wide cellular network. Histochemistry and Cell Biology 122(1):7–15

Langevin H M, Bouffard N A, Badger G J et al 2006 Subcutaneous tissue fibroblast cytoskeletal remodeling induced by acupuncture: Evidence for a mechanotransduction-based mechanism. Journal of Cell Physiology 207(3):767–774

Lee G S, Han J B, Shin M K et al 2003 Enhancement of electroacupuncture-induced analgesic effect in cholecystokinin-A receptor deficient rats. Brain Research Bulletin 62(2):161–164

Lewith G T, White P J, Pariente J 2005 Investigating acupuncture using brain imaging techniques: the current state of play. Evidence-Based Complementary and Alternative Medicine 2(3):315–319

Li A H, Zhang J M, Xie Y K 2004 Human acupuncture points mapped in rats are associated with excitable muscle/skin-nerve complexes with enriched nerve endings. Brain Research 1012(1–2):154–159

Li G, Liu H L, Cheung R T et al 2003 An fMRI study comparing brain activation between word generation and electrical stimulation of language-implicated acupoints. Human Brain Mapping 18(3):233–238

Li P, Pitsillides K F, Rendig S V et al 1998 Reversal of reflex-induced myocardial ischemia by median nerve stimulation: a feline model of electroacupuncture. Circulation 97(12):1186–1194

Litscher G 2006 Bioengineering assessment of acupuncture, part 1: thermography. Critical Reviews in Biomedical Engineering 34(1):1–22

Lo S Y 2002 Meridians in acupuncture and infrared imaging. Medical Hypotheses 58(1):72–76

Ma S X 2003 Enhanced nitric oxide concentrations and expression of nitric oxide synthase in acupuncture points/meridians. Journal of Alternative and Complementary Medicine 9(2):207–215

Ma S X 2004 Neurobiology of acupuncture: toward CAM. Evidence-Based Complementary and Alternative Medicine 1(1):41–47

Ma W, Tong H, Xu W et al 2003 Perivascular space: possible anatomical substrate for the meridian. Journal of Alternative and Complementary Medicine 9(6):851–859

Martinsen O G, Grimnes S, Morkrid L et al 2001 Line patterns in the mosaic electrical properties of human skin – a cross-correlation study. IEEE Transactions in Biomedical Engineering 48(6):731–734

Mayer D J, Price D D, Rafii A 1977 Antagonism of acupuncture analgesia in man by the narcotic antagonist naloxone. Brain Research 121(2):368–372

McCarroll G D, Rowley B A 1979 An investigation of the existence of electrically located acupuncture points. IEEE Transactions in Biomedical Engineering 26(3):177–181

Melzack R, Stillwell D M, Fox E J 1977 Trigger points and acupuncture points for pain: correlations and implications. Pain 3(1):3–23

Napadow V, Webb J M, Pearson N et al 2006a Neurobiological correlates of acupuncture: November 17–18, 2005. Journal of Alternative and Complementary Medicine 12(9):931–935

Napadow V, Kettner N, Ryan A et al 2006b Somatosensory cortical plasticity in carpal tunnel syndrome – a cross-sectional fMRI evaluation. NeuroImage 31(2):520–530

Newberg A B, Lariccia P J, Lee B Y et al 2005 Cerebral blood flow effects of pain and acupuncture: a preliminary single-photon emission computed tomography imaging study. Journal of Neuroimaging 15(1):43–49

Oleson T D, Kroening R J, Bresler D E 1980 An experimental evaluation of auricular diagnosis: the somatotopic mapping or musculoskeletal pain at ear acupuncture points. Pain 8(2):217–229

Oschman J 2003 Energy medicine: therapeutics and human performance, 3rd edn. Butterworth-Heinemann, Amsterdam

Ovechkin A, Lee S M, Kim K S 2001 Thermovisual evaluation of acupuncture points. Acupuncture Electro-therapeutics Research 26(1–2):11–23

Pariente J, White P, Frackowiak R S 2005 Expectancy and belief modulate the neuronal substrates of pain treated by acupuncture. NeuroImage 25(4):1161–1167

Pomeranz B 2001 Acupuncture analgesia – basic research. In: Stux G, Hammerschlag R (eds) Clinical acupuncture: scientific basis. Springer-Verlag, Berlin, p 1–28

Pomeranz B, Chiu D 1976 Naloxone blockade of acupuncture analgesia: endorphin implicated. Life Sciences 19(11):1757–1762

Ralt D 2005 Intercellular communication, NO and the biology of Chinese medicine. Cell Communication and Signaling 3(1):8

Research Group of Acupuncture Anesthesia PMC 1973 The effect of acupuncture on the human skin pain threshold. Chinese Medical Journal 3:151–157

Research Group of Acupuncture Anesthesia PMC 1974 The role of some neurotransmitters of the brain in finger-acupuncture analgesia. Scientia Sinica 17:112–130

Rubik B 2002 The biofield hypothesis: its biophysical basis and role in medicine. Journal of Alternative and Complementary Medicine 8(6):703–717

Saku K, Mukaino Y, Ying H 1993 Characteristics of reactive electropermeable points on the auricles of coronary heart disease patients. Clinical Cardiology 16(5):415–419

Sancier K M 2001 Search for medical applications of qigong with the Qigong Database. Journal of Alternative and Complementary Medicine 7(1):93–95

Schlebusch K P, Maric-Oehler W, Popp F A 2005 Biophotonics in the infrared spectral range reveal acupuncture meridian structure of the body. Journal of Alternative and Complementary Medicine 11(1):171–173

Shin H S, Johng H M, Lee B C et al 2005 Feulgen reaction study of novel threadlike structures (Bonghan ducts) on the surfaces of mammalian organs. Anatomical Record. Part B, New Anatomist 284(1):35–40

Simon J, Guiraud G, Esquerre J P 1986 La Methodologie des Radioisotopes Permet-elle de Justifier l'Existance de Meredians d'Acupuncture. Bulletin de l'Académie nationale de médecine 172:363–368

Tang N M, Dong H W, Wang X M et al 1997 Cholecystokinin antisense RNA increases the analgesic effect induced by electroacupuncture or low dose morphine: conversion of low responder rats into high responders. Pain 71(1):71–80

Tiller W 1988 On the evolution of electrodermal diagnostic instruments. Journal of Advanced Medicine 1(1):41–72

Tiller W A 1989 On the evolution and future development of electrodermal diagnostic instruments. Energy fields in medicine. John Fetzer Foundation, Kalamazoo, MI, p 258–328

Uchida S, Kagitani F, Suzuki A et al 2000 Effect of acupuncture-like stimulation on cortical cerebral blood flow in anesthetized rats. Japanese Journal of Physiology 50(5):495–507

Vogel W F 2001 Collagen-receptor signaling in health and disease. European Journal of Dermatology 11(6):506–514

White P 2006 A background to acupuncture and its use in chronic painful musculoskeletal conditions. Journal of the Royal Society of Health 126(5):219–227

Wisneski L A, Anderson L 2005 The scientific basis of integrative medicine. CRC Press, Boca Raton

Wu C C, Chen M F, Lin C C 1994 Absorption of subcutaneous injection of Tc-99 m pertechnetate via acupuncture points and non-acupuncture points. American Journal of Chinese Medicine 22(2):111–118

Zerhouni E A 2005 US biomedical research: basic, translational, and clinical sciences. Journal of the American Medical Association 294(11):1352–1358

Evidence overviews: the role of systematic reviews and meta-analyses

11

Klaus Linde, Richard Hammerschlag and Lixing Lao

INTRODUCTION

Every year more than two million articles are published in over 20 000 bio-medical journals (Mulrow 1994). Even in a speciality area like acupuncture it is impossible to keep up to date with all relevant new information. In this situation systematic reviews hold a key position to summarise the state of the actual knowledge. A review is called systematic if it asks a specific question, uses predefined and explicit methods to identify and select the research articles relevant to the question, and uniformly applies a pre-established set of criteria to critique the included articles. A systematic review is called a meta-analysis if it includes a pooled statistical analysis of a subset of the included studies assessed as uniform enough in quality and design.

A large number of systematic reviews of acupuncture have been published since the late 1980s. Systematic reviews are of crucial interest for decision-makers, can help to improve future research and should, in principle, also be relevant for practitioners. In this chapter we will present an overview of what performing a systematic review involves, what has been learned thus far from systematic reviews of acupuncture, where the main research challenges for the future lie, and how information distilled from such reviews might translate into practice.

HOW SYSTEMATIC REVIEWS ARE DONE (AND HOW READERS CAN ASSESS THEM)

Protocol

Whenever possible, the key methods to be used in a systematic review should be predefined in a protocol. However, compared to the protocol of a randomised trial which should regulate every detail, the initial protocol of a systematic review often can only provide a crude guideline of what will be done. This is due to the fact that reviewers have to work with the material available, similar to in a retrospective study. If, for example, the available studies do not provide sufficient detail a statistical meta-analysis planned in the protocol simply cannot be performed. The protocol of a systematic review should have subheadings similar to those listed below.

The research question

As in any research study, a clear and straightforward question is a precondition for a conclusive answer. Such a question could be for example whether acupuncture interventions improve function in patients with chronic low back pain better than sham interventions. If possible the question of a review already predefines broadly the group of patients (those with chronic low back pain), the type of experimental (acupuncture) and control intervention (sham acupuncture) as well as the outcome of interest (function). However, due to the limited number of trials, reviews of acupuncture often have broader questions, for example, is there evidence from randomised trials that acupuncture is effective for low back pain. Reviews with broader questions in general cannot test a hypothesis (as they do not explicitly state one) but should be considered primarily as descriptive overviews.

Most available systematic reviews on acupuncture have focused on treatment effects investigated in randomised trials. But of course, it is possible for systematic reviews to focus on other topics (safety, practice style, outcome under routine conditions, mechanisms, etc.) and include other types of primary studies or sources (case reports, surveys, observational studies, laboratory studies, etc.).

Searching the literature

A precondition for a good-quality systematic review is that the relevant literature is searched comprehensively. In conventional medicine the majority of research journals are listed in one or more of the electronic databases such as PubMed (free access at http://www.ncbi.nlm.nih.gov/entrez/query.fcgi), EMBASE (limited access at http://www.embase.com/), the Cochrane Controlled Trials Registry (limited access at http://www.thecochranelibrary.com/), etc. While many acupuncture studies are published in conventional medicine journals and some acupuncture (and complementary and alternative medicine) journals are listed in these databases, a significant number of acupuncture trials appear in journals not listed in these databases. There are a number of complementary medicine databases. Examples of well-accessible databases of interest to acupuncturists include AMED (for access information see http://www.bl.uk/collections/health/amed.html) or Acubriefs (http://www.acubriefs.com/). However, the majority of databases are specialised in certain areas, difficult to access and to search. Another problem for Western reviewers is the abundant, but hardly accessible, literature from China and other Asian countries. It has been shown that clinical studies from these countries report almost exclusively very positive results, which raises serious doubts about validity (Vickers et al 1998). Therefore, many Western researchers are reluctant to invest relevant resources into identifying, obtaining and translating such studies. Whether this approach is always justified is debatable. In general, it is reasonable to assume that most high-quality research on acupuncture is available through major databases.

A very effective and simple additional search strategy is to check the references of identified studies and reviews relevant to the topic. This method often also identifies studies that are published only as abstracts, in conference proceedings or books.

In practice, the comprehensiveness of the literature search will depend strongly on the resources available. Reviews that are based on literature searches in only one or two of the mentioned sources, for example, should be interpreted with caution keeping in mind that a number of relevant studies might have been missed. Reviews restricted to studies published in the English language might exclude a relevant proportion of studies published in other (non-Asian) languages. For all reviews, the problem of unpublished studies − particularly those with negative results (resulting in publication bias) − has to be kept in mind.

Selecting the relevant studies

Selecting the studies for detailed review from the often large number of references identified from the search is the next crucial step in the review process. Readers should check carefully whether this process was transparent and unbiased.

A good systematic review must explicitly define inclusion and exclusion criteria. In practice the selection process is commonly performed in two steps. In the first step all the obviously irrelevant material is discarded, for example articles addressing a completely different topic or not reporting original data. To save money this step is normally done by only one reviewer in a rather informal way. The remaining articles should then be checked carefully for eligibility by at least two independent (one does not know the decision of the other) reviewers. In the publication of a systematic review the potentially relevant studies that were excluded should be listed and the reasons for exclusion given. Readers should be aware that minor modifications of selection criteria can have a dramatic effect on the number of included studies and possibly on the conclusions (Linde & Willich 2003).

Extracting information and assessing quality

Once the eligible studies have been identified, obtained, and checked to be certain they have met the inclusion criteria, relevant information has to be extracted. This typically includes details of the patient sample, setting and therapist; design, outcome measurement criteria, and length of follow-up; details of the experimental and the control intervention; and finally the overall findings and most important data of the primary studies. If possible the extraction should be standardised, for example, by using a pre-tested form. Extraction and all assessments should be done by at least two independent reviewers.

Parallel to the extraction of information, the quality of a study should be assessed. Methodologists tend to define quality as the likelihood that the results of a study are valid. This dimension of quality is sometimes referred to as internal validity or methodological quality. There is widespread agreement that key criteria for the internal validity of treatment studies are random allocation to treatment group, blinding to treatment group, and adequate handling of drop-outs and withdrawals. Often these and other criteria are combined in scores (see Moher et al 1995, 1996 for overviews, and Box 11.1 for an example). But the validity of such scores is doubtful (Jüni et al 1999). Whether the criteria are combined in scores or applied separately the problems remain that the formalised assessment is often crude and that the reviewers have to rely on the information reported.

Obviously, a trial which is internally valid is not necessarily a good trial in other respects. The acupuncture intervention might be inappropriate, outcome measures might be irrelevant or the sample of patients may be inadequate for the clinical question. While the assessment of dimensions of quality for these parameters is desirable, it is extremely difficult to reach consensus on such subjective items. In the section on challenges, the challenges of assessing the adequacy of interventions and the external validity of a study will be discussed in detail. It is easier to assess whether the acupuncture intervention has been *described* adequately. The STRICTA (STandard of Reporting Interventions in Controlled Trials of Acupuncture) guidelines provide a comprehensive list of details which should be reported in any publication of a trial (MacPherson et al 2001).

Summarising the results

Since a major target audience for systematic reviews is clinicians, who are mainly interested in the 'bottom line' results, it can be argued that a straightforward narrative description of the findings for each of the included studies should be sufficient. However, if the number of studies is not very small, such summaries are tiring to read and the risk of selective reporting is considerable. Summarising results of studies as positive or negative (so-called vote counts) is attractive and has often been used in

Box 11.1 The Jadad scale: a widespread method for assessing the methodological quality of trials

The most widely used instrument for quality assessment in systematic reviews is the Jadad scale (Jadad et al 1996). This instrument was originally developed to 'measure the likelihood of bias in pain research reports'. In the first step of development of the instrument, the aim was defined and a preliminary list of items was established with the help of a panel of experts. The list was refined in a follow-up consensus process and tested on a set of trials to determine whether the items could be scored in a reliable manner (inter-rater agreement) and whether they were discriminative (separated better from worse trials). This process led to the development of a very simple instrument with only three questions: 1. was the study described as randomized?; 2. was the study described as double-blind?; 3. was there a description of drop-outs and withdrawals? Up to two points are given for questions 1 and 2, and one point for question 3 (so the maximum score is 5). For the rating a study is regarded as double-blind if neither the person doing the assessments nor the study participant knows the allocation group. This is interpreted to mean that trials in which blinded patients self-assess their outcomes are considered double-blind. This simple instrument works rather well on a pragmatic level to separate groups of studies with lower (less than 3 points) and higher methodological quality in larger study sets. However, the assessment of a single trial can be completely misleading. From a methodological point of view the scale misses the most important issue of concealment of allocation (making sure that at the moment of including a patient into a trial it cannot be predicted to which group the participant will be allocated). It has been shown that studies with inadequate concealment often yield over-optimistic results. A great variety of other instruments exist but it is unclear whether they are truly better than the Jadad scale.

the past. However, the findings of many studies are not easily summarised in such a simplistic manner and depending on definitions and perception/prejudices of reviewers the votes on the same study might differ. If possible it is always preferable to summarise the findings of primary studies with quantitative outcomes in so-called effect size measures. Typical effect size estimates are relative risks or responder ratios (proportion of responders in the acupuncture group/proportion of responders in the control group), or weighted or standardised mean differences (mean pain rating in the acupuncture group — mean pain rating in the control group). The effect size measures of the different studies are then typically plotted in a mixture of graph and figure (the so-called Forest plot — Box 11.2). The review only becomes a meta-analysis if the data of the single studies are subsequently pooled to create an overall effect size. Whether it is justified to do this is a difficult decision that depends mainly on whether the primary studies are considered sufficiently comparable regarding patients,

Box 11.2   Understanding Forest plots

Most systematic reviews or meta-analyses which summarise the results of single studies in a single figure (the effect size estimate) present a Forest plot. This mixture of tables and graphics allows any reader with basic knowledge of biostatistics to get an intuitive idea of the overall results. The example below has been extracted from ongoing work on the Cochrane review of acupuncture for idiopathic headaches. It shows the response (at least 50% reduction of headache frequency) observed in nine trials comparing acupuncture and sham interventions in patients with migraine.

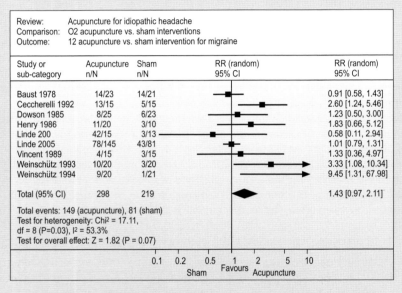

Example of a Forest plot taken from ongoing work on the Cochrane review of acupuncture for idiopathic headaches.

Each line reports the findings of one trial. The small 'n' gives the number of patients who responded while the big 'N' gives the total number of patients in the group. The effect size estimate in this case is the RR (originally relative risk, however, as we talk here about a positive event, responder ratio fits better). This is illustrated most easily by the trial of Weinschütz (1993): 10 of 20 patients (50%) receiving acupuncture responded compared to 3 of 20 (15%) in the sham group. Dividing 50% by 15% gives the RR of 3.33 (the square in the graph). If more patients respond to acupuncture than to sham the RR is always greater than 1; if more patients respond to sham it is smaller than 1. By looking at the squares the reader immediately sees whether the majority of squares are on the right or on the left side of 1 (no difference). The lines right and left to the small square indicate the 95% confidence interval (95% CI). The CI indicates to what extent chance might have influenced the results: in small trials, random error might have a large role and therefore CIs tend to be wide while large trials mostly have small CIs. If the 95% CI does not include 1 the difference between acupuncture and sham is statistically significant (a p-value smaller than 0.05). In the example this is the case for three trials (Ceccherelli 1992, Weinschütz 1992, 1993). Up until now we are still at the level of a systematic review. Only when the results of the single trials are pooled into a common effect estimate has the step to a full meta-analysis been taken (see the line 'total'). The pooled effect size estimate is often displayed as a diamond. In our example it is 1.43 with a CI from 0.97 to 2.11. This indicates that more patients responded to acupuncture than to sham treatment, however, this difference is not statistically different because the horizontal line crosses 1.0 (see the p-value for the overall effect which is 0.07). Z and Chi^2 are test statistics which are not discussed here.

The software used also performs a heterogeneity test. This checks whether the differences in the findings of the different studies can be explained by chance. In other words the tests check whether the findings of the different studies give a consistent picture or whether they do not fit together. In our example this test is significant (p = 0.03) and the heterogeneity estimator I^2 is over 50% (0% would mean that the differences in results can be explained fully by chance). This indicates that the findings of the trials are contradictory and that trials either do not address the same questions or differ in some other respect, in which case it should not be considered justifiable to calculate a pooled estimate.

The type of effect size estimate and details of the presentation differ between meta-analyses but the principle is always the same. For further details see textbooks for meta-analyses cited at the end of this chapter.

interventions, outcome and quality. If possible, a meta-analysis should include sensitivity analyses to check the robustness of the results. For example, one can check whether the overall effect size is different when only the best trials are included. Unfortunately, in the acupuncture research literature the number of trials is rarely sufficient to perform reliable sensitivity analyses.

A SHORT HISTORY OF SYSTEMATIC REVIEWS OF ACUPUNCTURE

A comprehensive collection of the Cochrane Complementary Medicine Field covering the period from 1989 to 2000 identified no less than 39 systematic reviews restricted to clinical trials of acupuncture (Linde et al 2001). We estimate that between 1989 and 2005, the effectiveness or safety of acupuncture has been addressed in more than 70 systematic reviews. While effectiveness for defined conditions remains by far the most frequently investigated subject, systematic reviews also exist on safety aspects (for example Ernst & White 1997, 2001), the description of treatment strategies in clinical trials (Linde et al 2001) or focusing almost exclusively on the methodological quality of trials (Rosted 1998).

Early systematic reviews on acupuncture have been strongly influenced by the pioneering work of Gerben ter Riet, Jos Kleijnen and Paul Knipschild from the University of Maastricht, Netherlands. Mainly in the early nineties of the last century this group of clinical epidemiologists produced a series of influential reviews on acupuncture, homeopathy, herbal medicines and food supplements. After a series of eight short papers on controlled (not necessarily randomised) clinical trials of acupuncture for different conditions in a Dutch family practice journal, two major summary papers on chronic pain and addiction were published in English-language journals in 1990 (ter Riet et al 1990a, 1990b). At that time the methodological rigour and transparency of the reviews produced by the Maastricht group were exceptional, and not only in the area of complementary medicine. Characteristics of the Maastricht reviews were a comprehensive coverage of the literature, a strong focus on the assessment of methodological quality using complex scoring systems, a very simplistic vote count approach to summarise study results combined with a great reluctance to pool heterogeneous studies in a statistical meta-analysis. Interestingly, this group of methodologists without any practical experience of acupuncture already tried to incorporate aspects of quality related to the acupuncture intervention into their assessments (avoidance of diffuse noxious inhibitory control for sham interventions, adequate description of the intervention, and mentioning of the 'good quality' of the acupuncturist). The Maastricht reviews had considerable impact on complementary medicine reviews in the following years: assessment of methodological quality became the major focus, with less emphasis on descriptions of study characteristics and results. And it was considered acceptable that reviews were primarily done by methodologists with little or no practical experience of the intervention and the condition addressed.

With very few exceptions the systematic reviews on acupuncture efficacy, performed in the first years after the Maastricht reviews, came to very similar conclusions regardless of the condition: the methodological quality of the majority of trials was considered insufficient, sample sizes too small, and study results were contradictory. An exception was the stimulation of P6 (not necessarily by needling) for nausea (Vickers 1996) where the findings were clearly positive.

In the late 1990s the Complementary Medicine Field of the Cochrane Collaboration was established. The Cochrane Collaboration is a worldwide network with the objective to perform, regularly update and disseminate systematic reviews in all areas of healthcare. The Complementary Medicine Field, which is coordinated by Brian Berman at the University of Maryland, has successfully facilitated numerous activities within the Collaboration. While some see the strong focus of the Cochrane Collaboration on randomised trials with mixed or negative feelings, its methodological influence as well as the growing experience of reviewers has contributed to a considerable shift in the methodology of overviews of acupuncture. Whenever possible review teams now also include (but still are rarely headed by) persons with practical expertise in the intervention and the clinical condition investigated. While assessment of methodology is still a relevant issue, summaries of the actual study results are considered the most important component of an overview (see for example, Manheimer et al (2005), Box 11.3). A critical assessment of the interventions and a careful look at the validity of sham procedures is becoming more and more frequent. Despite the progress in these areas there are still major methodological challenges facing systematic review of acupuncture (see below and Box 11.4).

While systematic reviews clearly state their selection and evaluation criteria, the absence of a generally accepted prescriptive format has led,

---

Box 11.3   Example of a recent review

Manheimer et al (2005) reported a systematic review on acupuncture for low back pain. They searched databases such as MEDLINE, Cochrane Central, EMBASE, AMED, CINAHL, CISCOM, and GERA and identified 33 randomised, controlled trials that met inclusion criteria which were sub-grouped according to acute or chronic pain, style of acupuncture, and type of control group used. Data were extracted for the outcomes of pain, functional status, overall improvement, return to work, and analgesic consumption by two independent investigators and entered onto a piloted spreadsheet. Differences between the two researchers were settled by discussion with reference to the original article. A meta-analysis using quantitative data synthesis was then performed. The principal measure of effect size was the standardised mean difference. They also assessed the quality of the studies using a scoring system for each item of research methods used in the trials. For example, they scored a maximum of 5 points in 3 categories: randomisation (2 points for an appropriate method, 1 point if method not described, or 0 points for an inappropriate method); blinding (1 point for patient blinding and 1 point if blinding was tested after treatment); and withdrawals and dropouts (1 point if a statement gave full details of withdrawals and dropouts or confirmed that no patient withdrew or dropped out). A score of 2 points or less was considered as poor quality. The quality assessment of each trial allows researchers to determine the effectiveness of treatment not only based on the results of outcome analysis, but also by taking the consideration of the quality of these studies.

The study shows that acupuncture is significantly more effective than sham treatment (standardised mean difference, 0.54 (95% CI, 0.35–0.73)) and no additional treatment (standardised mean difference, 0.69 (CI, 0.40–0.98)) in short-term relief of chronic pain. But for patients with acute low back pain, data are sparse and inconclusive. Data are also insufficient for drawing conclusions about acupuncture's short-term effectiveness compared with most other therapies. They concluded that acupuncture effectively relieves chronic low back pain but no evidence suggests that acupuncture is more effective than other active therapies.

Box 11.4   Discordant findings and interpretations in systematic reviews

Linde & Willich (2003) compared the conclusions on the same set of studies on acupuncture for low back pain included in two systematic reviews (van Tulder et al. (1999) and Smith et al. (2000)). Both reviews summarised the conclusions drawn by the study authors as well as their own conclusions. Van Tulder et al used a 3-step vote count (positive, neutral, negative) with an unclear option while Smith et al voted trials as positive or negative. Both reviews did not report exactly how reviewers decided on votes.

Trial	Author conclusion		Reviewer conclusion	
	Van Tulder	Smith	Van Tulder	Smith
Coan et al	Positive	Positive	Unclear	Positive
Duplan et al	Positive	Positive	Positive	Negative
Edelist et al	Neutral	Negative	Neutral	Negative
Garvey et al	Positive	Negative	Neutral	Negative
Gunn et al	Positive	Positive	Neutral	Positive
Lehmann et al	Positive	Negative	Neutral	Negative
Lopacz & Gralewski	Neutral	Negative	Neutral	Positive
Mendelson et al	Neutral	Negative	Unclear	Negative

on occasion, to reviews on the same topic arriving at somewhat differing conclusions (see Box 11.4 for an example). These inconsistencies make clear that despite the use of systematic methods there are many subjective judgements in the review process. Given these subjective elements it seems desirable, particularly in those cases where a relatively large literature exists, for more than one group to work on a specific question. Still, efforts should not be duplicated unnecessarily, even though the resources needed to perform a systematic review are clearly less than those for a major clinical study. This bears the risk that too many reviews are performed, instead of focusing resources on more primary studies based on the methodological recommendations of existing reviews.

In 2006, a team of sceptical researchers concluded that systematic reviews published between January 1996 and August 2005 do not provide robust evidence that acupuncture works for any condition (Derry et al 2006). While many researchers in the field would probably agree that apart from the stimulation of P6 for nausea (Lee & Done 2004) the evidence is not fully convincing, such a negative conclusion does not seem justified. In recent years more and more high-quality trials of acupuncture became available, and at least for some conditions the evidence is consolidating. For example, the conclusion of the update of the Cochrane review of acupuncture for low back pain is clearly more positive than that of the first version (Furlan et al 2005, Van Tulder et al 1999). Compared to usual care or waiting list controls, reviews integrating recent, large high-quality trials clearly show that acupuncture provides clinically relevant benefit in low back pain, headaches or osteoarthritis of the knee (Linde & Streng 2005, Manheimer et al 2006, Melchart et al 2001). However, they also show that effects over sham acupuncture interventions tend to be minor and highly variable (see Chapter 8 for possible explanations of these findings).

CHALLENGES

Systematic reviews are clearly the best tool to summarise the available evidence on defined research questions. The methodology has been improved both in general and in the area of acupuncture over the last two decades. Still, the considerable limitations must be kept in mind: although most systematic reviews proceed from predefined search strategies and evaluation criteria, subjective decisions and judgement are inevitable. For example, a small change in the inclusion criteria (for example, to include or exclude studies published in languages other than English) can greatly influence the number of studies included, or the use of different statistical methods can yield quite different results (for a list of examples see Linde & Willich (2003)). In our view there is a tendency to overrate the objectivity and conclusiveness of systematic reviews. Researchers performing a systematic review of acupuncture face multiple challenges in addition to issues related to subjectivity. We consider two challenges of particular relevance: the heterogeneity of trials and the assessment of the adequacy of interventions.

Heterogeneity of trials

Acupuncture is not applied in a uniform manner (see Chapter 9). Practice styles differ to a great extent and it is unclear whether different styles vary in their effects in general or for certain conditions. Outcomes may also depend on the skills of the acupuncturist. If a trial investigates one style of acupuncture it is unclear whether the results are also valid for other styles. To increase transparency and reproducibility, many clinical trials in acupuncture use standardised or semi-standardised treatments. In a trial with standardised treatment, all patients having a given (mostly Western) diagnosis are treated at the same points in the same way with the same frequency, etc. Trials using semi-standardised interventions often require the use of some points in all patients while allowing flexibility regarding additional points. Number of sessions, frequency, etc. are mostly standardised in such trials as well. Unless there are several trials from the same team the standardised formula used in a study is mostly unique, that is each trial uses more or less different interventions.

In principle, if such differences matter it is problematic to pool trials with different interventions in a meta-analysis. In a meta-analysis of drug treatment for depression, for example, it might be adequate to pool different selective serotonin inhibitors but mixing all available antidepressants does not seem a good option.

Diverse experimental interventions are only one source of heterogeneity in systematic reviews and meta-analyses of randomised trials (or other studies) of acupuncture. The main result of each randomised trial is the difference in the outcomes of the experimental and the control group. Therefore, differences in control group interventions between trials also influence effect size estimates. Chapter 8 describes the great variety of sham procedures used in clinical research. It is unclear whether different sham interventions have different effects but there are good reasons to assume that a procedure which uses deep needling 1 cm distant from true points might be more active than the use of a switched-off laser acupuncture pen in distant dermatomes. Further, if acupuncture is compared to another therapy the result may strongly depend on the type and adequacy of the specific therapy used. The types of co-intervention are also found to vary between trials. For example, acupuncture for chronic low back pain can be tested as part of a complex treatment programme involving physiotherapy, relaxation coping training, drugs, etc. or as sole treatment.

Acupuncture is often used in conditions with highly variable and subjective complaints as, for example pain. There is no straightforward single outcome measure which is clearly most important in such conditions. A great variety of instruments have been used in trials with findings often reported selectively and with insufficient detail (partly due to space constraints in journals).

Finally, the methodological quality of acupuncture trials is highly variable. Many older trials have, from our current perspective, unacceptable flaws such as biased allocation to group or selective exclusion of participants from the analysis.

In conclusion, reviewers who want to address a clinically relevant question are often confronted with a patchwork of evidence (see Box 11.5 for an example). As a result, and because of the desire of journal editors and readers to see clear messages, reviewers often oversimplify and draw conclusions that are premature.

In our opinion, systematic reviews and meta-analyses should be as transparent as possible and refrain from simplifying with regard to describing problems encountered when assessing the quality of the available literature. Obviously, critical decisions concerning patients and healthcare systems must be based in part on the conclusions of systematic reviews. However, on the scientific level informed uncertainty is clearly preferable to a wrong belief in putative facts. While reviewers are obligated to draw conclusions at the end of their work, it should be clear that conclusions strongly depend on subjective prejudices, judgements and interpretations even if the review is systematic or includes a

> **Box 11.5** Heterogeneity of acupuncture trials – an example of headache trials comparing acupuncture and a no-treatment/usual care control condition
>
> A systematic review performed for the German health authorities (Linde & Streng 2005) included six trials which compared acupuncture with a no treatment/usual care control condition in patients with headaches. Sample sizes ranged from 30 to 3182. Four trials focused on clearly defined headache diagnoses: one on therapy-resistant migraine, one on migraine without aura, one on migraine with and without aura, and one on episodic and chronic tension-type headache. Two trials included patients with either migraine or tension-type headaches, but one ended up predominantly with migraine patients while in the other diagnoses were more mixed. In three trials point selection was semi-standardised, in one it was standardised and in two it was individualised. Further details of the interventions like number of sessions or background of providers also varied considerably. In four trials patients only treated acute headaches while two trials used 'usual care' allowing a variety of other interventions in addition. Main outcome measures were number of headache days in three trials, number of days with headache of moderate or severe intensity in one trial, migraine days in one trial, and a headache score in one trial. Timing of outcome measurements also differed. Methodological quality was considered adequate in three studies, inadequate in one, and difficult to assess in two (insufficient information).
>
> Should these trials be pooled in a meta-analysis for calculating a single-effect size estimate? We think that the high degree of methodological heterogeneity would render such efforts uninterpretable. However, displaying the results from the different trials together in a Forest plot (Box 11.2) is certainly informative on a descriptive level.

meta-analysis. It might be a good way forward to include people with very different prior beliefs in a review team and, if necessary, report conflicting and controversial conclusions.

Assessing the adequacy of interventions

There can be little doubt that the acupuncture interventions in a significant proportion of trials have been inadequate (Birch 2004). For example, in a trial for patients with rheumatoid arthritis published in a leading rheumatology journal the treatment consisted of five sessions in which only the point Liver 3 was needled for four minutes (David et al 1999). Few acupuncturists would be surprised if trials with inadequate treatment yielded negative results. Conversely, if a trial with negative results is published there are always acupuncturists arguing about the adequacy of the treatment no matter how carefully it was chosen.

Several attempts have been made to include formalised assessments of the adequacy of acupuncture into systematic reviews. A review on asthma trials (Linde et al 1996) used a 16-point checklist on many details including depth, stimulation, etc. which was rated independently by four acupuncturists who were given only the introduction and methods sections of the original articles. Agreement between raters was not much higher than would be expected by chance alone. This might have been partly due to problems of the complex instrument. Later reviewers used much simpler instruments. For example, White and Ernst (1998) simply asked six (medical) acupuncturists to score the overall adequacy of the treatment on a visual analogue scale that ranged from 0 (complete absence of any evidence that the acupuncture was adequate) to 100 (total certainty that the acupuncture was adequate). Considerable variation was observed in the ratings. While the overall inter-rater reliability was low, a good correlation was seen among the ratings of four of the six assessors. Current reviews that include assessments of acupuncture quality use a variety of approaches. Most are rather simplistic and, as far as we know, none has been developed and tested in a truly systematic manner. But it is questionable whether a generally valid instrument can be developed at all (see Box 11.6).

Box 11.6 Why is it so difficult to assess the adequacy of interventions?

What is considered an adequate treatment varies considerably with the background and experience of an acupuncturist. A Japanese acupuncturist using superficial treatment, a practitioner trained in an orthodox Chinese approach and a physician trained to needle at trigger points consider different treatments as adequate. There is probably no 'absolute' standard of good acupuncture. Every trial investigates a specific treatment intervention and the findings are not generalisable to 'all acupuncture'. Whether a study intervention is adequate also depends on the objective of the study. If, for example, a trial aims to investigate whether the addition of acupuncture to standard care within the British National Health Service (NHS) is effective, it is necessary that the intervention is 'representative' for this setting: acupuncturists within the trial optimally should be a sufficiently large random sample of those providing acupuncture within the UK and the treatment process should mimic routine practice as much as possible. The results of such a trial might not be valid for another country in which providers have different training, practice style and where the regulatory framework is different. If a trial only aims to investigate whether it makes a difference to needle at P6 or 3 cm away to prevent postoperative nausea it might be sufficient to train a novice to exactly locate this point without knowing much about the background of Chinese medicine.

In summary, if an assessment of the adequacy of study interventions is included in a systematic review, the perspective must be made explicit. The criteria chosen in a specific review might not be useful if a different perspective is considered.

Some authors also discuss whether the appropriateness of control interventions, particularly in regard to sham controls, should be an item on a quality assessment instrument. This is another aspect of research design that has a large subjective component. As such, it has similar problems for 'scoring' as previously discussed regarding adequacy and appropriateness of the acupuncture treatment protocol. Whether a sham procedure is appropriate depends on the specific question addressed. If, for example, a trial aims to investigate whether point location matters, it makes little sense to use a non-penetrating sham. If instead a trial specifically aims to investigate if skin penetration matters the same points should be treated in both groups. The problem is less the adequacy of the control group but the often insufficient precision of the question. It should be noted that the literature reveals the use of a considerable variety of both penetrating and non-penetrating sham procedures (see Chapter 8). It has even been argued that an appropriate sham cannot be designed until the 'mechanism of acupuncture' is known (Hammerschlag & Zwickey 2006). This lack of agreement on the choice of sham control is likely to be reflected in reviewers' assessments of appropriateness. Probably the best cautionary note that can be introduced on this issue is that reviewers should not lump trials together that use different sham controls. If reviewers and readers would approach the body of evidence more as a large and complex puzzle to which single studies add (hopefully different but complementary) pieces this would lead to more helpful assessments of the current evidence of whether 'acupuncture works'.

CLINICAL RELEVANCE

There can be little doubt that systematic reviews are of great importance to healthcare decision-makers. For systematic reviews to impact on decisions affecting clinical care their conclusions need to be based on clinical trials that report rigorous as well as clinically relevant protocols. The latter cannot be stressed strongly enough. As discussed above, rigorous designs do not necessarily equate to clinically relevant designs, since inadequate and even inappropriate treatment can readily be provided within a rigorous trial design. It is also the case that outcomes found to be statistically significant may not be clinically significant. A 10%, or even less, difference between treatment group and control group may well be statistically significant, but marginally satisfactory for informing clinical decisions, if the sample size is sufficiently large. With acupuncture trials it can be argued that until fairly recently relatively few trials have met the twin standards of methodological rigour and clinical relevance. And, even in the single condition — stimulation of P6 for decreasing postoperative nausea and vomiting — where systematic reviews agree that both standards have been met and positive outcomes have generally been detected, this conclusion has not led to the implementation of the relatively simple intervention into routine post-surgical care.

The paucity of trials with clinically relevant protocols and designs is arguably also a major factor why many acupuncturists care little about the findings of systematic reviews in this field. For the acupuncturist who 'sees every day that it works', negative findings are only the consequence of flawed research methods. Despite the 'negative' findings of systematic reviews, smoking cessation as one example is still a major indication for acupuncture treatment.

Some of these problems will decrease with the inclusion of the increasing number of pragmatic but rigorous clinical trials in future reviews, since pragmatic trials are one approach to apply randomised controlled trial designs to real-world clinical practice. However, reviewers should also actively try to increase clinical relevance by approaching questions that are of direct interest to practitioners as, for example, the impact of the number of sessions on outcome or the comparison of different acupuncture interventions. Since systematic reviews will certainly retain their relevance for decision-making, it is important for acupuncturists with research experience to consider learning and becoming involved in the systematic review process. The lead authors of acupuncture reviews should not be methodologists but experienced acupuncturists who are also competent in clinical research. It is also of critical importance for acupuncturists to become involved in research so that future clinical trials of acupuncture can best reflect real-world clinical practice. In this way, the relatively few funding opportunities for acupuncture research will have greater assurance of producing trials that provide sound methodology and relevant interventions so their outcomes can, without qualifications, contribute to conclusions of future systematic reviews.

SUMMARY

Systematic reviews are of crucial interest for decision-makers, can help to improve future research and should, in principle, also be relevant for practitioners. A review is called systematic if it uses predefined and explicit methods for identifying, selecting and assessing the information (typically research studies) deemed relevant to answer the particular question posed. A systematic review is called a meta-analysis if it includes an integrative statistical analysis, i.e. pooling, of the included studies. Numerous systematic reviews of acupuncture have been published since the late 1980s, mainly evaluating randomised clinical trials designed to answer questions of efficacy and effectiveness. While the earlier reviews usually addressed methodological quality, the majority of recent reviews have focused on what the studies actually found. A major problem of systematic reviews is that acupuncture trials are very heterogeneous: experimental and control interventions, patients, outcomes and quality differ to a great extent making it very difficult to provide a consistent summary and to draw clear-cut conclusions. A further problem is that it is very difficult to assess the adequacy of acupuncture interventions, since reliable and valid instruments are lacking and different schools disagree about what constitutes adequate treatment. Since the systematic review is likely to remain high on the evidence hierarchy for decision-makers, it is imperative that the clinical relevance of such reviews, let alone the clinical trials on which they are based, should become a major priority in the future.

Research resources

Bain C, Colditz G, Glasziou P et al 2001 Systematic reviews in health care. A practical guide. Cambridge University Press, Cambridge

Cooper H, Hedges L V 1994 The handbook of research synthesis. Russell Sage Foundation, New York

Egger M, Smith G D, Altman D (eds) 2001 Systematic reviews in health care meta-analysis in context. BMJ Books, London

Green S, Higgins J (eds) 2006 Cochrane handbook for systematic reviews of interventions 4.2.6. Online. Available: http://www.cochrane.org/resources/ handbook/index.htm (accessed 15 May 2007).

Mulrow C, Cook D (eds) 1998 Systematic reviews — synthesis of best evidence for health care decisions. American College of Physicians, Philadelphia

References

Birch S 2004 Clinical research on acupuncture: Part 2. Controlled clinical trials, an overview of their methods. Journal of Alternative and Complementary Medicine 10:481–489

Ceccherrelli F, Altafini L, Rossato M et al 1992 Trattamento agopunturale dell' emicrania senz'aura. Studio in doppio cieco vs. placebo. Associazione Italiana per lo Studio del Dolore. XV Congresso Nazionale A.I.S.D., p 310–318

David J, Townsend S, Sathanathan R et al 1999 The effect of acupuncture on patients with rheumatoid arthritis: a randomized, placebo-controlled cross-over study. Rheumatology 38:864–869

Derry C J, Derry S, McQuay H J et al 2006 Systematic review of systematic reviews of acupuncture published 1996–2005. Clinical Medicine 6:381–386

Ernst E, White A 1997 Life-threatening adverse reactions after acupuncture? A systematic review. Pain 71:123–126

Ernst E, White A R 2001 Prospective studies of the safety of acupuncture: a systematic review. American Journal of Medicine 110:481–485

Furlan A D, van Tulder M, Cherkin D et al 2005 Acupuncture and dry-needling for low back pain: An updated systematic review within the framework of the Cochrane Collaboration. Spine 30:944–963

Hammerschlag R, Zwickey H 2006 Evidence-based complementary and alternative medicine: back to basics. Journal of Alternative and Complementary Medicine 12:349–350

Jadad A R, Moore R A, Carroll D et al 1996 Assessing the quality of reports of randomized clinical trials: is blinding necessary? Controlled Clinical Trials 17:1–12

Jüni P, Witschi A, Bloch R et al 1999 The hazards of scoring the quality of clinical trials for meta-analysis. Journal of the American Medical Association 282:1054–1060

Lee A, Done M L 2004 Stimulation of the wrist acupuncture point P6 for preventing postoperative nausea and vomiting. Cochrane Database of Systematic Reviews 2004, Issue 3. Art. No.: CD003281.pub2. DOI: 10.1002/14651858.CD003281.pub2

Linde K, Streng A 2005 Kapitel 6 — Komponente IV: Systematische Übersichtsarbeiten der randomisierten Studien. In: Melchart D (ed) Programm zur Evaluation der Patientenversorgung mit Akupunktur (PEP-AK) — Bericht zum Modellvorhaben Akupunktur der Ersatzkassen. Centre for Complementary Medicine Research, Technische Universität München, Munich, Germany, 2005. [Online] Available at: http://www.lrz-muenchen.de/~ZentrumfuerNaturheilkunde/pub/down/mvaku_ersatzkassen_kIV.pdf

Linde K, Willich S 2003 How objective are systematic reviews? Differences between reviews on complementary medicine. Journal of the Royal Society of Medicine 96:17–22

Linde K, Worku F, Stör W et al 1996 Randomized clinical trials of acupuncture for asthma — a systematic review. Forschende Komplementärmedizin 3:148–155

Linde K, Melchart D, Willich S 2001 Beschreibung der Therapie in klinischen Studien zur Akupunktur bei chronischen Kopfschmerzen. Deutsche Zeitschrift für Akupunktur 44:8–14

Linde K, Vickers A, Hondras M et al 2001 Systematic reviews of complementary therapies — an annotated bibliography. Part I: Acupuncture. BMC Complementary and Alternative Medicine 1:3

MacPherson H, White A, Cummings M 2001 Standards for reporting interventions in controlled trials of acupuncture: the STRICTA recommendations. Complementary Therapies in Medicine 9:246–249

Manheimer E, Linde K, Las L et al 2007 Metanalysis: Acupuncture for osteoarthritis of the knee

Manheimer E, White A, Berman B et al 2005 Meta-analysis: acupuncture for low back pain. Annals of Internal Medicine 142:651–663

Melchart D, Linde K, Fischer P et al 2001 Acupuncture for idiopathic headache (Cochrane review update).Cochrane Database System Review (1):CD001218

Moher D, Jadad A R, Nichol G et al 1995 Assessing the quality of randomized controlled trials: an annotated bibliography of scales and checklists. Controlled Clinical Trials 16:62–73

Moher D, Jadad A R, Tugwell P 1996 Assessing the quality of randomized controlled trials. International Journal of Technology Assessment in Health Care 12:195–208

Mulrow C D 1994 Rationale for systematic reviews. British Medical Journal 309:597–599

Rosted P 1998 The use of acupuncture in dentistry: a review of the scientific validity of published papers. Oral Diseases 4:100–104

Smith L A, Oldman A D, McQuay H J et al 2000 Teasing apart quality and validity in systematic reviews: an example from acupuncture trials in chronic neck pain. Pain 86:119–132

ter Riet G, Kleijnen J, Knipschild P 1990a A meta-analysis of studies into the effect of acupuncture in addiction. British Journal of General Practice 40:379–382

ter Riet G, Kleijnen J, Knipschild P 1990b Acupuncture and chronic pain: a criteria-based meta-analysis. Journal of Clinical Epidemiology 43:1191–1199

Van Tulder M W, Cherkin D C, Berman B 1999 The effectiveness of acupuncture in the management of low back pain. A systematic review within the framework of the Cochrane Collaboration Back Review group. Spine 24:1113–1123

Vickers A J 1996 Can acupuncture have specific effects on health? A systematic review of acupuncture antiemesis trials. Journal of the Royal Society of Medicine 89:303–311

Vickers A, Goyal N, Harland R et al 1998 Do certain countries produce only positive results? A systematic review of controlled trials. Controlled Clinical Trials 1998 19(2):159–166

Weinschütz T, Lindner V, Niederberger U et al 1993 In: Schimrigk K (ed) Verhandlungen der Deutschen Gesellschaft für Neurologie. Band 7. Springer, Berlin, p 533–534

Weinschütz T, Niederberger U, Johnsen S et al 1994 Zur neuroregulativen Wirkung der Akupunktur bei Kopfschmerzpatienten. Deutsche Zeitschrift für Akupunktur 37:106–117

White A R, Ernst E 1998 A trial method for assessing the adequacy of acupuncture treatments. Alternative Therapies in Health and Medicine 4:66–71

Engaging acupuncturists in research — some practical guidelines

12

Peter Wayne, Karen Sherman and Mark Bovey

INTRODUCTION

Acupuncture research requires the active collaboration of experienced acupuncture practitioners. Knowledgeable acupuncturists are needed not only to provide effective treatments in the context of clinical or mechanistic studies, but are needed to inform all aspects of research — from study conception and identification of relevant hypotheses to development of treatment interventions, choosing outcomes measures, and interpreting results. In addition to contributing to the scientific evidence base of acupuncture, participation in research can provide practitioners hands-on opportunities for professional development, additional sources of income to that earned in clinical practice, and increased visibility in the biomedical community that could improve patient referral streams. To date, only a small number of practising acupuncturists participate in research. This chapter summarises some of the more accessible methods of research relevant to acupuncture practitioners, including those with only limited research experience. It also explores some practical aspects related to engaging members of the acupuncture community in acupuncture and Oriental medicine research.

There are two questions that active acupuncture researchers regularly are asked by established practitioners, faculty or students at acupuncture schools, and staff at acupuncture and Oriental medicine clinics: 'How do we initiate research projects in environments with limited research infrastructure and resources?'; and 'How do I collaborate with established research groups/programs?'. Below we address these two related, yet distinct questions. For both questions, we discuss practical steps members of the acupuncture community can take to pursue these different initiatives, barriers they might encounter, and representative examples of successes.

INITIATING RESEARCH PROJECTS IN ACUPUNCTURE SCHOOLS AND CLINICS

Faculty and students at acupuncture schools, and practitioners at clinics have the potential to make significant and unique contributions to acupuncture research (Bovey et al 2005, Lao et al 2002, Sherman et al 2004). Both schools and established clinics often have large numbers of faculty with diverse clinical training and extensive experience in patient care. Clinics can also provide access to motivated patients, and schools can provide large numbers of student practitioners with graded levels of knowledge. These unique resources can be drawn upon to develop and undertake smaller clinical, methodological, and educational research studies that are of direct practical relevance to the acupuncture community. They can also be deployed to conduct pilot and feasibility studies that lay the groundwork for larger and more definitive controlled trials. However, for most schools and clinics, research-related infrastructure and financial support for research are limited, and access to faculty or staff with significant research experience is rare (Wayne et al 2007a). Consequently, the types and scale of studies conducted in acupuncture schools and clinics may be practically constrained. Nevertheless, even with these resource limitations, meaningful research can be conducted. In this section, we discuss some ways that acupuncture schools and clinics can engage in research, emphasising the use of case studies and case series, surveys, clinical outcomes studies, and pilot prospective studies. As the value and limitations of these approaches have been discussed in detail in prior chapters of the book, in this section we emphasise practical matters related to initiating and completing studies, and illustrate each with examples that were accomplished at acupuncture schools or clinics.

Case studies and case series

A case study documents in detail the response of an individual patient to a treatment. Case series generally document the responses of multiple patients that share common features (e.g. common medical condition, common treatment strategy) and that are treated by either a single practitioner or a group of associated practitioners (e.g. within a clinic). Case-based studies are an excellent and logical place for many acupuncture school faculty and clinicians to begin getting involved in research (Lukoff et al 1998, White 2005). These studies enable clinicians to engage in research that is centred on their own patients, making the research both practical and clinically relevant. Moreover, the process of learning all the stages that are involved in writing and publishing a peer-reviewed case study or case series serves as an excellent introduction to many of the key steps involved in other types of research studies.

With the support of a National Institutes of Health (NIH) grant to train faculty in research methods, the New England School of Acupuncture

(NESA) developed and implemented a course specifically designed to teach faculty how to write a publishable case series (Wayne et al 2007b). An outline of the course curriculum is presented in Table 12.1. The course was co-developed and administered by two NESA faculty members in collaboration with the Director of Education at the Harvard Medical School Osher Institute, and includes didactic lectures, interactive and independent exercises, and one-on-one mentoring. It is taught over a 12-month period, with one 2-hour meeting per month supplemented with one-on-one meetings with instructors and participants between sessions.

A number of observations that were made during the teaching of this course at NESA may be generally relevant to acupuncture practitioners

Table 12.1 Curriculum outline for a faculty course taught at the New England School of Acupuncture, 'How to write a publishable case report'

Modules	Examples of topics and questions considered
Case reports: overview	What is a case report and what is it used for? What is the place of case reports in evidence-based research?
Types of case reports	What are differences between prospective vs. retrospective reports? What are differences between case reports vs. case series vs. cohort studies?
Identifying, retrieving and critically evaluating peer-reviewed research literature	What is the process of conducting an electronic literature search? How does one retrieve full-text articles? How does one critically evaluate an already published case study and what are the key features to consider? What makes a case worthy of publishing?
Outcome measures	Why are outcome measures important for case reports? What are the categories of outcome measures? How do we choose the most appropriate outcome measure(s)?
Institutional review or ethics boards	What is the history and purpose of Institutional Review or Ethics Boards in protection of human subjects in research? What kinds of case studies require Institutional Review Board (IRB) approval? How does one complete an IRB protocol application?
Writing	What is the structure/format of a case report or case series? What is the function of the background, results, and discussion sections?
Publishing a case report	Why is publishing case reports of potential value to both researchers and clinicians? How is authorship of papers determined? How does one determine the most appropriate journal for submission? How does one find out about the instructions/guidelines for authors regarding formatting and submission of manuscripts for review? How does one evaluate and respond to reviewers' comments?

Adapted from Wayne et al 2007b

interested in writing publishable case studies. First, the process of developing and writing a case study introduces practitioners to a rich variety of research competencies. NESA faculty members benefited greatly from learning fundamental, yet key skills such as electronically locating, retrieving and critically reading already published case studies. The process of learning these skills in a group also provided practitioners with a forum for collegial and academic interactions; such opportunities are often lacking for acupuncture school faculty and practitioners, even in well-established acupuncture schools (Wayne et al 2007b). Second, the process of more formally developing a case study highlighted the importance of keeping good clinical records and including objective measures related to patient diagnosis and outcomes. While initially, all participants believed they had numerous 'interesting' retrospective cases worthy of developing, on closer inspection, lack of consistent and objective outcomes data became an obvious limitation for developing a compelling, evidence-based case. This informed practitioners about the value of maintaining good clinical records that include basic outcomes measures, not only for creating potentially publishable cases, but also for good clinical practice. Some course participants, for example, are now including simple outcomes instruments like the MYMOP scale in their clinical practice (Paterson 1996). The value of objective data also highlighted the benefits of collaborating with conventional clinicians who could provide such information related to both biomedical diagnoses and outcomes. Third, for practitioners with limited academic training, writing can be difficult and requires time and support. Course leaders actively maintained contact with participants, and peer support teams were set up so that participants could share drafts of papers with one another to help keep the process of writing moving along. Box 12.1 summarises a case series published by a NESA faculty member and acupuncture practitioner.

Surveys

Surveys are another form of research that may be suitable for acupuncture practitioners associated with clinics or schools. Survey research includes a diverse set of tools and approaches that can be employed to provide valuable information about patients, practitioners, and clinics. Surveys have been used to provide various kinds of information about the patients who seek acupuncture and related therapies, for example: socio-demographic characteristics of patients and the conditions they seek treatment for (Barnes et al 2004, Bullock et al 1997, Cassidy 1998a, Cherkin et al 2002, MacPherson et al 2006); prevalence of usage by specific groups such as physicians (Diehl et al 1997) or cancer patients (Swisher et al 2002, Vandecreek 1999); expectations, beliefs, and motivations of patients seeking treatments (Astin 1998, Sharples et al 2003); and satisfaction of patients with their treatments (Cassidy 1998a, Xing & Long 2006). Surveys have also been employed to ascertain practice behaviours

Box 12.1 Adolescent endometriosis-related pelvic pain treated with acupuncture: a peer-reviewed case series published by an acupuncture college faculty member (Highfield et al 2006)

Highfield et al published a case series describing the use of acupuncture to treat adolescent girls with endometriosis-related chronic pelvic pain (Highfield et al 2006). The decision to develop these cases into a peer-reviewed article was based on the fact that: 1) current standard of care does not adequately treat this condition for this population, and thus new therapies are warranted; 2) there are few published studies evaluating acupuncture for endometriosis, especially in young women; 3) little is known about the receptivity of adolescents to acupuncture; and 4) treatments were initiated following referrals from a prominent gynaecologist who provided objective, independent data on patients' diagnosis, and pre- and post-treatment measures of pain.

Two young women (ages 17 and 15 years old) with laparoscopically diagnosed endometriosis were administered 9 and 15 TCM-style acupuncture treatments over a 7- and 12-week period, respectively. Both patients experienced modest improvement in pain as measured by oral self-reports of pain on a scale from 1 to 10, as well as self- or family-reported improvement in headaches, nausea and fatigue. Also noteworthy were marked improvements in health-related quality of life, including increased attendance at school and participation in extra-curricular activities. No adverse effects were reported. These case reports provided preliminary evidence that acupuncture may be an acceptable and safe adjunct treatment therapy for some adolescents with endometriosis-related pelvic pain refractory to standard anti-endometriosis therapies. These observations also suggested that a prospective, randomised controlled trial to evaluate the safety and efficacy of acupuncture for this population is warranted. An NIH-funded trial addressing this topic was subsequently conducted.

and characteristics of acupuncturists, such as the fee structures employed for treatments (Cherkin et al 2002), and the TCM diagnostic categorisations and treatment strategies employed for common biomedical conditions (Kalauokalani et al 2005, Sherman et al 2001, 2006). Box 12.2 illustrates a survey study designed to characterise how a population of acupuncturists diagnose and treat chronic low back pain. Surveys of both patients and practitioners have also been used to characterise the prevalence of adverse events associated with treatments (Ernst 2003, MacPherson et al 2001, 2004, White & Ernst 2001). Finally, some surveys employ qualitative dimensions/approaches, which allow for open-ended responses — sometimes including lengthy stories or narratives — that enable respondents the freedom to answer queries in their own words. Such qualitative surveys have been employed to characterise both patients' (Cassidy 1998a, 1998b, Gould & MacPherson 2001, Paterson & Britten 2003) and practitioners' (Paterson & Britten 2003) perceptions of treatments.

> **Box 12.2** A survey to characterise how traditional Chinese medicine acupuncturists diagnose and treat chronic low back pain (Sherman et al 2001)
>
> As one step in the process of developing a valid standardised treatment protocol for a clinical trial evaluating acupuncture for chronic low back pain, Sherman et al undertook a survey to learn how traditional Chinese medicine acupuncturists diagnose and treat chronic low back pain in clinical practice (Sherman et al 2001). A randomly selected sample of 56 licensed acupuncturists practising in Washington State, USA, were surveyed regarding the styles of acupuncture they used for treating chronic low back pain, diagnoses made, and key features of treatment for this condition. Results of the survey indicated substantial variability among practitioners, but there was still agreement on several broad features of treatment including: the use of local and distal acupuncture points (86% of practitioners); the use of acupuncture points on meridians traversing the back (especially the Bladder meridian, 90%); the use of acupuncture points determined by palpation (82%); the importance of eliciting *de Qi* (60%); and the provision of up to eight treatments for achieving therapeutic results (79%). The results of this survey laid the foundation for the development of a protocol used in a subsequent prospective clinical trial (Sherman & Cherkin 2003).

While the basic concept of survey research – administering questionnaires and cataloguing responses – appears straightforward, there are many factors to consider to assure the results obtained from surveys are meaningful (Neuman 2003). Once a clear global research question or hypothesis is well articulated, key factors to consider relate to the survey instrument and the sample population. Regarding the survey instrument, when appropriate, using already developed and validated questionnaires is recommended. If such tools are not available, careful thought must be given to a number of issues including assuring that the wording of questions is clear/unambiguous, the response categories employed produce analysable data, and that the overall length of the survey is not burdensome as this may reduce response rates. Careful thought must also be given to the survey sample. Most surveys attempt to seek responses from a representative sample of a population; how well a sample reflects the larger population depends on the sample size and the methods used for selecting the sample. For these reasons, it is recommended that acupuncturists with limited research experience carefully review practical text books related to survey research (Alreck & Settle 2004, Fowler 2002) and/or partner with collaborators with survey research experience.

Clinical outcome studies

Clinical outcome studies measure changes in health status before and after an intervention (Thomas & Fitter 2002). They entail the systematic monitoring of the outcomes resulting from normal clinical practice. Once infrastructure is in place to properly collect such information, it requires relatively few resources. In addition to providing a means to evaluate the potential benefits and safety of interventions provided at clinics, outcome studies can be particularly useful for helping clinic practitioners and staff in creating profiles of the patients they treat, and in getting preliminary data exploring the correlations between treatment outcomes and the variety of characteristics related to patients, and practitioners, and treatment strategies. One recent study that nicely illustrates one application of this approach is summarised in Box 12.3.

Box 12.3 Patient characteristics and clinical outcomes in an acupuncture and Oriental medicine teaching clinic (Maiers et al 2006)

Maiers et al (2006) designed a clinical outcome study to characterise patients who seek treatment at the Edith Davis Acupuncture and Oriental Medicine Teaching Clinic associated with NorthWest Health Sciences University, and to measure patient response to treatment experience. Over a 3-month period, all new patients seen at the clinic were asked to participate in a data collection project. Initial data collected included demographics, type and severity of their primary complaint and health history. Patients who consented were followed up with a survey after 4 and 12 weeks of the initial clinic visit to measure changes in their primary conditions, and satisfaction with care.

Over a period of 3 months, 104 new patients consented to participate. Of these, 63% were female, 92% were Caucasian, and the mean age was 35 years. The most common reason for seeking treatment was pain (59%) and general wellness (49%). Of those patients who presented to the clinic with symptoms, 54% were seeking treatment for a chronic condition, while 17% reported symptoms of less than 6 weeks in duration. The mean severity of symptoms on the day of intake was 4.9 on an 11-point scale. When asked to indicate the percent of change in their conditions, 86% noted positive changes, with 44% stating they were over 75% improved. Satisfaction was generally high among this group of patients with 88% indicating they were satisfied with the care they received, and over half of the respondents reported they were continuing with TCM care for their condition.

An initial limitation reported by the authors in this pilot study was a high prevalence of missing data on outcomes instruments and significant loss to follow-up. After the initial pilot stage, the study team re-evaluated protocols and designed and implemented the following procedural modifications: 1) shortened and more focused intake survey; 2) more active role for front-desk staff in data collection and follow-up; 3) number of follow-up surveys decreased from 2 to 1; and 4) more assertive follow-up process including e-mail, scheduled phone reminders, and a second survey sent to those participants who failed to initially respond. Implementing these changes markedly improved subsequent quality and quantity of data collected.

Other examples of acupuncture and Oriental medicine clinical outcomes research include studies by MacPherson & Fitter (1998), Bovey et al (2005) and Hull et al (2006).

Well-structured databases maintained by acupuncture school clinics can be extremely valuable for addressing clinically relevant research questions that can be pursued for both teaching purposes, as well as for improving clinical services. Recognising this, Lao et al (2002) developed a list of research questions that can be addressed using clinic outcomes data. These questions are listed in Box 12.4.

Researching the procedures of Oriental medicine diagnosis and treatment

Studies on evaluating practical aspects of the clinical diagnostic and treatment methods are particularly relevant to acupuncture and

---

Box 12.4 Outcome studies well suited for acupuncture school clinics (Lao et al 2002)

1. How do different conditions respond to acupuncture treatments?
2. Do patients with different TCM patterns and a single biomedical condition respond differently to their TCM treatments?
3. What is the optimal dose of an acupuncture treatment (frequency and number of treatments) for a given biomedical condition or TCM pattern of disharmony?
4. What is the response rate of a given condition to different styles of acupuncture practice (e.g. TCM, Japanese, 5 element, etc.)?
5. What treatments are most cost-effective in different clinical settings?
6. What is the effectiveness of combination therapies, such as acupuncture combined with Chinese herbs, or with Western medicine?
7. What is contraindicated among co-interventions?
8. How important is practitioner's *Qi*/energy level when a treatment is rendered?
9. How important is the practitioner's level of training and experience?
10. How important is a practitioner's personal profile (e.g. emotional state, health status) in influencing the effectiveness of treatment?
11. What influences do selected patient personal characteristics (e.g. demographic, medical history, beliefs, emotional state) have on patient outcomes?
12. What are common side effects/adverse effects of acupuncture/TCM treatments?
13. What aspects of the relationship between patient and practitioner have a significant effect on the treatment response?
14. What are the effects of different needle depths/manipulation methods/retention times on outcomes?

Box 12.5 Comparing the accuracy of two methods of locating acupuncture points (Aird et al 2000)

Aird et al (2000) at the College of Traditional Chinese Medicine in Sydney, Australia undertook a study to evaluate the reliability of acupuncture point location. Twenty final-year students were randomly selected from a class of 42 and recruited to characterise how accurately they located the points LI 10 (Shousanli) and ST 40 (Fenglong) using two commonly used mechanical methods based on *cun* units, i.e. directional and proportional. The directional method locates points by counting *cun* units from a single anatomical landmark where the proportional method relies on subdividing the distance between two landmarks to locate points. All point assessments were made on a single volunteer. Accuracy of students' point location was based on their deviations to point locations determined by a single, experienced practitioner. Point locations were all recorded on transparent films and then transferred to a Cartesian grid system to enable quantitative estimates of distances from reference 'true' locations.

Analysis of the results found no significant difference in accuracy between the two methods for either acupuncture point, and both methods were found to be similarly and substantially inaccurate. The findings of this study demonstrated the serious limitations of both methods for accurate point location, and identified significant implications for acupuncture practice, training, and research. Subsequent studies explored the value of alternative methods for point location (Aird et al 2002).

More generally, this study demonstrates how a relatively simple, yet meaningful experiment can be conducted at acupuncture schools using limited resources.

Oriental medicine teaching institutions. Students (and practitioners) are often evaluated regarding their abilities in a number of clinical domains, for example, discrimination of radial pulses and tongue characteristics, accuracy of acupuncture point locations and needle placement, and overall identification of TCM diagnostic classes. As central as these skills are to training, and as critical as they are thought to be for effective treatment, surprisingly little research has been devoted to documenting their reliability, and the consequences that variability in their application may have on treatment outcomes. Some examples of clinically relevant questions that could form the basis for outcomes research projects in clinics or even classrooms include: what are the *De Qi* characteristics of patients and practitioners, and how does eliciting the *De Qi* response impact outcomes? (Bovey 2006); how much inter-practitioner variability is there in TCM diagnoses and treatment prescriptions for different biomedical conditions? (Zhang et al 2004, 2005); and how reliable are radial pulse and tongue assessments? (King et al 2002, Walsh et al 2001). Box 12.5

summarises an example of a methodology-related study that evaluated the accuracy of acupuncture point location among final-year acupuncture students.

GENERAL GUIDELINES FOR CONDUCTING RESEARCH STUDIES

The life cycle of any research study has a number of key stages that must all be carefully considered. Addressing these stages in detail is beyond the scope of this chapter, and many of these topics are covered elsewhere in this book. Below we briefly introduce and summarise a few key issues to keep in mind when developing small research studies. Helpful books related to clinical and epidemiological research methods include those by Kane (2004), Lewith et al (2002), and Portney & Watkins (2000).

Developing the research question

Having a clear research question is a critical and sometimes under-appreciated component in the research process. If significant time and resources are going to be invested in a project, it is important to conduct some preliminary ground work to assess the value of proposed questions. This might include reviewing the literature on the topic of interest and learning what has and has not already been done, and where there is room for improvement. Discussing your research questions with colleagues and other researchers can also help to sharpen them. Vickers (2002) provides a very useful framework for structuring medical research questions related to various approaches including surveys and outcomes research.

Building a team of collaborators

Even small research studies require a wide range of skills for successful completion. A typical study will involve many tasks, including: searching and retrieving relevant published literature, designing a protocol to answer the research question, choosing appropriate validated outcome measures, obtaining ethical approval, recruiting participants, developing and managing a database, statistical analysis of data, and interpretation and writing up of results. Even amongst experienced researchers, these skills are commonly divided among personnel with relevant expertise (e.g. medical specialists, librarians, statisticians, computer programmers, and project managers). It is highly recommended that novice researchers find experienced researchers to collaborate with, and that such collaborations begin right at the start of the study development process. Key considerations in looking for appropriate collaborators are their expertise in the type or focus of research being pursued (e.g. survey vs. clinical research, cardiovascular vs. cancer research), their interest in acupuncture and willingness to understand the complexities and challenges in the field, their time and availability to commit to your project, monetary resources they require for their participation, and their willingness to mentor/coach and teach you skills along the way.

Obtaining approval from an ethics committee

Ethics committees and Institutional Review Boards serve to ensure the protection of human subjects by independently approving, modifying, or rejecting research protocols. Typically, the ethical approval process involves the completion and submission of a structured application that includes a detailed description of the study protocol, subjects involved, and the risks and benefits to subjects for their participation. The requirement for ethics board approval can vary depending on the types of studies being conducted, the country research is being conducted in, and the sources of funding. While few schools or clinics may have formal ethics boards, this does not mean that research studies conducted in these environments are exempt from review. In such cases, researchers may often be able to purchase commercially available services, or take advantage of review boards or ethics committees of nearby medical institutions or universities, especially if a collaborating member of the research team has an appointment at these institutions. Ethical issues and requirements related to research continue to evolve. It is highly recommended that before embarking on any study, one consult with a local ethics board for advice on compliance. Failure to do so could be illegal, and could seriously jeopardise the completion of a study. Finally, in cases when ethical approval is required, adequate resources and time required for completing applications, and awaiting their approval (sometimes many months) should be considered.

THE ENGAGEMENT OF PRACTITIONERS IN ONGOING COLLABORATIVE RESEARCH

Independent practitioners not affiliated with clinics or schools, and faculty members of acupuncture schools and clinics that are not personally interested or prepared to undertake self-initiated research projects, can still get involved in research by collaborating with already established research groups. In addition to contributing to the evidence base, participation in collaborative research can provide practitioners with: 1) hands-on opportunities for professional development, adding new proficiencies in research and/or clinical practice and thereby improving one's credentials; 2) additional sources of income to that earned in clinical practice (especially valuable to recent graduates in the early stages of building private practices); and 3) increased visibility in the biomedical community, and consequently, the attraction of a potentially greater diversity and quantity of patient referrals. As this list of potential motivations indicates, the process of getting involved in research may be more closely related to the domain of business practice and career development than to the domain of 'doing science'. As such, to be successful in finding research opportunities, acupuncturists seeking collaborative research positions need to shift from wearing their clinical or practitioner thinking caps to wearing their job-seeking hats.

The job-seeking process involves a number of well-described and distinct phases/steps that are catalogued in career development books. These steps include: 1) assessing your interests and personal skill sets; 2) researching potential opportunities; 3) networking; 4) honing your interests and creating a strong communication strategy; 5) cultivating and pursuing opportunities; and 6) determining if you need to pursue additional training. Below we briefly discuss the most relevant of these steps as they specifically relate to acupuncture practitioners seeking opportunities in collaborative research.

Assessing your interests and personal skill sets

In the process of finding collaborative opportunities, it is important to give careful thought both to what aspects of research you wish to be involved in, and what unique skills you might have that qualify you for those roles. As an acupuncturist, you may simply wish to limit your role to providing treatments in the context of a clinical trial. However, depending on your interests and professional skills, you may also wish to participate in other aspects of research such as consulting in the development of treatment protocols, administering outcome instruments, or overseeing some aspects of project management and administration. Many practitioners come to acupuncture after prior careers in various disciplines and industries. Those with prior experience in nursing, mental health, or physical therapy, for example, may have valuable skills related to assessing outcomes in clinical research. Practitioners with backgrounds in fields not related to health (e.g. database administration, advertising and public relations, software development, and work team management) also possess skills that are critical to the success of many research studies. Thinking clearly about the professional skills you possess, in addition to those of an acupuncturist, can help inform your thinking about the ways you might get involved in research, and can also help you to position yourself more competitively as you seek opportunities in collaborative research.

Conducting research on potential opportunities

Perhaps the most important step in establishing a collaborative role in a research project is finding out what kind of research is going on in your community, where it is occurring, and who is doing it. There are a number of excellent internet-related resources to draw upon to help in this stage of the job-searching process. Websites of government funding agencies (e.g. NIH, NHS) often manage databases listing all active and completed trials (e.g. www.clinicaltrials.gov). These databases provide information on the types of research being pursued, as well as the names and contact information of principal investigators. These databases can often be searched using keywords related to, for example, geographic location (e.g. a city name) and research topics (e.g. acupuncture and/or cancer). Searching the websites of all hospitals, universities and other medical institutions in your area can be similarly valuable; many of these institutions will have specific pages dedicated to research highlighting recent grant awards, recipients and publications. Finally, most of the commonly used medical literature search engines such as MEDLINE, PubMed, EMBASE and CINHAL allow users to search for research publications using combinations of terms such as 'Acupuncture and San Francisco', or 'Electroacupuncture and London', which can help you identify the research going on in your community. In addition to these electronic resources, attending local medical conferences or seminars is a good way to learn about the research being conducted in your community.

Networking

Once you have learned in a more general sense the kinds of research taking place in your community, it is valuable to begin the 'networking' process, i.e. meeting face to face with those engaged in research to learn in more detail about the work they and their colleagues are doing, what skill sets and personnel they require to get their work done, and what opportunities currently exist. The early stages of networking should be focused much more on listening to those willing to meet with you and learning from them about what their needs are, rather than talking about yourself and asking for a position. Knowledge gained from these informational interviews will assist you in evaluating how your skills might be employed, what specific roles in research you are most attracted to, and how to most effectively present yourself when pursuing a particular position. More often than not, the person you are networking with cannot directly offer you an opportunity. Nevertheless, it is still valuable to find out what they are doing, and when appropriate, to share with them your relevant interests; this may then trigger their ideas of who they can refer you to that might, in turn, have opportunities that are fit for your skills and goals. While networking, the more people you talk with, the more likely you will eventually be referred to other opportunities or that you will be remembered for opportunities in the future. Throughout the networking process, keep in mind that most of the researchers you will contact have busy schedules. Even if your goal is only to have a 10–15-minute interview, it is preferable and courteous to request and arrange this interview with a brief introductory letter, email or phone call. It is also a good practice to follow up all meetings with thank you notes, both as a courtesy and as a reminder to your contact to follow-up on any referrals or networking ideas discussed.

Cultivating opportunities and pursuing additional research training

As is commonly the case for most individuals beginning any new career, practitioners seeking collaborative positions that begin with limited research experience may not land their 'dream' job right away. For example, one might identify a new clinical trial in which they ideally might want to help design acupuncture intervention protocols, however, the only paid opportunities available in the study are administrative ones. For some practitioners, pursuing these less-than-ideal research positions can be very valuable. Through participating in the research study, they will get exposed first hand to the culture and conduct of research, and will most likely be introduced to a number of new practical skills. In some cases where responsibilities do not provide significant exposure to broader research issues (e.g. data entry), it may be appropriate to ask permission to sit in (as a silent observer) on meetings with more scientific content. In situations when interesting studies are identified but there are no paid positions available, it may even be valuable to volunteer one's services in exchange for the opportunity to be involved in a study. Both for volunteers and those doing less-than-ideal jobs, the research experience gained and the contacts made with researchers on each study will increase the likelihood of eventually being considered for future positions.

For practitioners that become increasingly interested and engaged in research, and who may wish to expand the roles in research that they play, it may be valuable and necessary to pursue research-related training. The types of training that are most relevant will be dependent on the specific roles one wishes to play. For example, practitioners interested in developing manualised protocols for controlled trials might benefit from taking a basic clinical research course and reviewing the published literature on acupuncture protocol development. In contrast, those wishing to help design and possibly take a leading role in writing competitive grants and overseeing clinical studies may need to pursue additional advanced degrees such as an MSc, MPH, a PhD, or an OMD. Box 12.6 summarises how one practitioner integrated research into her career.

Box 12.6 From acupuncture student to practitioner and part-time researcher

After taking a required research course in her second year at the New England School of Acupuncture (NESA) and learning about an upper classmate's positive experience as a research assistant in a clinical trial, a student (MS) became interested in learning more about acupuncture research. MS approached the research director at NESA, and in exchange for the opportunity to learn about ongoing studies, volunteered to help with administrative responsibilities in the research department including retrieving articles from offsite libraries and electronic databases, scheduling and organising meetings, and recording and disseminating meeting minutes. Over a period of 6 months, MS demonstrated a sustained interest in research and proved to be a reliable, committed member of the research department who enjoyed learning new skills. Upon the departure of a key member of one of NESA's research studies, MS was formally hired as a part-time research assistant and trained by more experienced staff to help with an expanded set of responsibilities including assisting with writing and managing Institutional Review Board protocols, providing administrative support for submission of NIH reports and peer-reviewed manuscripts, and managing various databases. After graduating from NESA and becoming a licensed practitioner, MS's research responsibilities were further expanded to include providing treatments to patients enrolled in trials, monitoring the fidelity of treatment of other acupuncturists participating in trials, and giving presentations to groups of conventional medical practitioners about a new research study in order to stimulate patient recruitment. In the course of overseeing her diverse responsibilities, MS significantly increased her visibility and credibility in the Boston area as a responsible and bright fledging acupuncturist, which has begun to impact the success of her private practice. MS is currently helping to write and co-author what will be her first peer-reviewed paper.

SUMMARY

It is widely believed that in order for acupuncture to become more fully integrated into future healthcare, it must be evidence based, that is, it must be based on sound research. It is also increasingly appreciated that in order for research to be sound, it must be informed by the clinical experience and cultural context of seasoned practitioners. In the US, this appreciation has led to a number of recent NIH-funded initiatives to better engage complementary and alternative medicine practitioners in research (Wayne et al 2007a). Unfortunately, we are all still regularly disappointed by published and sometimes influential studies where the conclusions commonly reached, e.g. acupuncture is not shown to be effective for condition X, are based on study protocols or designs that have not appropriately included the expertise of the acupuncture community. Of course, like all medical interventions, we should not expect acupuncture to demonstrate positive benefits for all conditions and populations; but unless appropriate clinical interventions and outcomes are used, the conclusions of such studies are of limited value and can be misleading. Becoming frustrated by some aspects of the culture of acupuncture research may cause some practitioners to further distance themselves from research, thinking for example, that research can never capture what is relevant in clinical practice. This may be true and an appropriate stance for some practitioners. However, acupuncture research is likely to continue with or without the relevant contribution of practitioners. Consequently, not getting involved/abstaining from research and letting others determine what are the important questions to ask and how to address them, effectively means that acupuncturists will be giving up an important voice that will impact the future of their profession. We hope that the sum of the motivations and practical guidelines presented in this chapter will help to encourage a greater participation of the acupuncture community in research.

Research resources

Kane M. Research made easy in complementary and alternative medicine. London: Churchill Livingstone; 2004.

Lewith G, Jonas WB, Walach H. Clinical research in complementary therapies. London: Churchill Livingstone; 2002.

Portney LG, Watkins MP. Foundations of clinical research: applications to practice. 2nd ed. Upper Saddle River, NJ: Prentice Hall; 2000.

References

Aird M, Coyle M, Cobbin D M et al 2000 A study of the comparative accuracy of two methods of locating acupuncture points. Acupuncture in Medicine 18(1):15–21

Aird M, Cobbin D M, Rogers C 2002 A study of the relative precision of acupoint location methods. Journal of Alternative and Complementary Medicine 8(5):635–642

Alreck P L, Settle R B 2004 The survey research handbook, 3rd edn. McGraw Hill/Irwin, New York

Astin J A 1998 Why patients use alternative medicine: results of a national study. Journal of the American Medical Association 279(19):1548–1553

Barnes P M, Powell-Griner E, McFann K et al 2004 Complementary and alternative medicine use among adults: United States, 2002. Advance Data 343:1–19

Bovey M 2006 Deqi. Journal of Chinese Medicine. 81:18–29

Bovey M, Horner C, Shaw J et al 2005 Engaging in the audit of acupuncture practice. Journal of Alternative and Complementary Medicine 11(2):293–298

Bullock M L, Pheley A M, Kiresuk T J et al 1997 Characteristics and complaints of patients seeking therapy at a hospital-based alternative medicine clinic. Journal of Alternative and Complementary Medicine 3(1):31–37

Cassidy C M 1998a Chinese medicine users in the United States. Part I: Utilization, satisfaction, medical plurality. Journal of Alternative and Complementary Medicine 4(1):17–27

Cassidy C M 1998b Chinese medicine users in the United States. Part II: Preferred aspects of care. Journal of Alternative and Complementary Medicine 4(2):189–202

Cherkin D C, Deyo R A, Sherman K J et al 2002 Characteristics of visits to licensed acupuncturists, chiropractors, massage therapists, and naturopathic physicians. Journal of the American Board of Family Practice 15(6):463–472

Diehl D L, Kaplan G, Coulter I et al 1997 Use of acupuncture by American physicians. Journal of Alternative and Complementary Medicine 3(2):119–126

Ernst E 2003 Serious adverse effects of unconventional therapies for children and adolescents: a systematic review of recent evidence. European Journal of Pediatrics 162(2):72–80

Fowler F J 2002 Survey research methods. Vol 1. Sage Publications, Thousand Oaks, CA

Gould A, MacPherson H 2001 Patient perspectives on outcomes after treatment with acupuncture. Journal of Alternative and Complementary Medicine 7(3):261–268

Highfield E S, Laufer M R, Schnyer R N et al 2006 Adolescent endometriosis-related pelvic pain treated with acupuncture: two case reports. Journal of Alternative and Complementary Medicine 12(3):317–322

Hull S K, Page C P, Skinner B D et al 2006 Exploring outcomes associated with acupuncture. Journal of Alternative and Complementary Medicine 12(3):247–254

Kalauokalani D, Cherkin D C, Sherman K J 2005 A comparison of physician and nonphysician acupuncture treatment for chronic low back pain. Clinical Journal of Pain 21(5):406–411

Kane M 2004 Research made easy in complementary and alternative medicine. Churchill Livingstone, London

King E, Cobbin D, Ryan D 2002 The reliable measurement of radial pulse: gender differences in pulse profiles. Acupuncture in Medicine 20(4):160–167

Lao L, Sherman K, Bovey M 2002 The role of acupuncture schools and individual practitioners in acupuncture research. Clinical Acupuncture and Oriental Medicine 3:32–38

Lewith G, Jonas W B, Walach H 2002 Clinical research in complementary therapies. Churchill Livingstone, London

Lukoff D, Edwards D, Miller M 1998 The case study as a scientific method for researching alternative therapies. Alternative Therapies in Health and Medicine 4(2):44–52

MacPherson H, Fitter M 1998 Factors that influence outcome: an evaluation of change with acupuncture. Acupuncture in Medicine 16:33–39

MacPherson H, Thomas K, Walters S et al 2001 The York acupuncture safety study: prospective survey of 34 000 treatments by traditional acupuncturists. British Medical Journal 323(7311):486–487

MacPherson H, Scullion A, Thomas K J et al 2004 Patient reports of adverse events associated with acupuncture treatment: a prospective national survey. Quality & Safety in Health Care 13(5):349–355

MacPherson H, Sinclair-Lian N, Thomas K 2006 Patients seeking care from acupuncture practitioners in the UK: a national survey. Complementary Therapies in Medicine 14(1):20–30

Maiers M, McKenzie E, McKenzie M et al 2006 Data collection and outcome measurement in an Oriental medicine teaching clinic (abstract). Journal of Alternative and Complementary Medicine 12(2):205–215

Neuman W L 2003 Social research methods, 5th edn. Pearson Education, Inc., Boston

Paterson C 1996 Measuring outcomes in primary care: a patient generated measure, MYMOP, compared with the SF-36 health survey. British Medical Journal 312:1016–1020

Paterson C, Britten N 2003 Acupuncture for people with chronic illness: combining qualitative and quantitative outcome assessment. Journal of Alternative and Complementary Medicine 9(5):671–681

Portney L G, Watkins M P 2000 Foundations of clinical research: applications to practice, 2nd edn. Prentice Hall, Upper Saddle River, NJ

Sharples F M, van Haselen R, Fisher P 2003 NHS patients' perspective on complementary medicine: a survey. Complementary Therapies in Medicine 11(4):243–248

Sherman K, Cherkin D 2003 Developing methods for acupuncture research: rationale for and design of a pilot study evaluating the efficacy of acupuncture for chronic low back pain. Alternative Therapies in Health and Medicine 9(5):54–60

Sherman K J, Hogeboom C J, Cherkin D C 2001 How traditional Chinese medicine acupuncturists would diagnose and treat chronic low back pain: results of a survey of licensed acupuncturists in Washington State. Complementary Therapies in Medicine 9(3):146–153

Sherman K J, Cherkin D C, Connelly M T et al 2004 Complementary and alternative medical therapies for chronic low back pain: what treatments are patients willing to try? BMC Complementary and Alternative Medicine 4:9

Sherman K J, Cherkin D C, Deyo R A et al 2006 The diagnosis and treatment of chronic back pain by acupuncturists, chiropractors, and massage therapists. Clinical Journal of Pain 22(3):227–234

Swisher E M, Cohn D E, Goff B A et al 2002 Use of complementary and alternative medicine among women with gynecologic cancers. Gynecologic Oncology 84(3):363–367

Thomas K, Fitter M 2002 Possible research strategies for evaluating CAM interventions. In: Lewith G, Jacobs WB, Walach H (eds) Clinical research in complementary therapies. Churchill Livingstone, London, p 59–91

Vandecreek L 1999 Should physicians discuss spiritual concerns with patients? Journal of Religion and Health 38(3):193–201

Vickers A 2002 Inspiration and perspiration: what every researcher needs to know before they start. In: Lewith G, Jacobs W B, Walach H (eds) Clinical research in complementary therapies. Churchill Livingstone, London, p 47–58

Walsh S, Cobbin D, Bateman K et al 2001 Feeling the pulse. European Journal of Oriental Medicine 3(5):25–31

Wayne P M, Pensack L M, Connors E M et al 2007a Increasing research capacity at the New England School of Acupuncture: building grants management infrastructure as an NCCAM-funded Developmental Center for Research on Complementary and Alternative Medicine (DCRC). Alternative Therapies in Health and Medicine

Wayne P M, Buring J E, Davis R et al 2007b Increasing research capacity at the New England School of Acupuncture through NCCAM-supported faculty and student research training initiatives. Alternative Therapies in Health and Medicine

White A 2005 Conducting and reporting case series and audits: author guidelines for acupuncture in medicine. Acupuncture in Medicine 23(4):181–187

White A, Ernst E 2001 Adverse events associated with acupuncture reported in 2000. Acupuncture in Medicine 19(2):136–137

Xing M, Long A F 2006 A retrospective survey of patients at the University of Salford Acupuncture Clinic. Complementary Therapies in Clinical Practice 12(1):64–71

Zhang G G, Lee W L, Lao L et al 2004 The variability of TCM pattern diagnosis and herbal prescription on rheumatoid arthritis patients. Alternative Therapies in Health and Medicine 10(1):58–63

Zhang G G, Lee W, Bausell B et al 2005 Variability in the traditional Chinese medicine (TCM) diagnoses and herbal prescriptions provided by three TCM practitioners for 40 patients with rheumatoid arthritis. Journal of Alternative and Complementary Medicine 11(3):415–421

13

Future strategies for acupuncture research

George Lewith

THE STORY SO FAR

History always provides us with perspective and before launching into an exercise of crystal-ball-gazing in relation to what the future may hold for acupuncture research, it would be wise to reflect on the processes that have occurred over the last 30 years. My history comes very much from a practitioner perspective, having learned acupuncture in China in 1978 with my wife who is a physiotherapist. We were the first UK citizens to come to China as WHO-sponsored students since the Communist revolution. Like all practitioners the therapeutic power of the needle in my hands astonished me with the clinical response that I was able to obtain. I became academically curious and fairly swiftly began to take part in the development of acupuncture as an academic discipline. My first funded acupuncture research was in Southampton in 1979. While my interests have broadened into the wider field of complementary medicine the disciplines learnt in the context of acupuncture research have been essential to my academic development.

My vision in 1979 was to establish an academic centre of excellence that could inform decision-making about complementary medicine from the viewpoint of both patients and providers. In the early 1980s, that appeared to be a vision which would not be fulfilled; from the perspective of the early twenty-first century it seems prescient.

Research drivers; politics and public policy

The most important motivator for service provision has undoubtedly been the popularity of complementary medicine in general and acupuncture in particular. US President Richard Nixon's visit to China in 1972 heralded a new relationship between the West and China, with traditional Chinese medicine and table tennis providing the two main focal points. The West at that time was, and to some extent still is, in the thrall of privately owned pharmaceutical companies with respect to its healthcare provision. Many people were beginning to distrust their claims particularly after the thalidomide disaster. There is, and always has been, a strong counter-current to conventional medicine in the United States; lest we forget, the American Medical Association and its major publication, JAMA, was set up to 'defeat' the success of homeopathy in the early twentieth century when one in four American physicians were practising homeopaths and the major homeopathic *materia medicas* were American in origin. Eisenberg's seminal papers (Eisenberg 1993, 1998) served notice on the American medical establishment that patients were turning to complementary and alternative medicine (CAM) in increasing numbers, moving substantial out-of-pocket expenditure towards CAM practitioners. In the early 1990s the US National Institutes of Health (NIH) established the Office of Alternative Medicine, now the National Centre for Complementary and Alternative Medicine (NCCAM) as a consequence of political pressure, and began substantial research funding. CAM began to become integrated into healthcare provision. However, the cynics would argue that this was purely a commercial move by astute US healthcare providers to minimise the 'leakage' of patients and their ability to fund 'out-of-pocket expenditure' into the alternative healthcare system.

A consensus about funding emerges

The emergence of research funding streams in the early 1990s, particularly in the United States but also in Germany and the United Kingdom allowed the acupuncture research community to begin to develop sustainable academic groups within CAM. These activities were promoted politically and developed by charities and others such as the Foundation for Integrated Medicine in the UK. The Chinese, Japanese and Koreans also saw the development of research as essential for the integration of acupuncture into patient care, particularly in the context of the Japanese medical system (see Chapter 2). Some may argue that acupuncture research in China was politically biased and few would support the 'overclaiming', particularly during the Cultural Revolution and the immediate post-revolutionary period, while no one could doubt the academic excellence of the endorphin work carried out during this period by Han (Han & Terenius 1982, Han 1986). What has emerged from a number of governments in both the East and West is a consistent, if sometimes faltering, desire to investigate the mechanisms, effects and safety of acupuncture as a treatment modality. Research units have been established in the United States and Canada. There is a consistent drive for higher-quality research along with a requirement that research methodology is taught at undergraduate level in acupuncture courses. To some extent this development has been facilitated by the World Health Organisation which has promoted communication and understanding with respect to addressing the research issues and the underlying concerns of both patients and healthcare purchasers.

Research is sustained by patient demand

The demand for CAM, which is certainly patient driven, has enabled the patient's voice to become increasingly heard. The development of qualitative research designs within CAM, and acupuncture in particular (see Chapters 3 and 5), has helped us understand how and why patients seek and understand acupuncture treatment. Furthermore the voice of both patient and practitioner has meant that acupuncture has become part of conventional physiotherapy in the UK and is delivered through almost all UK NHS pain clinics; it became integrated into conventional care during the 1990s in spite of limited evidence. These political pressures have improved and enabled service delivery and effectively promoted the research agenda. What has emerged from the research so far is a Western academic view that acupuncture appears to be a safe and cost-effective intervention for pain (Endres et al 2004, MacPherson et al 2001, White et al 2001, Wonderling et al 2004); the evidence suggesting that acupuncture falls well within the UK's National Institute for Clinical Excellence guidelines for cost-effectiveness (Ratcliffe et al 2006, Willich et al 2006, Witt et al 2006). There is a growing and sustainable argument, particularly based on the large and recently published German studies, that acupuncture is as clinically effective, if not more effective, than conventional care for chronic painful conditions (Lewith et al 2006b, Witt et al 2006). Thirty years ago a practising doctor in the UK may have been struck off the medical register for referring patients for acupuncture, now it is acceptable and legitimate to provide acupuncture as a clinical service within the NHS.

The development of the randomised controlled trial

When I first began to develop randomised controlled trial (RCT) methodology for acupuncture (Lewith & Machin 1983), our understanding of RCTs and the statistics through which we could evaluate treatment effects were simplistic. Statisticians were not always involved in clinical trials and data were often handled and reported very poorly. Nested qualitative studies that might be used to explain the intervention from both the patient's and practitioner's perspective were unheard of (Paterson & Dieppe 2005). Lewith and Machin developed an appropriate and clinically relevant methodological framework for clinical trials in acupuncture and suggested that it was not possible to investigate techniques such as acupuncture as an 'alternative pharmaceutical' (Lewith & Machin 1983) but required new approaches. Primary care (family medicine) researchers are only too aware of the importance of the therapeutic relationship as a 'whole system' (Mercer & Howie 2006, Mercer & Reynolds 2002). The unique therapeutic relationships that we find in both acupuncture and complementary medicine in general may provide some fascinating insights into the run of the mill general practice consultation and its central role in effect size of any clinical intervention (Blasi et al 2001, Verhoef et al 2004).

Are acupuncture points therapeutically important?

Our initial assumptions about acupuncture centred around the idea that point specificity was an essential. In essence this means that 'it matters' where you needle. Acupuncturists will choose a specific point prescription based on their training, understanding of acupuncture, acupuncture diagnosis, experience and the patient's previous response to treatment. As a trained and registered acupuncture professional one would assume that random or non-point-specific needling, anywhere on the body, would be an ineffective therapy. If, as acupuncturists, we focus on the importance of point prescription and stimulation during our training it seems obvious that practising clinicians will consider that 'finding and treating' the 'correct' acupuncture point is one of the most essential parts of effective therapy. It comes as a shock to find that whilst point specificity may be relevant in the treatment of some internal disease such as nausea (Ezzo et al 2006, Lewith & Vincent 1995, Lewith et al 2006b), this is certainly not an assumption that can be made in the context of chronic pain (Lewith et al 2006b). It might be both disillusioning and threatening for a practising acupuncturist to think that all those years of learning about 'how to formulate the ideal prescription' at a particular consultation for an individual may be threatened, when it is possible that in some conditions, based on the preliminary evidence available, it may not matter where you put the needles or even if you put them into known acupuncture points (Willich et al 2006). Acupuncturists can become very threatened and uneasy about these suggestions, yet we need to continually remind ourselves that it may be the therapeutic process and safety (Endres et al 2004, MacPherson et al 2001, White et al 2001) of acupuncture that underpins our clinical success (Paterson & Dieppe 2005) rather than needling specific points. This is certainly the case for many conventional interventions for chronic benign illness (Kirsch 2000, Weidenhammer et al 2006). Much clinical trial work in the past has served the practice of acupuncture poorly by claiming that a particular acupuncture intervention for a specific condition may be ineffective because of the lack of point specificity while entirely failing to evaluate the whole context of the intervention. It may be that an acupuncture-based intervention, even a treatment considered by some to be placebo, could be much more efficacious than the standard conventional intervention (Willich et al 2006, Witt et al 2006). This implies that contrary to much of our teaching within this field, acupuncture points may have only limited clinical and therapeutic specificity in the treatment of commonly evaluated problems such as headache and musculoskeletal pain but acupuncture as a whole may be a very effective intervention.

Is the process of consultation the most effective treatment?

There are many similarities between complementary medicine and primary care. The power and major effects of conventional medicine in the prescription of modern antidepressants, and the processes and protocols (rituals) that surround that, are largely within the consultation (80–90% of the clinical effect) and, to a much lesser extent, dependent on the presence of a specific chemical versus placebo (10–20% of the clinical effect) (Kirsch 2000, Kirsch & Sapirstein 1999). It is clear that the growth of evidence-based medicine in primary care has made us much more sceptical of the relevance of the RCT in a real-world clinical setting (Little 2006, Little et al 2005) and has allowed us to begin to consider evidence within the more contextual and pragmatic format of day-to-day clinical care (Fønnebø et al 2007, Walach et al 2006). It is becoming increasingly clear that the clinical decision-making process within conventional, and by implication complementary medicine, is a complex process that involves evidence, political priorities from healthcare providers and purchasers and a process of peer group consensus that exists within any given clinical and/or professional environment (Gabbay & le May 2004). Reviewing clinical trial evidence systematically and solely focusing on the point specificity of acupuncture has led to many substantive misunderstandings as conventional physicians may assume that acupuncture is point specific and therefore may fail to consider the overall effect size of treatment or compare acupuncture with the effect size and safety of conventional care for the same condition (Derry et al 2006, Lewith et al 2006a). People don't come to acupuncturists asking for placebos, they come with the expectation of effective treatment and ask for acupuncture. If it works they don't really seem to mind which points are used!

Patient centredness

The whole process within complementary medicine has been based on an approach that is patient centred and individualised. This can appear to stand in direct opposition to the practice of conventional medicine which is purportedly based on large clinical trials involving relatively homogeneous groups of individuals with subsequent evidence-based advice. In reality, the majority of good primary care is very individualised and frequently based on what doctors think the patient may or could be able to achieve and how a particular intervention might (or might not) 'fit' into their overall treatment plan and lifestyle. Good conventional physicians will claim that this has always been so but the patient-centred and individualised approach emphasised by all CAM therapies, including acupuncture, has served as an important cultural counterpoint in the development of the evidence-based matrix within acupuncture (Barry 2006). Research into acupuncture has enabled a far more explicit understanding of perceptions of health and a greater understanding of how such cultures view (philosophically) medical interventions (see Chapter 2) rather than simply accepting that clinical science is the only truth. Acupuncture is an example of an approach that is perceived as a whole system involving therapy, practitioner and patient rather than divorcing the therapy from those who provide it in a way that many have tried to do with conventional clinical bioscience (Paterson & Dieppe 2005). Perhaps through these 'cross-cultural' perceptions we may begin to consider the relative balance of various 'truths' and develop a truly integrated understanding of the sociology and anthropology of medical practice.

THE EMERGENCE OF THE ACUPUNCTURE RESEARCHER

Initially most clinical research was quite beyond the experience and skill of practising acupuncturists. However, papers evaluating acupuncture began to appear in the early 1970s and involved eminent medically qualified acupuncturists such as Felix Mann (1973). With increasing funding, academics with an interest and sometimes a clinical skill in acupuncture have begun to emerge as informed researchers. This has involved physicians, sociologists, psychologists, epidemiologists, anthropologists, statisticians and professional acupuncturists. Inevitably this has been led historically by medically qualified acupuncturists as the academic disciplines within medicine have been stronger and better funded than those within non-medical acupuncture. However, the current training in many acupuncture schools encourages a critical understanding of research among professional acupuncturists, enabling the development of appropriate appraisal and research skills. Research is not for everyone, but it will certainly continue to attract a small number of enthusiasts.

Building research capacity

Acupuncture research has been one of the many 'poor relations' of 'proper' medical research, but we have seen over the last decade an increasing number of high-quality publications involving RCTs and pragmatic studies, as well as health economic analyses in high-quality, medical, peer-reviewed journals (Berman et al 2004, Brinkhaus et al 2006, Linde et al 2005, Melchart et al 2005, Witt et al 2005). As Wonderling et al (2004) suggest, acupuncture's time has come. In an academic sense the acupuncture research community and acupuncture as a whole systems treatment modality appears to have obtained some consistent degree of academic respectability in association with a growing and considerable body of hard evidence that suggests acupuncture has much to offer, particularly in pain (Willich et al 2006). This of course must be set against the observation that we have as a community been very academically productive with limited resource. In the USA, NCCAM, while a generous funder within a CAM context, represents only a tiny proportion of NIH funding. In the UK the whole of CAM research received 0.0085% of the total medical research budget during 2005 (UK Clinical Research Collaboration 2006).

FUTURE STRATEGIES

As far as CAM research is concerned, acupuncture has found itself in a unique position. Possibly because of the Nixon visit in 1972 and as a consequence of the discovery of endorphins and a possible mechanism which might explain the effects of acupuncture (see Chapter 10), it has become an attractive and acceptable 'target therapy' for those wishing to develop a research agenda within CAM. There are therefore many lessons that we can begin to learn from the 'acupuncture research experience', not only for acupuncture but also for many other CAM interventions.

Patients lead and doctors follow

It is quite apparent that CAM has been a patient-led revolution over the last two decades, one that has received huge support from the general public in all the Western industrialised nations (Eisenberg et al 1993, 1998, MacLennan et al 1996, Thomas et al 2001). However the value of the same factual evidence has often been interpreted differently by patients. The epidemiologist and systematic reviewer may look at the difference between placebo and real treatment as the basis upon which to define whether a treatment 'works', whereas patients do not really understand (or perhaps wish to understand) the process of placebo intervention. What they perceive is overall treatment effects and this appears to be the basis upon which they make treatment decisions (Lewith & Chan 2002, Verhoef et al 2002). The patient's view of what 'works' is therefore very different to the systematic reviewer's. Consequently for patients, defining 'what works' is a pointless debate and a much more pragmatic and less hierarchical strategy will be required if we are to evaluate the evidence that applies to whole systems such as acupuncture (Gabbay & le May 2004, Walach et al 2006). As Chapter 11 on systematic reviews clearly outlines, when RCTs are combined in an evidence synthesis (a systematic review) we are able, in a conventional epidemiological context, to arrive at the best available evidence for a specific intervention (Lewith et al 2002). In the pragmatic context of clinical practice treatment, decisions are made with reference to evidence from outcome studies, peer-group opinion, patient preference and safety as well as systematic reviews – a more 'circular' than hierarchical approach. Complete or whole medical systems such as acupuncture practised in a traditional context, are complex interventions and are difficult to evaluate and dissect using a reductionist approach thus making the process of evidence-based medicine, based on RCTs within CAM, much more complicated than conventional medicine (see Table 13.1).

Table 13.1 Assumptions made in conducting randomised controlled trials	
Equipoise	Patient and provider do not have a preference for a treatment
Lack of knowledge	It is truly unknown which of two alternatives is 'better' and there is insufficient evidence about treatment effects from other sources
Preference for specificity	Only specific effects attributable to the intervention are therapeutically valid
Context independence	There is a 'true' magnitude of efficacy, or a stable effect size independent of context
Ecological and external validity knowable	The knowledge about a therapeutic effect extracted from an RCT is readily transferable into clinical practice, if exclusion and inclusion criteria of the trial match the characteristics of a given patient

Reproduced with kind permission from Walach et al 2006.

The issues raised in Table 13.1 assume a stable effect size, equipoise, an effect that is independent of context and an outcome which will be readily transferable to clinical practice. None of this is necessarily the case. Furthermore, comparing real versus sham acupuncture should in theory be 'enough' to define whether a treatment works, yet we are only too aware, as we have highlighted in Fig. 13.1 and discussed in Chapter 8, that treatment X may be insignificantly better than placebo X, but significantly better than an effective treatment Y. This is best described as the efficacy paradox. Therefore, progress towards a more circular and less hierarchical view of evidence will mirror both the medical and patient decision-making processes far more completely (Walach et al 2006).

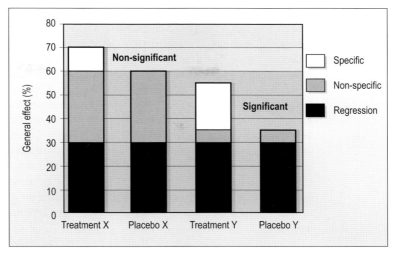

Fig 13.1 Illustration of the efficacy paradox. Treatment X can have a larger overall effect than treatment Y, although only treatment Y shows a sizeable and significant specific treatment effect. Specific = specific component of treatment; non-specific = non-specific component of treatment; regression = regression to the mean, natural regression of the disease. Placebo effects are often considered as a combination of non-specific effects and regression. (Adapted with kind permission from Walach et al 2006.)

Observing the effect: the case for observational studies

All too often within acupuncture we have rushed to clinical trials based on non-systematic observations of clinical effects within our practice. There is an emerging argument that systematic observational studies may provide us with the same effect size as clinical trials (Walach et al 2005). Even if that does not ultimately prove to be the case, it is essential that we develop a strategy which allows a process of careful observation and piloting before we launch into expensive and potentially ill-considered and inappropriate large-scale studies. Evidence can be seen as less hierarchical and more circular; clinicians (including conventional physicians) build evidence for their practice from a whole range of environments and this is influenced and reinforced by cost, safety, personal experience and randomised studies but is certainly not based solely on a hierarchy that is ultimately determined by systematic reviews.

Equipoise and research priorities

The essence of any clinical trial, as we have already suggested, is that of equipoise. Practitioners and patients have opinions about complementary medicine and, as Fønnebø et al (2007) have pointed out eloquently, the research strategies required to evaluate a system of medicine already in widespread use may involve entirely different political and health priorities to those involved in the development of rigorous prospective RCTs that evaluate new treatments. The specific research expertise required to evaluate safety or to conduct a qualitative study is not different 'just because you are evaluating CAM', however, the context and priority in which specific research questions are both asked and answered may be very different for a treatment that is 'out there' like acupuncture as compared to the development of a new pharmaceutical agent which in general has far more potential to 'do harm' and whose effects are genuinely unknown. Fig. 13.2 highlights some of the differences in method and priority between CAM and conventional drug trials that will influence research priorities and also effect patient and practitioner equipoise.

It seems sensible to assume that an available treatment will be perceived and considered differently by patients when compared to a new drug in development. Practitioners and physicians and thus both research priorities and equipoise may be challenged within the whole process of trial design if we fail to make appropriate allowances for these differences.

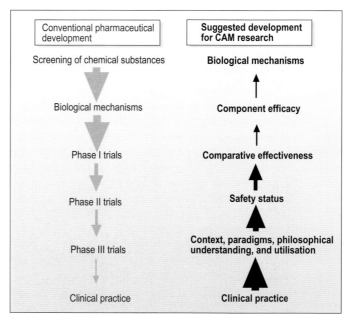

Fig 13.2 Phases that contrast the proposed phased research strategy in CAM (dark arrows) with that conventionally used in drug trials (light arrows). (Reproduced with kind permission from Fønnebø et al 2007.)

The placebo

Acupuncture research has been 'dogged' by the search for an adequate placebo so that it can mirror the pharmaceutical development process involved in drug trials. In all probability the development of a true acupuncture placebo may remain an enigma and differentiating specific from non-specific treatment effects may not be possible in the same way as one can for a discreet and well-characterised pharmaceutical agent. While most clinical researchers recognise that the substantial effects obtained in most chronic benign illnesses are non-specific (Baum 2006), it is still necessary to not only understand the mechanisms that underpin specific responses to treatments but also those that underpin the non-specific responses. Therefore, understanding and maximising treatment response for minimal expense, intervention and risk are laudable and important research aims. As with surgery, physio-therapy, and indeed all clinician-based physical interventions, acupunc-turists will struggle with the concept of placebo and defining a pure placebo with which to compare real treatment. The debate within con-ventional medicine has to date largely been about point specificity (Derry et al 2006, Lewith et al 2006a). Imaging studies have brought this debate to the fore (Lewith et al 2005) but sometimes serve to confuse rather than enlighten. Acupuncture may have a specific and well-defined effect (Pariente et al 2005), but we are currently unaware of whether the observed neurological effects correlate appropriately with clinical outcome. We are not yet able to define placebo so we can't define a convincing acupuncture placebo and consequently cannot define what is 'real' treatment and what is 'non-specific'; what is related to expectancy and the consultation and what is the 'real specific effect' of acupuncture.

Does it work over a long period of time?

We are beginning to develop an understanding that CAM interventions can have increasingly beneficial effects the longer we follow up our patients. The suggestion within the whole of complementary medicine is that we can empower our patients, helping them to manage their own difficulties and issues, the Alexander Technique being a case in point (Hollinghurst et al submitted, Little et al submitted). If we can demonstrate long-term clinical effects with appropriate economic benefits (for example the Quality Adjusted Life Years gained) and diminished long-term consul-tation with primary care, then this will have benefit for the management of chronic benign illness in primary care. The evidence for the economic benefit of acupuncture is becoming more convincing (Ratcliffe et al 2006, Willich et al 2006, Wonderling et al 2004), but it is not yet compelling and not well established for all the therapeutic claims that acupuncturists might like to make.

Pragmatic trials

While placebo-controlled RCTs may represent a gold standard for the pharmaceutical industry as they answer quite specific questions about efficacy for medicines, they may not address the practical issues that healthcare purchasers and providers (and indeed patients) really wish to ask and have answered about acupuncture. Comparing acupuncture with a supposed placebo does not answer whether it's cheaper and safer than a conventional treatment for back pain or headache (Thomas et al 2005, Vickers et al 2004, Wonderling et al 2004). These issues are certainly more important than asking whether one set of points selected either individually or by prescriptive formula provides a more immediate sustained or cheaper clinical outcome than sham acupuncture, a presumed placebo. Such questions are often best answered within a pragmatic study that may compare acupuncture to conventional treatment (Ratcliffe et al 2006, Vickers et al 2004).

Mixed methods

The concept of using randomised clinical trials in conjunction with economic and qualitative work is beginning to emerge within acupuncture both in the US and in Europe. These 'mixed methods approaches with nested studies' are complex to organise and difficult to deliver, but research funders are being increasingly persuaded by researchers to work with practitioners and patients in delivering more pragmatically relevant models for acupuncture. We will continue to improve our methodology with respect to these complex studies and will begin to balance the more medical quantitative view with a patient-centred qualitative approach while evaluating the economic component of the intervention simultaneously.

CREATING A RESEARCH DISCIPLINE

We are beginning to create a research discipline within acupuncture but it would be very dangerous for us to use that research expertise in an attempt to 'prove that we are right'. There is a danger among acupuncturists in that they may consider acupuncture research not as a tool for their own self-development, but rather a tool to prove that their pre-existing assumptions have always been correct and that they can legitimately challenge the hegemony of conventional medicine through research. This may have some basis if the evidence can support our clinical observations but it is more likely to challenge our bias and belief. The truth of the matter is that good research is a learning process from which we will develop a different understanding and context for the practice of acupuncture. We may have to consider that the learning process through which we develop a very specific and individualised point prescription may be an important component of the consultation, but when evaluated therapeutically may have far less impact than we may wish to believe. We may need to become sceptical about some of the 'traditional Chinese wisdom' that appears to have been handed down so dogmatically but all of this does not mean that acupuncture doesn't 'work'. The uninformed may reject a 'negative' research study, the manipulative will try and construct the research so that it provides the answers they wish to obtain and the arrogant will reject negative research as being biased in much the same way that conventional medicine tends to reject research into homeopathy because it 'simply couldn't work' (Shang et al 2005). Research is a process of genuine discovery, both for the individual, and for the discipline and profession as a whole. Fortunately, it is not possible to predict where that may lead.

What will acupuncture research teach us?

There are many things that we may learn from our multilevel approach to acupuncture research which involves pragmatic and fastidious clinical trials, imaging, economic and qualitative work, as well as consensus development around best practice and surveys of patient and practitioner use. Acupuncture now presents us with a research process and a requirement for research skills that mirror conventional primary care. However, it is perhaps more legitimate to ask (within acupuncture) questions that may be very difficult if asked in a conventional medical context; for instance, is the acupuncture consultation the key to its therapeutic effect? If that is the case, then how might that translate into primary care and will evidence-based medicine, driven by explanatory RCTs, really be the economic and clinical saviour of managed care systems such as the NHS? Acupuncture research brings many professional acupuncturists into direct contact with conventionally trained academic colleagues from a variety of different backgrounds. That allows for the development of a questioning and balanced research environment which will provide further challenges for healthcare purchasers and professionals. Understanding the reasons behind the substantial demand for CAM and its apparent clinical effectiveness may also begin to challenge the conventional medical process.

SUMMARY

There is no doubt that acupuncture research is beginning to come of age. It has diversified into many of the clinical and epidemiological disciplines currently practised within conventional medical research and involves clinical trials, basic mechanisms and a range of other research methods. Its academic infrastructure is fragile but hopefully development has gone too far for us to be able, or willing, to 'turn the clock back'. This research process will challenge clinical acupuncturists substantially and require them to manage their assumptions and expectations. It will also allow for the integration of acupuncture into conventional medicine within the Western industrialised nations and what will emerge over the next 20 years may only have a limited and tenuous connection with what practitioners feel they may now define as 'acupuncture'.

References

Barry C A 2006 The role of evidence in alternative medicine: contrasting biomedical and anthropological approaches. Social Science & Medicine 62:2646–2657

Baum M 2006 Paying a complement: should the NHS fund alternative medicine? The New Generalist 4:26–27

Berman B M, Lao L, Langenberg P et al 2004 Effectiveness of acupuncture as adjunctive therapy in osteoarthritis of the knee. Annals of Internal Medicine 141:901–910

Blasi Z, Harkness E, Ernst E et al 2001 Influence of context effects on health outcomes: a systematic review. Lancet 357:757–762

Brinkhaus B, Witt C, Jena S et al 2006 Acupuncture in patients with chronic low back pain. Archives of Internal Medicine 166:450–457

Derry C J, Derry S, McQuay H J 2006 Systematic review of systematic reviews of acupuncture published 1996–2005. Clinical Medicine 6:381–386

Eisenberg D M, Kessler R C, Forster C et al 1993 Unconventional medicine in the United States. New England Journal of Medicine 328:246–252

Eisenberg D M, Davis R B, Ettner S L 1998 Trends in alternative medicine use in the United States. Journal of the American Medical Association 280:246–252

Endres H G, Molsberger A, Lungenhausen M et al 2004 An internal standard for verifying the accuracy of serious adverse event reporting: the example of an acupuncture study of 190,924 patients. European Journal of Medical Research 9:545–551

Ezzo J M, Richardson M A, Vickers A et al 2006 Acupuncture-point stimulation for chemotherapy-induced nausea or vomiting. Cochrane Database Systematic Review CD002285

Fønnebø V, Grimsgaard S, Walach H et al 2007 Researching complementary and alternative treatments – the gatekeeper is not at home. BMC Medical Research Methodology 7:7

Gabbay J, le May A 2004 Evidence based guidelines or collectively constructed 'mindlines'? Ethnographic study of knowledge management in primary care. British Medical Journal 329:1013–1017

Han J S 1986 Electroacupuncture: an alternative to antidepressants for treating affective diseases? International Journal of Neuroscience 29:79–92

Han J S, Terenius L 1982 Neurochemical basis of acupuncture analgesia. Annual Review of Pharmacology and Toxicology 22:193–220

Hollinghurst S, Sharp D, Ballard K et al submitted Economic evaluation of the MRC ATEAM randomised controlled trial of Alexander Technique lessons, exercise, and massage for chronic or recurrent back pain.

Kirsch I 2000 Are drug and placebo effects in depression additive? Biological Psychiatry 47:733–735

Kirsch I, Sapirstein G 1999 Listening to Prozac but hearing placebo: a meta-analysis of antidepressant medication. In: Kirsch I (ed) How expectancies shape behavior. American Psychological Association, Washington DC, p 303–320

Lewith G T, Chan J 2002 An exploratory qualitative study to investigate how patients evaluate complementary and conventional medicine. Journal of Alternative and Complementary Medicine 8:777–786

Lewith G T, Machin D 1983 On the evaluation of the clinical effects of acupuncture. Pain 16:111–127

Lewith G T, Vincent C 1995 The evaluation of the clinical effects of acupuncture. A problem reassessed and a framework for future research. Pain Forum 4:29–39

Lewith G T, Walach H, Jonas W B 2002 Balanced research strategies for complementary and alternative medicine. In: Lewith G T, Jonas W B, Walach H (eds) Clinical research in complementary therapies. Churchill Livingstone, Edinburgh, p 3–27

Lewith G T, White P, Pariente J 2005 Investigating acupuncture using brain imaging techniques: the current state of play. Evidence-based Complementary and Alternative Medicine 2:315–319

Lewith G T, Berman B, Cummings M et al 2006a Systematic review of systematic reviews of acupuncture published 1996–2005. Letter Clinical Medicine 6(6):623–625

Lewith G T, White P, Kaptchuk T 2006b Developing a research strategy for acupuncture. Clinical Journal of Pain 22(7):632–638

Linde K, Streng A, Jurgens S et al 2005 Acupuncture for patients with migraine. A randomized controlled trial. Journal of the American Medical Association 293:2118–2125

Little P 2006 Delayed prescribing — a sensible approach to the management of acute otitis media. Journal of the American Medical Association 296:1290–1291

Little P, Rumsby K, Kelly J et al 2005 Information leaflet and antibiotic prescribing strategies for acute lower respiratory tract infection. Journal of the American Medical Association 293:3029–3035

Little P, Lewith G, Webley F et al submitted The MRC ATEAM randomised controlled trial of Alexander Technique, exercise and massage for chronic and recurrent back pain: hope for chronic back pain sufferers?

MacLennan A H, Wilson D H, Taylor A W 1996 Prevalence and cost of alternative medicine in Australia. Lancet 347:570–573

MacPherson H, Thomas K, Walters S et al 2001 The York acupuncture safety study: prospective survey of 34,000 treatments by traditional acupuncturists. British Medical Journal 323:486–487

Mann F 1973 Acupuncture anaesthesia. Lancet 2:563–564

Melchart D, Streng A, Hoppe A et al 2005 Acupuncture in patients with tension-type headache: randomised controlled trial. British Medical Journal 331:376–379

Mercer S W, Howie J G R 2006 CQ1-2 A new measure of holistic interpersonal care in primary care consultations. British Journal of General Practice 262–268

Mercer S W, Reynolds W J 2002 Empathy and quality of care. British Journal of General Practice S9–S12

Pariente J, White P, Frackowiak R S J et al 2005 Expectancy and belief modulate the neuronal substrates of pain treated by acupuncture. NeuroImage 25:1161–1167

Paterson C, Dieppe P 2005 Characteristic and incidental (placebo) effects in complex interventions such as acupuncture. British Medical Journal 330:1202–1205

Ratcliffe J, Thomas K, MacPherson H et al A randomised controlled trial of acupuncture care for persistent low back pain: cost effectiveness analysis. British Medical Journal 333:626–631

Shang A, Huwiler-Muntener K, Nartey L et al 2005 Are the clinical effects of homoeopathy placebo effects? Comparative study of placebo-controlled trials of homoeopathy and allopathy. Lancet 366:726–732

Thomas K, Nicholl P, Coleman P 2001 Use and expenditure on complementary medicine in England. Complementary Therapies in Medicine 9:2–11

Thomas K J, MacPherson H, Thorpe L et al 2005 Longer term clinical and economic benefits of offering acupuncture care to patients with chronic low back pain. Health Technology Assessment 9(32):1–109

UK Clinical Research Collaboration 2006 UK Health Research Analysis

Verhoef M J, Casebeer A L, Hilsden R J 2002 Assessing efficacy of complementary medicine: adding qualitative research methods to the 'gold standard'. Journal of Alternative and Complementary Medicine 8:275–281

Verhoef M J, Lewith G T, Ritenbaugh C et al 2004 Whole systems research: moving forward. FACT 9:87–90

Vickers A J, Rees R W, Zollman C E et al 2004 Acupuncture for chronic headache in primary care: large, pragmatic, randomised trial. British Medical Journal 328:744

Walach H, Sadaghiani C, Dehm C 2005 The therapeutic effect of clinical trials: understanding placebo response rates in clinical trials – a secondary analysis. BMC Medical Research Methodology 5:26

Walach H, Falkenberg T, Fonnebo V et al 2006 Circular instead of hierarchical: methodological principles for the evaluation of complex interventions. BMC Medical Research Methodology 6:29

Weidenhammer W, Streng A, Linde K et al 2006 Acupuncture for chronic pain within the research program of 10 German Health Insurance Funds – basic results from an observational study. Complementary Therapies in Clinical Practice 10.1016/j.ctim.2006.09.005

White A, Hayhoe S, Hart A et al 2001 Adverse events following acupuncture: prospective survey of 32,000 consultations with doctors and physiotherapists. British Medical Journal 323:485–486

Willich S N, Reinhold T, Selim D et al 2006 Cost-effectiveness of acupuncture treatment in patients with chronic neck pain. Pain 125:107–113

Witt C, Brinkhaus B, Jena S et al 2005 Acupuncture in patients with osteoarthritis of the knee: a randomised trial. Lancet 366:136–143

Witt C M, Jena S, Brinkhaus B et al 2006 Acupuncture for patients with chronic neck pain. Pain 125:98–106

Wonderling D, Vickers A J, Grieve R et al 2004 Cost effectiveness analysis of a randomised trial of acupuncture for chronic headache in primary care. British Medical Journal 328:747

Index